S0-ALL-399

A SOCIOLOGY OF
FOOD & NUTRITION

Dedication

We dedicate this book to our respective parents, Jan Williams and the late Ivan Germov, for fostering our intellectual and gastronomic development

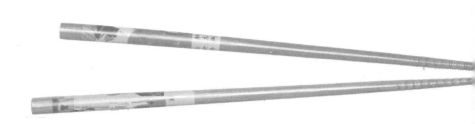

A SOCIOLOGY OF
FOOD & NUTRITION
The Social Appetite
Third Edition

Edited by John Germov & Lauren Williams

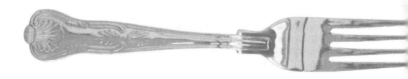

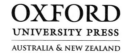

OXFORD
UNIVERSITY PRESS
AUSTRALIA & NEW ZEALAND

OXFORD
UNIVERSITY PRESS
AUSTRALIA & NEW ZEALAND

253 Normanby Road, South Melbourne, Victoria 3205, Australia

Oxford University Press is a department of the University of Oxford.
It furthers the University's objective of excellence in research,
scholarship, and education by publishing worldwide in

Oxford New York

Auckland Cape Town Dar es Salaam Hong Kong Karachi
Kuala Lumpur Madrid Melbourne Mexico City Nairobi
New Delhi Shanghai Taipei Toronto

With offices in

Argentina Austria Brazil Chile Czech Republic France Greece
Guatemala Hungary Italy Japan Poland Portugal Singapore
South Korea Switzerland Thailand Turkey Ukraine Vietnam

OXFORD is a trademark of Oxford University Press
in the UK and in certain other countries

Copyright © John Germov and Lauren Williams 2008
First published 1999
Reprinted 2000, 2001
Second edition published 2004
Reprinted 2005, 2006
Third edition published 2008
Reprinted 2009 (twice)

Reproduction and communication for educational purposes
The Australian *Copyright Act 1968* (the Act) allows a maximum of one
chapteror 10% of the pages of this work, whichever is the greater,
to be reproduced and/or communicated by any educational institution
for its educational purposes provided that the educational institution
(or the body that administers it) has given a remuneration notice to
Copyright Agency Limited (CAL) under the Act.

For details of the CAL licence for educational institutions contact:

Copyright Agency Limited
Level 15, 233 Castlereagh Street
Sydney NSW Australia 2000
Telephone: (02) 9394 7600
Facsimile: (02) 9394 7601
E-mail: info@copyright.com.au

Reproduction and communication for other purposes
Except as permitted under the Act (for example, any fair dealing
for the purposes of study, research, criticism or review) no part of this
book may be reproduced, stored in a retrieval system, communicated or
transmitted in any form or by any means without prior written permission.
All enquiries should be made to the publisher at the address above.

National Library of Australia Cataloguing-in-Publication data

A sociology of food and nutrition : the social appetite/
edited by John Germov and Lauren Williams.

ISBN 978 0 19 555150 1

1. Food habits-Social aspects. 2. Food-Social aspects.
3. Nutrition-Social apects.

Germov, John
Williams, Lauren.

394.12

Edited by Anne Mulvaney
Cover design, text design and typeset by Kerry Cooke, eggplant coomunications
Proofread by Liz Filleul
Indexed by Russel Brooks
Printed in Hong Kong by Sheck Wah Tong Printing Press Ltd.

Contents

Preface

A Sociology of Food and Nutrition: The Social Appetite introduces readers to the field of food sociology. It presents 'sociologies of food', that is, it is not dominated by one thesis or one theory or method, but rather presents a 'potlatch' of topics organised under key sociological themes. This third edition expands on the successful format of earlier editions, with new chapters, updated material and new online resources. The book is designed to be used both as a general reader, bringing together many of the key authors in the field and focusing on topics that dominate the literature, and as a teaching resource. To fulfil this second function, each chapter has:

- an overview section containing a series of questions and a short summary of the chapter, designed to encourage a questioning and reflective approach to the topic
- key terms (concepts and theories) listed at the start of the chapter, highlighted in bold in the text, and defined in a glossary at the end of the book
- a summary of the main points
- sociological reflections (new to this edition)
- questions for tutorial discussion
- further investigation (essay-style) questions
- further reading
- recommended chapter-specific web links.

What's new in this edition?

The book has been completely revised in response to user feedback and the latest research findings to ensure that it is completely up to date with current developments in the field. Specifically, the third edition includes:

- **New chapters from leading international authors:** 'World Hunger' (now authored by Frances Moore Lappé); 'The Politics of Government Dietary Advice' (Jennifer Lisa Falbe and Marion Nestle); and 'Culinary Cultures of Europe: Food, History, Health and Identity' (Stephen Mennell).
- **A substantially revised and updated chapter on dieting:** 'Constructing the Female Body: Dieting, the Thin Ideal and Body Acceptance' (Lauren Williams and

John Germov with updated findings that combine our previous two chapters on these topics from the second edition).

- **Sociological reflection exercises:** New to this edition, these can be used as self-directed or class-based activities that assist readers to apply their learning.
- **An expanded Social Appetite website (http://www.oup.com.au/orc/resources/ sociology_of_food_and_nutrition.aspx):** Provides access to relevant web links, books, teaching resources, journals, associations, documentaries and films. In addition, readers can access:
  — PowerPoint slides of all tables, graphs and figures in the book
  — chapters from previous editions of the book ('Setting the Menu' by John Duff, and 'Culture, Food, and Nutrition in Increasingly Culturally Diverse Societies' by Joanne P. Ikeda).

The interdisciplinary nature of studying food and nutrition

The central importance of food in social life means that its study is the province of diverse academic disciplines. In such a field as the study of food and nutrition, there is much that we can learn through interdisciplinary exchange. This book aims to draw together readings from what might be seen as opposing disciplines: sociology and nutrition. Interdisciplinary collaboration is a lengthy and challenging process involving active debate over philosophical assumptions and methodologies, as well as the overcoming of jargon and territorial defences, not to mention the academic structures of universities.

As editors, we have worked through the challenges of interdisciplinary collaboration in compiling this book. John Germov is a sociologist and Lauren Williams is a dietitian with a science background, and we both work as university academics. Our interdisciplinary collaboration resulted from having to share an office because of a lack of university office space. Our office became a place of daily intellectual exploration as we probed the perspectives of sometimes opposing disciplines through discussion and debate. This debate informed the development of a new undergraduate sociology subject in 1996 at the University of Newcastle (Australia) called 'The Sociology of Food'. Originally designed for students of nutrition and dietetics, it was subsequently extended to arts and social science students. In 2006 the course was also redeveloped into a postgraduate subject called Food Sociology: Understanding the Social Appetite. The original and continuing aim of the book was to make the sociological study of food relevant to readers across health, nutrition and social science disciplines.

Part of the value of our collaboration has been the extension of our networks, reflected in the range of people who have contributed to this book. Most are either sociologists or dietitians and all share an interest in the sociology of food and nutrition. Many of the contributing authors have published widely in the field and are based in the United Kingdom, the USA or Australia. The chapters provide a review of the relevant literature and some present original empirical findings.

Our aim in writing this book is to reach a broad readership so that those interested in food, nutrition, and wider issues of consumption and social regulation can discover the relevance of studying the social context of food; this, we hope, will lead to future interdisciplinary collaboration. We encourage readers interested in the social context of food and nutrition—both inside and outside the discipline of sociology—to break down disciplinary barriers and to facilitate the coalescence of a variety of perspectives through ongoing debate and discussion of the issues presented in this book. Despite our enthusiasm for food sociology and interdisciplinary collaboration, it would be folly to claim that this book contains all the answers for understanding food and eating. The study of food is rightly the province of many disciplines. Had the university placed a geographer in our office, there would no doubt have been more input from that discipline in this text.

We hope that *A Sociology of Food and Nutrition* inspires people from many disciplines to add a sociological perspective to their understanding of why we eat the way we do.

Suggestions, comments and feedback

We are always interested in receiving feedback on the book and suggestions for future editions. You can contact us at the Social Appetite website at http://www.oup.com.au/orc/resources/sociology_of_food_and_nutrition.aspx.

Bon appetit!

John Germov and Lauren Williams
University of Newcastle, Australia
January 2008

Acknowledgments

We would like to thank the contributing authors for being so professional in their dealings with us and for their high-quality chapters. Our gratitude to the book's earlier publishers, Jill Henry (1st edition) and Debra James (2nd edition), for their belief in the book. For this third edition, we record our thanks to Lucy McLoughlin, Katie Ridsdale, Rachel Saffer, Tim Campbell and all the OUP staff. We also thank Annette Murphy for assistance with the third edition.

We are grateful to our students, whose interest in and enthusiasm for food sociology was the original stimulus for this book. And we thank the academics who have used earlier editions for providing feedback and encouraging us to produce subsequent editions.

On a personal note, thanks go to our support team: John thanks his wife Sue Jelovcan, daughter Isabella (already an active food sociologist!), sister Roz, and late parents Ivan and Ivanka; Lauren thanks her husband Greg Hill for the thousands of cups of coffee, parents Jan and Merve, sisters, Julie and Kim, and her niece and nephew Georgia and Ben, who have given her new insights into food sociology through infancy and childhood.

*   *   *   *   *

Unless otherwise stated, all quotations used in the Part openings are from Ned Sherrin's *Oxford Dictionary of Humorous Quotations* (1995, Oxford University Press, Oxford).

The editors and publisher are grateful to the following copyright holders for granting permission to reproduce various extracts and photographs in this book: The Body Shop International PLC for the photograph of the 'Ruby' advertising campaign; *Cleo* magazine for the covers of the January 1973, 1983, and 1993 issues; *Who Weekly* magazine for the cover of the 27 May 1996 issue. Every effort has been made to trace the original source of all material reproduced in this book. Where the attempt has been unsuccessful, the author and publisher would be pleased to hear from the copyright holder to rectify any omission.

John Germov and Lauren Williams
University of Newcastle, Australia
January 2008

Contributors

John Coveney is Associate Professor in the Department of Health at Flinders University in Adelaide, South Australia. He is coordinator of the primary health care and public health program. His research projects examine social, economic and environmental influences on the food supply and on eating habits.

Jane Dixon is a public health social scientist at the National Centre for Epidemiology and Population Health, ANU. Her PhD was published by UNSW Press in 2002 as *The Changing Chicken: Chooks, Cooks and Culinary Culture*. She continues to undertake research on transformations in the food system, with a focus on the role of supermarkets. In addition, she is researching the socio-cultural trends underlying the rise in obesity and this is the subject of another two co-edited books, *The Seven Deadly Sins of Obesity* (UNSW Press 2007) and *The Weight of Modernity* (under research).

Jennifer Lisa Falbe is from Community Health and Human Development in the School of Public Health at the University of California. She has a BA (public health) and an MPH from the University of California, Berkeley. Her research interests are in food policy and chronic disease prevention.

John Germov is an Associate Professor of Sociology and Head of the School of Humanities and Social Science at the University of Newcastle, Australia. He has published widely in the areas of food sociology, health sociology, workplace change, and general sociology. John's books include *Public Sociology: An Introduction to Australian Society* (with M. Poole; Allen & Unwin 2007); *Australian Youth: Social and Cultural Issues* (with P. Nilan and R. Julian; Pearson 2007); *Histories of Australian Sociology* (with T. McGee; Melbourne University Publishing 2005); *Second Opinion: An Introduction to Health Sociology* (Oxford University Press 2005, 2002, 1998), *Get Great Marks for Your Essays* (Allen & Unwin 2000 1996), *Surviving First Year Uni* (with L. Williams; Allen & Unwin 2001) and *Get Great Information Fast* (with L. Williams; Allen & Unwin 1998).

Janet Grice is Senior Research Fellow with the Centre for the Study of Agriculture, Food and the Environment (CSAFE) at the University of Otago, Dunedin, New Zealand. Janet was awarded her PhD in 2000 for her study of Australian consumer perceptions and acceptance of genetically engineered foods. Before joining CSAFE, she held a Postdoctoral Research Fellowship within the School of Social Science, The University of Queensland. She is a principal investigator on the ARC-funded project 'The Social Construction of Safe Foods: Uncertainty, Risk and Trust in Agri-food Applications of Genetically Modified Organisms' and also works with the Cooperative Research Centre for Innovation in Sugar Cane on the project 'Evaluation of Knowledge and Attitudes to Biotechnology and Genetic Engineering in Sugarcane Among Industry Stakeholders'. Janet is co-editor of *Altered Genes: Reconstructing Nature: The Debate* (Allen & Unwin 1998).

Julie Hepworth is an Associate Professor of Psychology in the College of Psychology and Behavioural Sciences, Argosy University, USA, and is a Chartered Health Psychologist with the British Psychological Society. Her research includes the theory and practice of health psychology in public health and medicine, gender and health, and research methodology. She is author of the book *The Social Construction of Anorexia Nervosa* (Sage 1999) and a number of articles including 'Public Health Psychology: A Conceptual and Practical Framework' (*Journal of Health Psychology* 2004, vol. 9, no. 1, pp. 41–54) and 'The Emergence of Critical Health Psychology: Can it Contribute to Promoting Public Health?' (*Journal of Health Psychology* 2006, vol. 11, no. 3, pp. 331–41).

Roger Hughes is Associate Professor of Public Health Nutrition and Deputy Head of the School of Public Health at Griffith University, Australia. For the last 10 years he has been at the forefront of public health nutrition workforce development research and practice in Australia as principal investigator in the Australian public health nutrition workforce development project; a foundation faculty member of the Australian Public Health Nutrition Collaboration; and the architect of Australia's public health nutrition competencies. At an international level he is a visiting scholar at the Karolinska Institutet's (Stockholm) Unit for Public Health Nutrition, Deputy Editor of the journal *Public Health Nutrition* and part of the international research collaboration leading the EU-based JobNut project. He is one of a group of 10 public health nutritionists internationally selected in 2006 to develop the constitution of the World Public Health Nutrition Association.

Karen S. Kubena is Associate Dean for Academic Affairs at the College of Agriculture and Life Sciences, and Professor of Nutrition and Food Science at Texas A&M University. Her research interests include nutrition throughout the life span, dietary intake, social, and other factors that impact on health and nutrition.

Frances Moore Lappé is a social entrepreneur and co-author of the 1971 bestseller *Diet for a Small Planet* (Tarcher/Penguin) as well as the recent *Hope's Edge* (Tarcher/

Penguin, 2002) and *Democracy's Edge* (Jossey Bass, 2006) and the upcoming *Getting a Grip* (2007). Lappé is currently co-founder of the Small Planet Institute, and previously co-founded the Center for Living Democracy (1990–2000) and the California-based Institute for Food and Development Policy (Food First). Her television, radio and media appearances are extensive, and she lectures widely to university audiences, community groups and professional conferences. Lappé is a recipient of the Right Livelihood Award and a founding councillor of the World Futures Council.

Geoffrey Lawrence is Professor of Sociology and Head of the School of Social Science at The University of Queensland. He has had over 25 years' involvement in agri-food research, teaching and researching in: Australia (Central Queensland University, Charles Sturt University and The University of Queensland); the USA (Cornell and Madison-Wisconsin); and the United Kingdom (University of Essex). He is an associate editor of the *Journal of Environmental Policy and Planning* and is on the board of the *Journal of Sociology*. Recent co-authored/co-edited books include: *Supermarkets and Agri-food Supply Chains: Transformations in the Production and Consumption of Foods* (Edward Elgar 2007); *Rural Governance: International Perspectives* (Routledge 2007); *Going Organic: Mobilising Networks for Environmentally Responsible Food Production* (CABI 2006); *Agricultural Governance: Globalization and the New Politics of Regulation* (Routledge 2005); and *Recoding Nature: Critical Perspectives on Genetic Engineering* (UNSW Press 2004). He is a Fellow of the Academy of Social Sciences in Australia.

Mark Lawrence is Associate Professor in Public Health Nutrition at Deakin University, Australia. He has over 20 years' experience working in food policy at the local, state, national and international levels. His research focus is the analysis of food fortification, food labelling, nutrient reference values and dietary guidelines. Mark is a steering committee member of the New Nutrition Science project; committee member of the World Public Health Nutrition Association; council member of the Victorian Food Safety Council; and advisor to the World Health Organization. Recently, he co-edited an international reference book entitled *Public Health Nutrition: From Principles to Practice* (Allen & Unwin 2007).

Terry Leahy is currently employed as a Senior Lecturer in the Sociology and Anthropology Discipline of the University of Newcastle. Among other things he teaches the subject 'Environment and Society'. He has recently completed a study of the attitudes of Australians to environmental issues and to environmental politics. He has a long-standing interest in permaculture and is working on a book on sustainable agriculture for rural communities in South Africa.

Wm. Alex McIntosh is a Professor in the Department of Sociology and the Department of Recreation, Park, and Tourism Science – Rural and Community

Studies at Texas A&M University; he is also a member of the Faculty of Nutrition. His book *Sociologies of Food and Nutrition* was published in 1996 by Plenum. Recent publications include 'Rural Eating, Diet, Nutrition and Body Weight' with Jeffery Sobal (in *Critical Issues in Rural Health* edited by Nina Glasgow, Lois Wright Morton and Nan E. Johnson; Blackwell Publishing 2004) and 'Food Safety Risk Communication and Consumer Food-Handling Behavior' (in *Preharvest and Post Harvest Food Safety*, edited by Ross Bier and others; Wiley 2004). McIntosh recently completed a three-year study of 'Parental Time, Income, Role Strains, and Children's Diet and Obesity' funded by the US Department of Agriculture.

Stephen Mennell is Professor of Sociology at University College Dublin, Ireland. From 1990 to 1993 he was Professor of Sociology at Monash University, Melbourne. His many books include *All Manners of Food: Eating and Taste in England and France from the Middle Ages to the Present* (University of Illinois Press 1985, 1996), *Norbert Elias: Civilisation and the Human Self-image* (Blackwell 1989, 1992), *The Sociology of Food: Eating, Diet, and Culture* (with A. Murcott and A.H. van Otterloo; Sage 1992) and *The American Civilising Process* (Polity Press 2007).

Elizabeth Murphy is Professor of Medical Sociology and Head of the School of Sociology and Social Policy, at the University of Nottingham, England. Her empirical research covers a wide range of topics in health and social care, including chronic disease, lifestyle change, infant feeding, motherhood, nutritional health and learning disabilities. These are drawn together by a common interest in the relationship between individuals, families, professionals and the state. In particular, this research has been concerned with the ways in which, in contemporary liberal states, power operates through discourses that define what is good, moral, responsible and legitimate. It explores the possibilities of resistance that exist for clients and professionals who are caught up in such discourses in relation to the delivery of health and social care. Her methodological scholarship focuses upon the applications of social science methods to policy-relevant research. This includes extended work on the application of qualitative methods to health policy research and a current interdisciplinary collaborative study identifying optimal methods for eliciting professional and end-user requirements in the design and development of medical devices.

Marion Nestle is the Paulette Goddard Professor of Nutrition, Food Studies, and Public Health, and Professor of Sociology at New York University. She is the author of *Food Politics: How the Food Industry Influences Nutrition and Health* (2002; University of California Press, revised edition 2007), *Safe Food: Bacteria, Biotechnology, and Bioterrorism* (University of California Press 2003), and *What to Eat* (North Point Press 2006).

Jeffery Sobal is a nutritional sociologist who is a Professor in the Division of Nutritional Sciences at Cornell University, New York, where he teaches courses that apply social science concepts, theories and methods to food, eating and nutrition. His research interests focus on the sociology of obesity and body weight, the food and nutrition system, and food choice processes. His recent work on body weight focuses on the relationship between marriage and weight and the construction of body weight as a social problem. He has co-edited several books with Donna Maurer: *Eating Agendas: Food and Nutrition as Social Problems* (Aldine de Gruyter 1995), *Weighty Issues: The Construction of Fatness and Thinness as Social Problems* (Aldine de Gruyter 1999) and *Interpreting Weight: The Social Management of Fatness and Thinness* (Aldine de Gruyter 1999).

Deidre Wicks, formerly Senior Lecturer in Sociology at the University of Newcastle, is an independent social researcher with connections as an Honorary Scholar to the Sociology discipline at the University of Newcastle and the National University of Ireland, Galway. She has published widely in the areas of health sociology, including *Nurses and Doctors at Work: Rethinking Professional Boundaries* (Allen & Unwin 1999). Her current research and writing interests are centred on the sociology of food as it relates to vegetarianism.

Lauren Williams is a Senior Lecturer and Program Convenor of Nutrition and Dietetics at the University of Newcastle. She holds tertiary qualifications in science, dietetics, social science, health promotion and public health. Lauren has published journal articles and book chapters on her quantitative and qualitative research into weight gain, weight control practices and body acceptance in women. Along with this edited book, she has also co-authored study skills books with John Germov. With over 20 years of experience in the field of public health nutrition, Lauren is an Advanced Accredited Practising Dietitian, and an associate editor for the journal *Nutrition and Dietetics*.

Acronyms and Abbreviations

ABS	Australian Bureau of Statistics
ACMF	Australian Chicken Meat Federation
ANZFA	Australia New Zealand Food Authority
APHNAC	Australian Public Health Nutrition Collaboration
BMI	body mass index
BSE	bovine spongiform encephalopathy
Bt	*Bacillus thuringiensis*
CAC	Codex Alimentarius Commission
CHD	coronary heart disease
CJD	Creutzfeld-Jakob disease
CSA	Commodity Systems Analysis
CSIRO	Commonwealth Scientific and Industrial Research Organisation (Australia)
DAA	Dietitians Association of Australia
DES	diethyl stilboestrol
DGs	dietary guidelines
DNA	deoxyribonucleic acid
EC	European Community
EPOS	electronic point of sales
FAO	Food and Agriculture Organization (United Nations)
FDA	Food and Drug Administration (USA)
FSANZ	Food Standards Australia New Zealand
g	gram
GM	genetically modified
GMO	genetically modified organism
HFCS	high fructose corn syrup
HVFs	high-value foods
IMF	International Monetary Fund
IT	information technology
JIT	just-in-time
JSCRS	Joint Select Committee on the Retailing Sector
mg	milligram

ml	millilitre
MRC	Medical Research Council (UK)
NAFTA	North American Free Trade Agreement
NFA	National Food Authority (Australia)
NGO	non-government organisation
NHMRC	National Health and Medical Research Council (Australia)
NLEA	Nutrition Labeling and Education Act (USA)
NTDs	neural tube defects
OST	Office of Science and Technology (UK)
PHN	public health nutrition
RDA	recommended dietary allowance
RDI	recommended dietary intake
USDA	US Department of Agriculture
WHO	World Health Organization
WTO	World Trade Organization

PART 1
An Appetiser

We were compelled to live on food and water for several days.

W.C. Fields, *My Little Chickadee* (1940 film)

Beulah, peel me a grape.

Mae West, *I'm No Angel* (1933 film)

Good to eat, and wholesome to digest, as a worm to a toad, a toad to a snake, a snake to a pig, a pig to a man, and a man to a worm.

Ambrose Bierce, *The Enlarged Devil's Dictionary* (1967)

The aim of this book is to introduce a multidisciplinary readership to sociological enquiries into food and nutrition, regardless of whether or not they have a sociology background. The first chapter maps the field of food sociology and provides an overview of the chapters in the book. It also provides a sociology overview for those with little or no sociology background, highlighting the distinctive features of the sociological perspective through the analytical framework of the sociological imagination template and giving numerous examples of the application of sociology to the study of food and nutrition. We trust that this section, by providing a taste of things to come, will whet your social appetite for exploring the sociology of food and nutrition.

CHAPTER 1

Exploring the Social Appetite: A Sociology of Food and Nutrition

John Germov and Lauren Williams

OVERVIEW

* Why do we eat the way we do?
* What is sociology and how can it be applied to the study of food and nutrition?
* What are the major social trends in food production, distribution and consumption?

This chapter provides an overview of the sociological perspective as it applies to the study of food and nutrition by introducing the concept of the social appetite. We explain how food sociology can help to conceptualise the connections between individual food habits and wider social patterns to explore why we eat the way we do. The chapter concludes by reviewing the major themes discussed in this book, highlighting the social context in which food is produced, distributed and consumed.

Key terms

agency
agribusiness
body image
civilising process
cosmopolitanism
culinary tourism
dietary guidelines
eating disorders
food security

functional foods
genetic modification
globalisation
identity
McDonaldisation
muscular ideal
public health nutrition
reflexive modernity
risk society

social appetite
social construction
social differentiation
social structure
sociological imagination
structure/agency debate
thin ideal

Introduction: The social construction of food and appetite

> But food is like sex in its power to stimulate imagination and memory as well as those senses—taste, smell, sight … The most powerful writing about food rarely addresses the qualities of a particular dish or meal alone; it almost always contains elements of nostalgia for other times, places and companions, and of anticipation of future pleasures.
>
> Joan Smith, *Hungry for You* (1997, p. 334)

We all have our favourite foods and individual likes and dislikes. Consider the tantalising smell of freshly baked bread, the luscious texture of chocolate, the heavenly aroma of espresso coffee, the exquisite flavour of semi-dried tomatoes, and the simple delight of a crisp potato chip. In addition to these sensory aspects, food is the focal point around which many social occasions and leisure events are organised. While hunger is a biological drive and food is essential to survival, there is more to food and eating than the satisfaction of physiological needs. 'Social drives', based on cultural, religious, economic and political factors, also affect the availability and consumption of food. The existence of national cuisines, such as Thai, Italian, Indian and Mexican (to name only a few), indicates that individual food preferences are not formed in a social vacuum. The link between the 'individual' and the 'social' in terms of food habits begins early: 'While we all begin life consuming the same milk diet, by early childhood, children of different cultural groups are consuming diets that are composed of completely different foods, [sometimes] sharing no foods in common. This observation points to the essential role of early experience and the social and cultural context of eating in shaping food habits' (Birch et al. 1996, p. 162).

Therefore, despite similar physiological needs in humans, food habits are not universal, natural or inevitable; they are **social constructions**, and significant variations exist, from the sacred cow in India, to kosher eating among the orthodox Jewish community, to the consumption in some countries of animals that are kept as pets in other countries, such as dogs and horses. In Australia, the kangaroo may be on the coat of arms, but it is also a highly prized meat that is increasingly eaten in restaurants. Many indigenous peoples continue to consume traditional food; Australian Aboriginals, for example, consume 'bush foods' not often eaten by white Australians, such as witchetty grubs, honey ants, galahs and turtles. Some cultures prohibit alcohol consumption, while others drink alcohol to excess, and many cultures have gendered patterns of food consumption (see Box 1.1). As Claude Fischler (1988) notes, food is a bridge between nature and culture, and food habits are learnt through culturally determined notions of what constitutes appropriate and inappropriate food, and through cultural methods of preparation and consumption, irrespective of the nutritional value of these foods and methods (Falk 1994).

Gendered food habits

BOX 1.1

Gendered patterns of food habits can be observed in many cultures (DeVault 1991; Counihan 1999). Daily examples can be found in the widespread use of gender stereotypes in the advertising of certain food products. In Australia, over many years, the 'Meadowlea mum' commercials depicted a blissful mum who prepared home-cooked meals with margarine to serve her happy family. The Meat and Livestock Australia (MLA) Corporation regularly runs highly gendered advertising campaigns, such as the 'feed the man meat' campaign complete with sing-a-long jingle, which depicted dutiful mothers preparing hearty meat-based meals for their growing sons and hard-working husbands. In preparing these advertisements, the advertising companies are cashing-in on, and reinforcing, existing gendered eating habits. Red meat tends to be perceived as a masculine food, while fruit and vegetables are perceived as being feminine (Charles & Kerr 1988).

The sociology of food and nutrition, or food sociology, concentrates on the myriad sociocultural, political, economic and philosophical factors that influence our food habits—what we eat, when we eat, how we eat and why we eat. Sociologists look for patterns in human interaction and seek to uncover the links between social organisation and individual behaviour. Food sociology focuses on the social patterning of food production, distribution and consumption—which can be conceptualised as the **social appetite**. The chapters in this book explore the various dimensions of the social appetite to show the ways in which foods, tastes and appetites are socially constructed. However, the sociological perspective does not tell the whole story, which is rounded out by many other disciplines, including anthropology, history, economics, geography, psychology and **public health nutrition**. Sociological approaches are a relatively recent addition to the study of food. Despite the delayed interest, since the 1990s there has been a significant surge in food sociology literature.

Studying food via the sociological imagination template

Before we discuss how sociology can contribute to the study of food and nutrition, we need to provide an overview of the sociological perspective (with which some readers will already be familiar). In brief, sociology examines how society is organised, how it influences our lives, and how social change occurs. It investigates social relationships at every level, from interpersonal and small-group interactions to public policy formation and global developments. Sociology critiques explanations that reduce complex social phenomena to biological, psychological or individualistic causes.

A sociological study of food habits examines the role played by the social environment in which food is produced and consumed. This does not mean that individual choice and personal taste play no role. Rather, because social patterns in food habits exist, a sociological explanation is helpful in understanding the social determinants of why we eat the way we do. If food choice were totally based on individual or natural preferences for certain tastes, few people would persevere with foods such as coffee or beer, which are bitter on first tasting. These foods are said to be an 'acquired taste', and we 'acquire' them through a process of repetition that is socially, rather than biologically, driven.

Charles Wright Mills (1959) coined the term **sociological imagination** to describe the way that sociological analysis is performed. Interpreting the world with a sociological imagination involves establishing a link between personal experiences and the social environment—that is, being able to imagine or see that the private lives of individuals can have a social basis. When individuals share similar experiences, a social pattern emerges that implies that such experiences have a common, social foundation. For example, food and eating are imbued with social meanings and are closely associated with people's social interaction in both formal and informal settings. Box 1.2 provides some everyday examples of the social construction of food, especially food symbolism, to highlight the value of exploring the social appetite.

BOX 1.2

The social construction of food and taste

Food is central to social life and it is perhaps this centrality that has resulted in potent food symbolism and connections with key social events. That foods are imbued with social meaning is evident when we examine well-known books and films. The film *Eat, Drink, Man, Woman* (1994) explores the importance of food to family life and personal **identity**. *Babette's Feast* (1987) contrasts a pious lifestyle of moral austerity with the sensuality and carnality of food as a feast of sight, aroma, texture and taste—a spiritual experience of worldly pleasure. *The Wedding Banquet* (1993) conveys the social meaning of food in the context of marriage rituals. Other films have comically explored cannibalism, such as *Delicatessen* (1991) and *The Cook the Thief His Wife & Her Lover* (1989); and who can forget the vomit scene in *Monty Python's The Meaning of Life* (1997)? The film *La Grande Bouffe* (1973) and Linda Jaivin's book *Eat Me* (1995) mixed erotica with the sensuality of food in what could be termed a genre of 'food porn' if it were not for the long tradition of food advertisements that conflate the pleasures of sex and food—just think of any number of adverts about chocolate or ice-cream. More recently the passion of food

▶

BOX 1.2

has been explored in films like *Dinner Rush* (2000) and *No Reservations* (2007), while the manipulative power of the food industry has been exposed in *Fast Food Nation* (2006), a fictionalised account of Eric Schlosser's (2001) journalistic exposé. Food is often used as a metaphor in daily speech, through expressions such as 'sweetheart', 'honey', 'bad seed', 'couch potato', 'breadwinner' and 'cheesed off', to name a few. Imagine some of the food rituals and food symbolism involved in the following social situations:

- a birthday celebration
- a wake
- a wedding banquet
- a religious feast or fast
- an occasion when you might exercise virtue and restraint in eating
- an occasion when you crave 'naughty but nice' food, your favourite food, or comfort food.

Drawing on the work of Mills (1959) and Giddens (1986), Evan Willis (2004) conceptualises the sociological imagination as consisting of four interlinked factors: historical, cultural, structural and critical. When these four interrelated features of the sociological imagination are applied to a topic under study, they form the basis of sociological analysis. We have visually presented this approach in Figure 1.1 as a useful template to keep in mind when you want to apply a sociological perspective to an issue—simply imagine superimposing the template over the topic you are investigating and consider the following sorts of questions:

- **Historical factors:** How have past events influenced the contemporary social appetite (that is, current social patterns of food production, distribution and consumption)?

Figure 1.1   The sociological imagination template

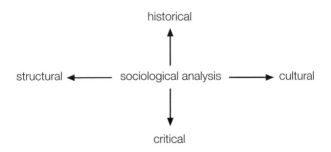

John Germov and Lauren Williams

- **Cultural factors:** What influence do tradition, cultural values and belief systems have on food habits in the particular country, social group or social occasion you are studying?
- **Structural factors:** How do various forms of social organisation and social institutions affect the production, distribution and consumption of food?
- **Critical factors:** Why are things as they are? Could they be otherwise? Who benefits?

Applying the sociological imagination template can challenge your views and assumptions about the world, since such 'sociological vision' involves constant critical reflection. By using the template, the social context of food can be examined in terms of an interplay between historical, cultural, structural and critical factors. It is important to note, however, that the template necessarily simplifies the actual process of sociological analysis, because, for example, there is a wide variety of research methods and social theories through which sociological analysis can be conducted. In practice, there can be considerable overlap between the four factors, and so they are not as distinctly identifiable as is implied by Figure 1.1. For instance, it can be difficult to clearly differentiate between historical factors and cultural factors, or structural factors and cultural factors, as they can be interdependent. Cultural values are often intricately intertwined with historical events and may also be the product of, or at least be reinforced by, structural factors. Nevertheless, the sociological imagination template is a useful reminder that the four factors—historical, cultural, structural and critical—are essential elements of sociological analysis (see Box 1.3).

BOX 1.3

Aboriginal food and nutrition: Applying the sociological imagination template

Until the colonisation of Australia by Europeans, Aboriginal and Torres Strait Islander people lived a hunter-gatherer lifestyle. However, today they suffer from disproportionately high rates of many nutrition-related health conditions, such as type 2 diabetes, iron-deficiency anaemia, low birthweight and restricted child growth, cardiovascular disease, and overweight and obesity (Lee 2003). Applying the sociological imagination template highlights the relationship between their social situation and food.

Historical factors

Many indigenous communities were dispossessed of their hunting and fishing areas and forced to live on missions and reserves, where they were provided with rations of highly processed Western foods low in nutrient value such as white flour and

▶

BOX 1.3

sugar. The historical legacy of these developments was a change from a traditional nutrient-dense diet (bush foods) to a Westernised diet high in saturated fat and sugar and low in fruit and vegetables.

Cultural factors

While bush foods such as galahs, turtles, goannas, honey ants and witchetty grubs represent only a small proportion of the food consumed by Aboriginal people today, they remain an important part of indigenous culture, identity and food preferences, particularly in rural and remote regions. Maintaining this cultural heritage and incorporating bush foods into nutrition-promotion strategies could help ameliorate nutritional problems in indigenous communities.

Structural factors

Unemployment, low education levels and poverty are experienced by a disproportionately high percentage of indigenous people. The limited food supply in rural and remote areas (particularly in terms of access to fresh foods such as fruit and vegetables), management of food stores and transport all provide challenges for **food security** in indigenous communities.

Critical factors

The *National Aboriginal and Torres Strait Islander Nutrition Strategy and Action Plan* (NATSINSAP), released in 2001 as part of the *Eat Well Australia* public health nutrition framework, documented indigenous food and nutrition problems and proposed a range of food supply, food security and nutrition promotion initiatives (SIGNAL 2001a, 2001b; for good overviews of this topic see NHMRC 2000; Lee 2003). Beyond public health nutrition approaches, a number of employment-generation schemes for indigenous communities have been attempted. For example, in recent years a 'bush tucker' industry has developed, marketing traditional foods (such as bush tomatoes and indigenous oils and spices) to the general community. While still in its infancy, the industry has received some government funding support, though considerably more funds are needed for industry development, which could result in it becoming a significant source of employment for indigenous people.

Food sociology and the structure/agency debate

A key sociological question concerns the relative influence over human behaviour (in this case food choice) of personal preferences and social determinants. To what extent are our food choices the result of social shaping as opposed to individual likes and dislikes? This represents a central concern of any sociological study, and is

John Germov and Lauren Williams

often referred to as the **structure/agency debate**. The term **social structure** refers to recurring patterns of social interaction by which people are related to each other through social institutions and social groups. In this sense we are very much products of our society, in that certain forms of social organisation, such as laws, education, religion, economic resources and cultural beliefs, influence our lives. However, as self-conscious beings, we have the ability to participate in and change the society in which we live. The term **agency** refers to the potential of individuals to independently exercise choice in, and influence over, their daily lives and wider society. Clearly, we are not simply automatons responding to preordained social outcomes. Human agency produces the scope for difference, diversity and social change.

It is important to note that structure and agency are inextricably linked—they should not be viewed as representing an either/or choice or as inherently positive or negative. The social structure may liberate individuals by ensuring access to inexpensive food, while the exercise of agency by some individuals may be constraining on others—for example, someone may steal your food!

What's on the menu?

A walk down the aisle of any supermarket reveals food products that were not widely available even two decades ago. French cheese, Russian caviar, Indian spices, Thai coconut cream, Belgian chocolate and Australian macadamia nuts are a small indication of the extent of social change in food habits. In restaurants and cafes in major urban areas of any country, people can now partake of global cuisines such as Chinese, Indian, Thai, Italian, Greek and French. In fact, **culinary tourism**, the promotion of gastronomic experiences and events as a key feature of tourism (such as regional food festivals and foodstuffs), has become increasingly popular (Rojek & Urry 1997), particularly amid calls for a return to authenticity and regionality in food and cooking (Symons 1993).

The processes of mass production and **globalisation** have resulted in such a pluralisation of food choices and hybridisation of cuisines that a form of food **cosmopolitanism** is emerging (Tomlinson 1999; Beck 2000). The popular description of modern Australian cuisine as 'Australasian' is just one example of this cosmopolitan trend. Anthony Giddens and Ulrich Beck both argue that contemporary social life is characterised by **reflexive modernity** (Beck et al. 1994). According to Giddens (1991), people's exposure to new information and different cultures undermines traditions. For Claude Fischler this can result in the omnivore's paradox, whereby when faced with such food variety and novelty 'individuals lack reliable criteria to make … decisions and therefore they experience a growing sense of anxiety' (1980, p. 948), or what he playfully refers to as gastro-anomie. In the face of food-borne diseases, such as 'mad cow disease' and Avian bird flu, resulting from modern agricultural processes, the wide variety of food choices coexist with increased risk and anxiety over what to eat (Lupton 2000), the constant management of which Beck (1992) describes as characteristic of a **risk society**.

The following chapters in this book have been grouped into four parts that represent major themes in the sociological literature:

- Part 2: Food systems, globalisation and agribusiness
- Part 3: Food and nutrition discourses, politics and policies
- Part 4: Food consumption, **social differentiation** and identity
- Part 5: Food and the body.

We do not propose that this classification scheme is an exhaustive or static depiction of the food sociology field, nor do we dispute that there are grey areas, and areas of overlap between the themes. Nonetheless, we believe these to be the dominant themes in the social appetite. The themes are discussed briefly here to provide an overview of the structure and content of the book.

Food systems: Globalisation and agribusiness

If commercial interests make people's tastes more standardised than they conceivably could in the past, they impose far less strict limits than did the physical constraints to which most people's diet was subject … the main trend has been towards *diminishing contrasts and increasing varieties* in food habits and culinary taste.

Stephen Mennell, *All Manners of Food* (1996, pp. 321–2)

The increasing mass production and commodification of food over the last century has resulted in food being one of the largest industries across the globe, with world food exports estimated to be over US$612 billion in 2005 (DAFF 2007; see Table 1.1).

Food is a major source of profit, export dollars and employment, and thus concerns a range of stakeholders, including corporations, unions, consumer groups, government agencies and health professionals. To conceptualise the size of the food industry or food system, various models have been proposed, such as food chains, food cycles and food webs (see Sobal et al. 1998 for an excellent review). Jeff Sobal and colleagues (1998) prefer to use the term 'food and nutrition system' to acknowledge the important role of public health nutrition in any food model, which they define as:

the set of operations and processes involved in transforming raw materials into foods and transforming nutrients into health outcomes, all of which functions as a system within biophysical and sociocultural contexts (Sobal et al. 1998, p. 853, *original italics*).

Food system models invariably simplify the operations involved in the production, distribution and consumption of food, often failing to take account of the global, political, cultural and environmental concerns, or the related stakeholders and industries, such as the media, waste-management, advertising, transport and health sectors. The model devised by Sobal and colleagues (1998) addresses most of these sociological concerns, though the issue of globalisation remains absent.

Table 1.1   Share of export food trade by country, in value terms (2005)

Rank	Country	Share (%)
1	USA	9.6
2	France	7.5
3	Netherlands	6.6
4	Germany	6.1
5	Brazil	4.7
6	Spain	4.4
7	Canada	3.9
8	China	3.9
9	Belgium	3.9
10	Italy	3.8
11	Argentina	2.9
12	UK	2.7
13	Australia	2.4

Source: Adapted from DAFF (2007, p. 13)

BOX 1.4 The McDonaldisation of the world

The **McDonaldisation** of food is a global phenomenon and represents the expansion of **agribusiness** through the standardisation of food production and the homogenisation of food consumption. Ritzer, in *The McDonaldization of Society*, first published in 1993, used the term 'McDonaldisation' as a modern metaphor for *'the process by which the principles of the fast-food restaurant are coming to dominate more and more sectors of American society as well as the rest of the world'* (2000, p. 1, italics in original). McDonald's is a prototype organisation that has been able, through rigid methods of managerial and technical control, to achieve a highly rationalised form of food production: no matter where in the world you come across a McDonald's restaurant, you can be assured of encountering the same look, the same service, the same products and the same tastes. Not only are there now many other food chains based on the same formula, but there are also fewer and fewer places where you can avoid the McDonald's experience.

Part 1 of the book explores some of the key sociological issues affecting the food system, particularly the impact of globalisation (see Box 1.4) and agribusiness (see Schlosser 2001). Specifically, this part investigates the inequitable distribution of food as the basis of world hunger, the environmental impact of current agricultural practices, the increasing power of food corporations stemming from the **genetic modification** of food, and the dominating influence of supermarket chains on how food is produced and consumed.

Food and nutrition discourses, politics and policies

The only way to keep your health is to eat what you don't want, drink what you don't like, and do what you'd rather not.

Mark Twain, *Following the Equator* (1897)

Given that food is a major industry and source of profit, it should come as little surprise that it is also an area rife with politics and debates over public policy, particularly over food regulation relating to hygiene standards, the use of chemicals, pesticide residues, the legitimacy of advertising claims, and various public health nutrition (PHN) strategies. PHN focuses on the population as a whole and aims to ensure the availability of safe and nutritious food, to improve the health and nutritional status of the general community as well as vulnerable subgroups of the population (such as the poor, indigenous groups and children) (SIGNAL 2001a). PHN strategies range from addressing food hygiene and food security to promoting improved nutritional knowledge and dietary behaviours among the population at large (SIGNAL 2001a, 2001b).

There has been a vast array of national and international PHN developments in the last two centuries. Australia was an early leader in the field, with a number of pioneering food laws, such as the *Pure Food Act 1905* (Vic.), which was used as a model by other countries to address food hygiene problems, set production standards and regulate the adulteration of food. Recent decades have seen a significant increase in PHN developments at the international level, such as the *World Declaration and Plan of Action for Nutrition*, issued jointly by the World Health Organization (WHO) and the United Nations' (UN) Food and Agriculture Organization (FAO). This was followed by the UN Millennium Development Goals in 2000, and the WHO *Global Strategy on Diet, Physical Activity and Health* in 2004. These measures aim to address global food security and lessen the impact of diet-related illness, though there has been little progress; for example, over 854 million people are estimated to be undernourished in developing countries in 2006 (FAO 2006).

Dietary guidance is another area where governments involve themselves in regulating food and nutrition. **Dietary guidelines** are statements of recommendations for the way in which populations are advised to alter their food habits. The ability of this advice to be influenced by powerful corporate interests is demonstrated in Chapter 6. An examination of the development and implementation of food policy exposes some of the individualistic assumptions and corporate interests that have swayed the good intentions of government authorities and health professionals attempting to address public health nutrition. An example of the influence of the food industry can be seen in the development of regulations governing food composition and labelling. For example, the food regulatory body Food Standards Australia New Zealand (FSANZ) was the subject of intense political lobbying regarding the labelling of genetically modified (GM) food (see Chapter 4). After initial indications from regulatory agencies that GM food would not need to be labelled in Australia and New Zealand, a public backlash ensued and the decision was overturned, with a similar policy adopted to that of the European Union (EU); however, the opposite has occurred in the United States of America, where labelling of GM food is not mandatory.

Food regulations are often the outcome of a compromise between the interests of the food industry and public health. Take, for example, the humble meat pie in

BOX 1.5

The Aussie meat pie and the definition of 'meat'

The quintessentially Australian meat pie—one of the earliest fast foods in Australia—was actually inherited from the British. Its popularity reflected the wide availability of meat in Australia, its simple flavours (meat and gravy encased in pastry), and its ability to be eaten with the hands, which made it a popular convenience food, especially at sporting occasions such as the football. The industrialisation and mass production of the meat pie has caused much speculation about its actual ingredients, particularly about how much meat and what types of meat it contains. The Australian Consumers' Association (2002) reported in its magazine, *Choice*, that meat pies may contain a minimum of 25 per cent actual meat. However, it is the definition of 'meat' that is of particular interest. Standard 2.2.1 (Meat and Meat Products) of the Australian New Zealand Food Standards Code defines meat as 'the carcass of any buffalo, camel, cattle, deer, goat, hare, pig, poultry, rabbit or sheep, slaughtered other than in a wild state'. So not only can a meat pie include very little actual beef or red meat, but it can include animal rind, fat, gristle, connective tissue, nerve tissue, blood and blood vessels under the label of 'meat' (offal must be listed separately in the ingredients list). This means that muscle meat—what people normally consider to be meat—may not even be included in a meat pie. Furthermore, meat content is measured by the presence of protein and this can be 'beefed up' by adding soy products (ACA 2002).

Australia and how FSANZ adopted a definition of 'meat', which makes it possible for buffalo, camel and deer, and gristle, animal rind and connective tissue to find their way into a meat pie (see Box 1.5). The chapters in this part of the book examine the role of food regulations in relation to the corporate influences on dietary guidelines, **functional foods**, public health nutrition as an influential field of professional practice, and food discourses and policies relating to the feeding of infants and children.

Food consumption, social differentiation and identity

Tell me what you eat, and I shall tell you what you are.

Jean Anthelme Brillat-Savarin, *The Physiology of Taste* (1825)

People in Western societies are presented with a large number of consumption choices, which can be used to construct their self-identity. As Deborah Lupton has described, food is often defined as 'good or bad, masculine or feminine, powerful or weak, alive

---

The 'slow food' and 'true food' social movements

BOX 1.6

The Slow Food Movement began in Italy in 1986 as a response to the mass production and globalisation of food. It claims to have over 80 000 members worldwide and it aims to 'counter the tide of standardization of taste' by promoting and cataloguing traditional, regional and national cuisines, including endangered animal breeds, vegetable species and cooking techniques. Using the emblem of the snail and calling themselves 'eco-gastronomes', members take a stand against the fast-food industry and work to protect food traditions, historic sites (cafes and bistros) and agricultural heritage (biodiversity, artisan techniques and sustainable agriculture). The Slow Food Movement promotes its aims by funding research, conferences and festivals, by publishing material, and by lobbying governments and corporations. Along similar lines but for vastly different reasons, the 'True Food Network', coordinated by Greenpeace, campaigns specifically against genetically engineered food and, in addition to its lobbying efforts, produces consumer guides on obtaining food free of genetic modification. For more information about these social movements and their food ideologies, see the following websites:

- Slow Food: www.slowfood.com/
- True Food Network: www.greenpeace.org.au/truefood/

John Germov and Lauren Williams

or dead, healthy or non-healthy, a comfort or punishment, sophisticated or gauche, a sin or virtue, animal or vegetable' (1996, pp. 1–2). These opposing attributes illustrate the social meanings, classifications and emotions that people can attach to food and, therefore by choosing certain foods above others, define who they are. Pierre Bourdieu (1979/1984) maintains that traditional modes of social distinction based on class persist through consumption practices, particularly food habits. The theme of this section of the book encapsulates food habits that are influenced by various forms of social group membership, whether based on traditional social cleavages or new social movements (see Box 1.6).

In 2005, the 'Save Toby' website (www.savetoby.com/) was launched on which it was claimed that Toby, a cute little rabbit, was being held for ransom. Unless visitors donated a certain sum of money, Toby would die. According to the site author: 'I am going to take Toby to a butcher to have him slaughter this cute bunny. I will then prepare Toby for a midsummer feast.' The website included pictures of Toby on a chopping board and in a saucepan, along with an updated diary of Toby's activities. What started as a bad taste joke gained global media attention and soon people sent money to save Toby or buy mugs, T-shirts and a book sold through Amazon.com. Eventually Toby was saved. Meanwhile, rabbits remain widely available from butchers and restaurants in many countries. The 'Save Toby' campaign exposed the contradictions inherent in meat consumption, particularly when some animals are socially constructed as pets, often with human-like attributes. The line between 'normality' and taboo foods is often fragile—never more so than when it concerns eating animals.

Ordering a vegetarian meal, eating a meat pie, dining at a trendy cafe or eating an exotic cuisine may be used and interpreted as social 'markers' of an individual's social status, group membership or philosophical beliefs. This part of the book addresses the relationship between social groups, food consumption and identity formation, with chapters on class-based food habits, vegetarianism, culture and ethnicity, and ageing.

Food and the body: Civilising processes and social embodiment

You are what you eat.

Anonymous

The adage 'you are what you eat' was originally intended as a nutrition slogan to encourage healthy eating, but today the meaning has changed as the focus has moved away from the internal health of the body to the external 'look' of the body. The final theme explored in the book concerns the impact of health, nutrition and beauty discourses on body management. The name of the well-known company Weight

Watchers symbolises the body discipline and surveillance that is now commonly practised in Western societies in efforts to conform to a socially acceptable notion of beauty and **body image**—a process that can be referred to as 'social embodiment', whereby the body is both an object and a reflective agent (Connell 2002). Attempts to regulate the body are gendered through the social construction of the **thin ideal** for women, and the **muscular ideal** for men. While external pressures from the media and corporate interests play a key role in the construction and maintenance of such discourses, they are also internalised and reproduced by individuals—an example of what Norbert Elias (1978) termed **civilising processes**, whereby social regulation of individual behaviour is no longer achieved through external coercion but through moral self-regulation.

Attempts to rationally manage and regulate the human body mean that for many people the pleasures of eating now coexist with feelings of guilt. While food companies encourage us to succumb to hedonistic temptations, health authorities proclaim nutritional recommendations as if eating is merely an instrumental act of health maintenance. The social-control overtones of such an approach are clearly evident in the'lipophobic'(fear of fat) health advice given by some health professionals. Changes in the advice of health authorities over the decades and the simplification of

'Lite' foods, balance and increasing obesity rates

BOX 1.7

Despite the increasing consumption of low-fat foods, rates of overweight and obesity continue to rise in many Western countries—a fact that should caution against any simplistic beliefs that low-fat foods can be used to control weight (Allred 1995). The latest estimates suggest that over 400 million adults worldwide are obese, and on current trends, by 2015 around 700 million adults will be obese and a further 2.3 billion will be overweight (WHO 2006).

While so-called 'light foods' are marketed for weight control purposes, Claude Fischler (1995) argues that people seek increased pleasure through the inclusion of light foods in addition to, rather than as a replacement for, other foods in the diet (possibly allowing them to eat more). For example, it is not uncommon for people to use artificial sweetener in their coffee so that they can have a slice of chocolate mud cake, or to purchase diet cola with a hamburger, giving a sense of dietary 'balance'. The commonsense notion of a 'balanced' diet is highly variable, but may be defined as a balance between 'good' and 'bad' choices, hedonism and discipline, healthy and unhealthy food (Fischler 1988).

John Germov and Lauren Williams

scientific findings into media slogans, mixed with the contra-marketing efforts of food companies, have served to create confusion over whether certain foods, particularly those marketed as 'low fat' or 'lite', are in fact health-promoting (see Box 1.7). While some people have become disciplined adherents to the new health propaganda, others have become increasingly sceptical of nutrition messages—particularly in light of the 'French paradox', or the fact that the French have lower rates of cardiovascular disease than Australians and Americans despite having a higher intake of saturated fat, which undermines simple causative links between fat consumption and heart disease (Renaud & de Logeril 1992; Drewnowski et al. 1996). This part of the book discusses the discourses related to eating and the disciplining of the body in the context of gender, dieting, body image, **eating disorders** and obesity stigmatisation.

A preliminary conclusion

There is no sincerer love than the love of food.

George Bernard Shaw, *Back to Methuselah* (1930)

While this book represents an academic enquiry into food, we would like to acknowledge the passion, delight and pure hedonism with which food is intimately associated. In that light and in the spirit of cosmopolitanism, we end this chapter with the following excerpt from Marcel Proust, which encapsulates the central role of food as part of *la dolce vita*:

> She sent for one of those squat, plump little cakes called 'petites madeleines', which look as though they had been moulded in the fluted valve of a scallop shell. And soon, mechanically, dispirited after a dreary day with the prospect of a depressing morrow, I raised to my lips a spoonful of the tea in which I had soaked a morsel of the cake. No sooner had the warm liquid mixed with the crumbs touched my palate than a shiver ran through me and I stopped, intent upon the extraordinary thing that was happening to me. An exquisite pleasure had invaded my senses, something isolated, detached, with no suggestion of its origin. And at once the vicissitudes of life had become indifferent to me, its disasters innocuous, its brevity illusory—this new sensation having had the effect, which love has, of filling me with a precious essence; or rather this essence was not in me, it *was* me. I had ceased now to feel mediocre, contingent, mortal. Whence could it have come to me, this all-powerful joy? I sensed that it was connected with the taste of the tea and the cake, but that it infinitely transcended those savours, could not, indeed, be of the same nature. Where did it come from? What did it mean? How could I seize and apprehend it?

Marcel Proust, *Swann's Way* (1913/1957)

SUMMARY OF MAIN POINTS

- The sociology of food and nutrition challenges individualistic accounts of people's eating habits that assume that personal likes and dislikes primarily govern food choice.
- The 'social appetite' refers to the social context in which food is produced, distributed and consumed, the context that shapes our food choices.
- Sociology examines how society works, how it influences our lives and how social change occurs. It adopts a critical stance by asking questions such as these: Why are things as they are? Who benefits? What are the alternatives to the status quo?
- Evan Willis suggests that the sociological imagination—or thinking sociologically—is best put into practice by addressing four interrelated facets of any social phenomena: historical, cultural, structural and critical factors.
- The way we eat reflects an interplay between social structure and human agency.
- Food cosmopolitanism is an increasing feature of contemporary social life in developed societies.

SOCIOLOGICAL REFLECTION

Think of the influences that have shaped your own food habits and likes and dislikes by imagining a social occasion at which food is consumed (such as a birthday party or Christmas celebration). Apply the sociological imagination template to explore the significance of the occasion, noting for each factor the influences on your food consumption:

- Historical: When did you first eat that way? What past events have influenced the social occasion?
- Cultural: What customs or values are involved? Who prepares and serves the food, and with whom is it consumed? Why?
- Structural: In what setting does the food event occur? What role do wider social institutions or organisations play?
- Critical: Has the particular event changed over time or not? Why?

DISCUSSION QUESTIONS

1. How can food and taste be socially constructed? Give examples.
2. What is meant by the term 'social appetite'?
3. Consider the social meanings and symbolism in the examples of the social appetite in Box 1.2. What other examples can you think of?

John Germov and Lauren Williams

Further investigation

1. Food choice is not simply a matter of personal taste, but reflects regional, national and global influences. Discuss.
2. Given that social patterns of food production, distribution, and consumption exist, to what extent are individuals responsible for their food choices?

FURTHER READING AND WEB RESOURCES

An extensive list of books and websites can be found on the companion website for this book.

Books

Beardsworth, A. & Keil, T. 1997, *Sociology on the Menu*, Routledge, London.

Belasco, W. 2006, *Meals to Come: A History of the Future of Food*, University of California Press, Berkeley.

Brownell, K.D. & Horgen, K.B. 2004, *Food Fight: The Inside Story of the Food Industry, America's Obesity Crisis, and What We Can Do About It*, McGraw-Hill, New York.

Burch, D. & Lawrence, G. 2007, *Supermarkets and Agri-food Supply Chains: Transformations in the Production and Consumption of Foods*, Edward Elgar, Cheltenham.

Charles, N. & Kerr, M. 1988, *Women, Food and Families*, Manchester University Press, Manchester.

Coveney, J. 2006, *Food, Morals, and Meaning: The Pleasure and Anxiety of Eating*, 2nd edition, Routledge, London.

Crotty, P. 1995, *Good Nutrition? Fact and Fashion in Dietary Advice*, Allen & Unwin, Sydney.

Dixon, J. 2002, *The Changing Chicken: Chooks, Cooks and Culinary Culture*, University of New South Wales Press, Sydney.

Lang, T. & Heasman, M. 2004, *Food Wars: The Global Battle for Mouths, Minds, and Markets*, Earthscan Publications, London.

Lupton, D. 1996, *Food, the Body and the Self*, Sage, London.

Maurer, D. & Sobal, J. (eds) 1995, *Eating Agendas: Food and Nutrition as Social Problems*, Aldine de Gruyter, New York.

Mennell, S. 1996, *All Manners of Food: Eating and Taste in England and France from the Middle Ages to the Present*, Revised edition, University of Illinois Press, Chicago.

Mennell, S., Murcott, A. & van Otterloo, A.H. 1992, *The Sociology of Food: Eating, Diet and Culture*, Sage, London.

Nestle, M. 2003, *Safe Food: Bacteria, Biotechnology, and Bioterrorism*, University of California Press, Berkeley.

Nestle, M. 2007, *Food Politics: How the Food Industry Influences Nutrition and Health*, Revised edition, University of California Press, Berkeley.

Pollan, M. 2006, *The Omnivore's Dilemma: The Search for a Perfect Meal in a Fast-food World*, Bloomsbury, London.

Schlosser, E. 2001, *Fast Food Nation*, Penguin, London.

Shepherd, R. & Raats, M. (eds) 2006, *The Psychology of Food Choice*, CABI Publishing, Cambridge MA.

Singer, P. & Mason, J. 2006, *The Ethics of What We Eat*, Text, Melbourne.

Symons, M. 2007, *One Continuous Picnic: A Gastronomic History of Australia*, Revised edition, Melbourne University Press, Melbourne.

Websites

Key sites can be accessed from the companion website for this book:
www.oup.com.au/orc/highereducation.aspx?ContentID=729&MasterID=18

REFERENCES

ACA—*see* Australian Consumers' Association.

Allred, J. 1995, 'Too Much of a Good Thing?', *Journal of the American Dietetic Association*, vol. 95, pp. 417–18.

Australian Consumers' Association 2002, 'Meat Pies? Well, sort of …', *Choice*, April, pp. 8–10.

Beck, U. 1992, *Risk Society: Towards a New Modernity*, Sage, London.

—— 2000, 'The Cosmopolitan Perspective: On the Sociology of the Second Age of Modernity', *British Journal of Sociology*, vol. 51, pp. 79–106.

——, Giddens, A. & Lash, S. 1994, *Reflexive Modernization: Politics, Tradition and Aesthetics in the Modern Social Order*, Polity Press and Blackwell Publishers, Cambridge.

Belasco, W. 2000, 'Future Notes: The Meal-in-a-Pill', *Food and Foodways*, vol. 8, no. 4, pp. 253–71.

Birch, L.L., Fisher, J.O. & Grimm-Thomas, K. 1996, 'The Development of Children's Eating Habits', in H.L. Meiselman and H.J.H. MacFie (eds), *Food Choice, Acceptance and Consumption*, Blackie Academic and Professional, London.

Bourdieu, P. 1979/1984, *Distinction: A Social Critique of the Judgement of Taste* (trans. by R. Nice), Routledge, London.

Charles, N. & Kerr, M. 1988, *Women, Food and Families*, Manchester University Press, Manchester.

Connell, R.W. 2002, *Gender*, Polity Press, Cambridge.

Counihan, C.M. (ed.) 1999, *The Anthropology of Food and Body: Gender, Meaning and Power*, Routledge, New York.

DAFF—*see* Department of Agriculture, Fisheries and Forestry.

Department of Agriculture, Fisheries and Forestry 2007, *Australian Food Statistics 2006*, Department of Agriculture, Fisheries and Forestry, Canberra.

DeVault, M.L. 1991, *Feeding the Family: The Social Organization of Caring as Gendered Work*, University of Chicago Press, Chicago.

Drewnowski, A., Henderson, S.A., Shore, A.B., Fischler, C., Preziosi, P. & Hercberg, S. 1996, 'Diet Quality and Dietary Diversity in France: Implications for the French Paradox', *Journal of the American Dietetic Association*, vol. 96, pp. 663–9.

Elias, N. 1978, *The Civilizing Process* (trans. by E. Jephcott), Blackwell, Oxford.

Falk, P. 1994, *The Consuming Body*, Sage, London.

FAO—*see* Food and Agricultural Organization.

Fischler, C. 1980, 'Food Habits, Social Change and the Nature/Culture Dilemma', *Social Science Information*, vol. 19, pp. 937–53.

—— 1988, 'Food, Self and Identity', *Social Science Information*, vol. 27, no. 2, pp. 275–92.

—— 1995, 'Sociological Aspects of Light Foods', in P.D. Leathwood, J. Louis-Sylvestre and J.-P. Mareschi (eds), *Light Foods: An Assessment of their Psychological, Sociocultural, Physiological, Nutritional, and Safety Aspects*, International Life Sciences Institute Press, Washington, DC.

Food and Agricultural Organization 2006, *State of Food Insecurity in the World 2006*, FAO, Rome.

Giddens, A. 1986, *Sociology: A Brief but Critical Introduction*, 2nd edition, Macmillan, London.

—— 1991, *Modernity and Self-identity: Self and Society in the Late Modern Age*, Stanford University Press, Stanford, California.

Lee, A. 2003, 'The Nutrition of Aboriginal and Torres Strait Islander Peoples', in National Health and Medical Research Council (NHMRC), *Dietary Guidelines for Adult Australians*, NHMRC, Canberra.

Lupton, D. 1996, *Food, the Body and the Self*, Sage, London.

—— 2000, 'Food, Risk and Subjectivity', in S.J. Williams, J. Gabe and M. Calnan (eds), *Health, Medicine and Society*, Routledge, London, pp. 205–18.

Mennell, S. 1996, *All Manners of Food: Eating and Taste in England and France from the Middle Ages to the Present*, 2nd edition, University of Illinois Press, Chicago.

Mills, C.W. 1959, *The Sociological Imagination*, Oxford University Press, New York.

National Health and Medical Research Council 2000, *Nutrition of Aboriginal and Torres Strait Islander Peoples: An Information Paper*, NHMRC, Canberra.

NHMRC—*see* National Health and Medical Research Council.

Proust, M. 1913/1957, *Swann's Way* (trans. by C.K. Scott Moncrieff), Penguin Books, Harmondsworth.

Renaud, S. & de Logeril, M. 1992, 'Wine Alcohol, Platelets, and the French Paradox for Coronary Heart Disease', *Lancet*, vol. 339, pp. 1526–32.

Ritzer, G. 2000, *The McDonaldization of Society*, 3rd edition, Pine Forge Press, Thousand Oaks, California.

Rojek, C. & Urry, J. (eds) 1997, *Touring Cultures: Transformations of Travel and Theory*, Routledge, London.

Schlosser, E. 2001, *Fast Food Nation*, Penguin, London.

SIGNAL—*see* Strategic Inter-Governmental Nutrition Alliance.

Smith, J. (ed.) 1997, *Hungry for You: From Cannibalism to Seduction—A Book of Food*, Vintage, London.

Sobal, J., Khan, L.K. & Bisogni, C. 1998, 'A Conceptual Model of the Food and Nutrition System', *Social Science & Medicine*, vol. 47, no. 7, pp. 853–63.

Strategic Inter-Governmental Nutrition Alliance 2001a, *National Aboriginal and Torres Strait Islander Nutrition Strategy and Action Plan, 2000–2010*, National Public Health Partnership, Canberra.

—— 2001b, *Eat Well Australia: A Strategic Framework for Public Health Nutrition 2000–2010*, National Public Health Partnership, Canberra.

Symons, M. 1993, *The Shared Table: Ideas for an Australian Cuisine*, Australian Government Publishing Service, Canberra.

Tomlinson, J. 1999, *Globalization and Culture*, Polity, Cambridge.

Willis, E. 2004, *The Sociological Quest*, 4th edition, Allen & Unwin, Sydney.

WHO—*see* World Health Organization.

World Health Organization 2006, *Obesity and Overweight (Fact sheet 311)*, WHO, Geneva.

PART 2

The Food System: Globalisation and Agribusiness

We are who we are because we are all things to all people all the time everywhere.

Ike Herbert, head of Coca-Cola USA, 1990, quoted in
Mark Pendergrast, *For God, Country and Coca-Cola* (1993, p. 398; Phoenix, London)

People often feed the hungry so that nothing may disturb their own enjoyment of a good meal.

Somerset Maugham, *A Writer's Notebook* (1949)

In this part of the book we examine why something as innocuous as choosing certain foods can be a politicised act with global consequences. Food is a highly profitable commodity and the pursuit of profit has significant implications for the way food is produced and distributed. Yet food is also an essential commodity—people must literally eat to live—and it therefore has fundamental humanitarian value. In developed countries, the wide availability of food is taken for granted by most, except those living in poverty. The unequal distribution of food is also played out on a global scale, and for a large proportion of the world's population, hunger is a way of life, with acute periods of starvation occurring in times of famine or political unrest.

The chapters in Part 2 cover the major influences on the food system, in terms of globalisation and agribusiness, by focusing on world hunger, the environment, the development of genetically modified food, and the power of supermarkets in the food commodity chain.

Specifically, this section consists of four chapters:

- Chapter 2 outlines a range of perspectives that attempt to explain the persistence of world hunger, and discusses the viability of proposed strategies for ensuring that every human has enough food.
- Chapter 3 explains how the dominant mode of agricultural production in developed countries, driven by the profit imperative, causes environmental degradation; it also examines a number of environmentally sustainable alternatives.
- Chapter 4 highlights the global nature of agribusiness by exploring the use of biotechnology to develop genetically modified foods.
- Chapter 5 examines the increasing power of supermarket chains over Australia's food system and their influence on culinary culture and food habits via a case study of the rise in popularity of chicken meat.

CHAPTER 2

World Hunger: Its Roots and Remedies

Frances Moore Lappé

OVERVIEW

- What is the extent of world hunger?
- What is the conventional explanation for explaining and alleviating hunger and what are its shortcomings?
- What are the real causes and remedies of world hunger?

To the question 'Why hunger?' the prevailing answer has long been 'scarcity', and the solution has seemed equally clear: we end hunger by alleviating scarcity as we extend the West's proven economic model to hungry people. Yet, despite more than enough food in the world to feed us all well (UN FAO 2002) and world economic output multiplying almost fivefold per person over the last 60 years (De Long 1998, pp. 1–12), hunger still plagues humanity and is worsening in many parts of the world (UN FAO 2006a, p. 6). In response to such failure, awareness is growing that scarcity is not the cause of hunger but a symptom of deeper causes. Hunger results from a set of beliefs governing human relationships that in turn generate artificial scarcity.

Historically, a range of belief systems have contributed to deprivation; one belief system prevailing today is that economies best operate outside democratic accountability and according to one rule: highest return to existing wealth (i.e. company shareholders). As a result, wealth and decision-making power inevitably concentrate to serve a minority, depriving many of life necessities, including food.

Thus, ending hunger is less about supplying missing 'things' — seeds, water, fertilisers — to increase supply than about letting go of a failing ideology and embracing a values-driven approach that aims to achieve greater equity and creativity in human relationships. This emergent approach re-embeds economic life in networks of relationships shaped by shared human needs and values: fairness, efficacy and regard for future generations.

Key terms

cooperative	genetically modified (GM)	participatory budgeting
food sovereignty	Green Revolution	sustainable farming/
frame	microcredit	agriculture
Global South, Global North	one-rule economics	

Introduction: What is the prevailing frame for explaining and alleviating hunger and what are its shortcomings?

The scarcity frame

'Within a decade no man, woman or child will go to bed hungry,' declared Henry Kissinger at the first World Food Conference of government and business leaders in Rome. That was 1974. Yet, more than a quarter century later, 854 million people are undernourished (UN FAO 2006a, p. 8). More recent initiatives set specific hunger-ending goals. In 1996, at the World Food Summit, also in Rome, national leaders from 186 countries pledged to halve the number of hungry in the world by 2015 (World Food Summit 1996). Then, in 2000, world leaders committed to Millennium Development Goals (see Box 2.1), with specific targets for reducing the scourges of poverty and hunger by 2015 (UN Development Programme 2003, p. 1).

BOX 2.1

UN Millennium Development Goals

1. Eradicate extreme poverty and hunger
2. Achieve universal primary education
3. Promote gender equality and empower women
4. Reduce child mortality
5. Improve maternal health
6. Combat HIV/AIDS, malaria and other diseases
7. Ensure environmental sustainability
8. Develop a global partnership for development

Source: UN Millennium Development Goals (2007)

Such global initiatives and much of the vast literature about the roots of hunger assume one cause—scarcity. People go hungry because something (usually a lot) is lacking: fertile soils, modern technologies, quality seeds, irrigation, roads, know-how and, therefore, food itself. From this **frame**, the solution is clear. We must alleviate these scarcities by extending the industrial countries' successful economic model to those left behind.

Over the last half century, this diagnosis has stayed remarkably consistent. Only the face of scarcity has changed. In the 1970s it was Bangladesh, the 'basket case' that for many people proved humanity had overrun the earth's capacities (see Box 2.2). Today, the face of scarcity is Africa. Sub-Saharan Africa now suffers the highest prevalence of chronic hunger in the world, afflicting roughly one-third of the population (UN FAO 2006a, p. 23), and we are encouraged to believe the primary reason to be due to the physical geography of the region. Observers emphasise the region's deficiencies—its lack of fertile soils and irrigation resulting in grain yields just one-third of what Asia and Latin America produce; 'its lack of medicine, medical care and education resulting in a disease burden that cuts three decades off life expectancy compared to the industrial countries' (Sachs 2005, pp. 204–8).

Taking population seriously

BOX 2.2

Despite the evidence, many people see high birth rates and hunger in the **Global South** and arrive at what seems like commonsense: just too many mouths to feed. But scanning the globe, no correlation between people density and undernourishment is to be found. High birth rates are best understood not as a cause of hunger but as a symptom. Along with hunger, they are a symptom of powerlessness, especially of women denied control over their fertility. Mounting evidence from around the world suggests that as people, especially women, gain education and income, fertility rates decline. Thus, to move human numbers into balance with ecological limits requires an end to poverty and hunger (Lappé et al. 1998, pp. 25–41).

The most commonly proposed solution has also held steady. In 1960 American economist W.W. Rostow released *Stages of Economic Growth: A Non-Communist Manifesto*, a title that captured well his cure for poverty; and soon the approach became gospel for a generation of development theorists. Four decades later, Jeffrey Sachs (2005), champion of the UN's Millennium Development Goals, saw the solution as the 'dynamism of self-sustaining economic growth' and called on the industrialised societies to fulfil their obligation to help the poor get their 'foothold on the ladder'. Sachs emphasised the need for more aid, more effectively given (Sachs 2005, pp. 73, 329–46).

Paralleling the overall growth prescription, the message about how to improve agriculture echoes through the decades: feeding the world requires 'modernising' agriculture by making it more like industry. Practices of over a billion poor farmers must become more and more standardised through global corporate chains supplying inputs—fertilisers, pesticides, seeds, machines—and buying and distributing outputs. In this model, farmers become links in an ever more uniform, commercial and global system (Sharma 2005).

Appealing to the belief that inadequate production is the root of hunger, in the 1990s multinational agribusinesses began to claim that their **genetically modified (GM)** seeds, in which genes from another species have been inserted, were the answer. In 2006, two large US foundations announced a major initiative to address

Africa's scarcity crisis through improved commercial seed and fertiliser distribution (Rockefeller Foundation and Bill and Melinda Gates Foundation 2006). Their goal was to jump-start a **Green Revolution** in Africa like the one centred in Asia that has almost tripled grain output in 40 years.

Within this frame, China and India are toasted as development 'miracles'. The focus is on China's success in cutting the number of hungry people by a quarter, to 146 million, in the period 1990–92 to 1995–97 (UN FAO 2006b). Regarding India, the international press has focused on grain production increases associated with the Green Revolution and its strong economic growth rates.

Shortcomings of the prevailing frame

We breathe in like invisible ether this scarcity-as-cause and economic-growth-as-cure framing, making it difficult even to register the contradictory evidence that is all around us. Worldwide, agricultural production per person has grown by 20 per cent since 1980 (UN FAO 2006c, p. 1). Yet, 'far from decreasing, the number of hungry people in the world is currently increasing—at the rate of four million a year', noted UN Food and Agriculture Organization (FAO) director-general Jacques Diouf in 2006 (UN FAO 2006d). Yet, because Diouf's alarming words did not fit the prevailing frame, they seemed to slip by with little media coverage.

Similarly, given India's much-touted development 'miracle', few seem to register that India is home to 212 million undernourished people, more than in all of Sub-Saharan Africa. Or that India's progress in reducing hunger came to a halt during the booming 1990s (UN FAO 2006a, pp. 32–3), and today almost half of India's children suffer malnutrition (World Bank 2005). These realities run counter to the popular image of India as an emerging region for 'call centres' and software developers.

Turning to China, the prevailing market frame also lacks explanatory power. There, productive advances have come less from a Western market model than from a form of 'state interference and violence', writes Wang Hui, research professor at Qinghua University in Beijing (Schell 2004). While statistics show a dramatic reduction in hunger in the first part of the 1990s, the number of hungry people rose during the periods 1995–97 and 2002–04 (UN FAO 2006c). Moreover, much of China's growth is being created, with staggering ecological damage, by the 120 to 130 million people surviving on less than US$1 a day with no protection of their labour rights (China Daily 2006).

Through the scarcity frame, Sub-Saharan Africa suffers hunger because of every sort of deficiency. But how does this view sit with the reality that 11 Sub-Saharan countries have reduced the prevalence of hunger to less than the 20 per cent still found in 'booming' India (UN FAO 2006a)? Or that the West African country of Ghana has made more rapid progress than any country in the Global South—already surpassing the World Food Summit goal of reducing the number of undernourished by half by

2015 (UN FAO 2006a, p. 24)? And how does the view of Africa as devoid of wealth hold up against the fact that it is home to one-third of the world's mineral reserves and is among the top five exporters of key agricultural products, including coffee, tea, cocoa and cotton? Further, in diverse settings African farmers are achieving striking improvements in agricultural productivity and general well-being by working with local endowments. Their successes, to which we turn later, belie the premise of lack.

Finally, viewing poor countries as simply lacking resources blinds solution-seekers to the systematic undervaluing and depletion of indigenous wealth that has occurred over centuries of colonial control and through subsequent externally driven 'development' strategies. One consequence of colonialism, for example, was the neglect, and in some cases, suppression, of roughly 2000 African native grains, roots, fruits and other food plants to the point that some scholars call them the 'lost crops of Africa' (National Research Council 1996; see also Rodney 1973). Solutions depend on acknowledging such losses so that they can be reversed.

Additional pitfalls of the dominant frame concern the ecological viability of its prescriptions. The prevailing view assumes humanity can continue increasing food output by spreading fossil-fuel-based fertilisers and pesticides, and other technologies, including GM seeds, and can feed the hungry via long-distance, corporation-created supply chains. Yet this approach has already wrought vast ecological damage, virtually none of which is registered in the price of food (see Chapter 3 for further details). Over time, such **one-rule economics** shifts diets towards processed foods that are high in fat, salt and sugar because these bring higher returns to food industry shareholders than do healthier, whole foods. Thus, worldwide, diet-related diseases, including heart disease and obesity, worsen even among the poor (Gardner & Halweil 2000). Furthermore, some GM foods have been linked to increased ecological and health risks (see Chapter 4; Smith 2007).

It is assumed that the dominant market-driven growth solution has already proven it can conquer hunger. But where the model is most firmly entrenched, in the United States of America, over five pounds (or two kilograms) of food (imagine eight loaded dinner plates) are available each day for each person. Yet, 38 million Americans live in households suffering from hunger or on the precipice of hunger, a number that has risen since 2000 by about a million a year (Nord et al. 2005, p. 6).

In the dominant frame, agricultural progress means less government involvement and greater farmer dependence on technologies purchased from global corporations, where control is increasingly concentrated. One company, Monsanto, for example, is the source of over 80 per cent of GM seeds (ETC Group 2005). Consider what India teaches about the viability of this approach for poor farmers with no economic 'cushion'. In the 1960s, millions of poor Indian farmers began taking on debt to buy costly inputs, including hybrid seeds. While these seeds are typically called 'high-yielding' varieties, they are more accurately 'high-responding'—producing more in response to irrigation and fertilisers if protected by pesticides, all of which cost farmers

Frances Moore Lappé

money. Rice and wheat displaced diverse, often highly nutritious food production. For many farmers costs rose and yields flagged over time as pests acquired resistance and soil became degraded. At the same time, prices sank, and, beginning in the 1980s as international lending agencies insisted on anti-government, pro-market policies, the Indian government cut its farm (and consumer) protections. As a result, many poor Indian farmers were bankrupted and lost their land (Shiva 1991, 1993; Shiva et al. 2002), and 150 000 have committed suicide since 1993 (BBC 2007). Even the world's richest country, the USA, lost 15 000 farms per year on average between 1999 and 2003 (National Agricultural Statistics Service 2005). An approach that destroys healthy rural communities is not socially viable.

In the dominant frame, as farm technology progressively replaces human labour, farmers and rural workers migrate to urban centres (Sachs 2005, p. 36). Yet, mega-cities in poor countries are already miserably overcrowded and lack basic services. Moreover, by 2015, two-thirds of the world's largest cities are projected to be coastal, where rising sea levels due to global warming could severely disrupt life (Worldwatch Institute 2007, p. 120). More generally, the dominant frame's economic formula leads to a deepening wealth divide that growth itself does not close. Even during the booming 1990s, every 100 dollars in economic growth worldwide brought just *60 pennies* to reducing the poverty of the world's billion poorest people (Woodward & Simms 2006, p. 3). As the world economy has grown over the past 40 years, the income chasm separating the top fifth and the bottom fifth of the world's people has more than doubled (UN Development Programme 1999, p. 36) and 80 per cent of people now live in societies where inequality is increasing (UN Development Programme 2005, p. 36).

The dominant frame suggests that increased foreign aid is a viable solution to world hunger. While greater resources transferred to poor communities could help people build power over their lives, aid does not necessarily touch many of the deepest roots of hunger (see below) that rob poor people of power in the first place. Plus, the realism of counting on markedly increased aid from the industrial nations as a primary solution must be weighed against the historical record. While the industrial nations pledged almost four decades ago to increase foreign development assistance to 0.7 per cent of Gross National Income, today this assistance is at 0.25 per cent, or US$79 billion annually, still only a third of the way towards their goal (Hirvonen 2005).

Focusing on official foreign assistance also ignores how much of it functions not to end poverty but to promote a donor's foreign policy goals. Half of US aid is considered military and 'economic, political/security' assistance; and almost three-quarters of total US foreign aid goes to Middle Eastern countries that the USA sees as strategically vital, especially Iraq and Israel (Nowels & Tarnoff 2004). Among nations, the USA makes the largest absolute contribution, but only 30 per cent of total US aid is development assistance (Nowels & Tarnoff 2004, p. 5), and less than half of that goes to the world's poorest counties (NetAid.Org 2007). For aid to be effective, it needs to reject the scarcity frame. Alternatives are outlined in Box 2.3.

Empowering aid

BOX 2.3

Despite the limits on the effectiveness of aid because of how donors define their interests, some nations use foreign aid to get at the roots of hunger. They see their interests in the advancement of poor people and grasp that aid passed through anti-democratic elites will not serve that goal. So they directly support local nongovernmental groups in poor countries working to empower their own communities.

Among nations with reputations for supporting social movements attacking the roots of hunger are the Scandinavian countries, the Netherlands, Germany, Belgium and Canada. Some have backed effective social movements, highlighted below, particularly in their take-off stages. Moreover, certain organisations that began as charities—Oxfam, for example, whose name derives from its 1942 founding as Oxford Committee for Famine Relief—have continued to evolve. Their strategies now include not only direct aid but public education and lobbying campaigns in the **Global North** to change the policies mentioned above that impoverish the Global South.

Other broad citizen anti-poverty movements like the Jubilee Debt Campaign and the Make Poverty History Campaign, both based in the United Kingdom, focus citizens' attention not on saving the pitiful, bereft poor abroad, but rather on removing obstacles—onerous debt repayment and discriminatory trade rules—that deplete the resources of poor countries. The Debt Campaign is calling for a complete cancellation of the debts of poorest counties. When such efforts help citizens in the Global North question the prevailing economic rules that work to generate poverty from plenty, they help not just the poor abroad but themselves as well.

What are the real roots of hunger?

To begin to make sense of this confusing picture, we have to dig deeper. While the proximate cause of hunger is that a person lacks food, we must ask—why? There is no absolute lack of food; the world produces more than enough food for all to thrive, even after subtracting the third of world grain fed to livestock, which return in meat only a fraction of the nutrients fed them (UN FAO 2002). Even where millions go hungry—from Brazil to India to Africa—food is exported. Hunger is a symptom of a deeper lack—it is a lack of power.

Taken to its Latin root *posse*, power means simply our capacity to act. It is a dynamic quality in all human relationships. Since all life seeks to sustain itself, life-destroying hunger is proof that people have been denied power, denied the capacity

Frances Moore Lappé

to protect themselves and their offspring. In other words, since the world's supply of food is more than adequate, and no one *chooses* to go hungry, the very existence of hunger is a sign of power imbalances so extreme that some people have been made powerless even to meet their survival needs.

While most attention to hunger focuses on *things*, to end hunger we must refocus on *relationships among people* for it is these relationships that determine people's capacities, their power to create and to access those things humans need to thrive. Immediately, attention shifts from better seeds or new roads, and moves to how power operates from the village level to the level of international commerce. Consider the following ways in which hunger-causing power imbalances are manifested.

Concentrating control over land. Since arable land is necessary to grow food, rural people without land are vulnerable to hunger. Power at the root of hunger shows up, therefore, in land ownership. In Guatemala, for example, 2 per cent of the population controls 72 per cent of the land (Krznaric 2005, p. 5). In Brazil, 1 per cent of the population owns almost half the arable land, leaving much of it idle (Kingstone 2004). In South Africa, 80 per cent of arable land is still owned by a white minority that is just 10 per cent of the population (BBC 2005).

Shrinking share of profits for poor producers. Over a billion of the world's poorest people are small farmers, many producing for export. Their livelihoods, and thus whether their families go hungry, depend on the prices they receive for their crops. Yet, the 'global commodity markets' on which they depend 'are increasingly dominated by fewer global transnational corporations', writes Special Rapporteur on the right to food, Jean Ziegler (2004, pp. 9, 13), of the UN's Commission on Human Rights, adding that global corporations 'have the power to demand low producer prices, while keeping consumer prices high, thus, increasing their profit margins'.

The real prices farmers received for their agricultural commodities fell almost 80 per cent in 40 years (UN FAO 2004b, p. 10). The consequence is that farmers themselves retain a shrinking share of economic benefit to be made from exports. Among them are 25 million coffee producers, working only a few acres (Oxfam America 2006). A decade ago the countries in which they live—from Guatemala to Vietnam—retained roughly 30 per cent of coffee revenue. Today they keep about 10 per cent. The winners aren't consumers but the four largest coffee companies, Nestlé, Philip Morris-Kraft Foods, Procter & Gamble and Sara Lee/Douwe Egberts, which together control almost half of the market (Vorley 2003, pp. 24, 25). In addition to controlling and thus benefiting most from agricultural exports, multinational corporations often work with powerful local interest groups to profit from extracting other resources—from tropical woods to diamonds to plant germplasm (Mgbeoji 2006).

Trade rules favouring the already wealthy. World trade flows have tripled over the last two decades, but the share of exports from the world's 48 poorest countries has dropped by almost half, to a negligible 0.4 per cent (Oxfam Great Britain 1999, p. i).

If all poor countries increased exports by merely 5 per cent, the additional revenue earned, US$350 billion a year, would be seven times larger than the foreign aid they receive. Yet, industrial nations, beholden to corporate interests, maintain barriers against imports from the Global South are on average four times greater than from other wealthy nations (Oxfam International 2002, pp. 7, 50).

Two further examples illustrate how distant power relationships directly generate hunger in the Global South. In the USA, just 10 per cent of farms have come to produce two-thirds of agricultural products (Public Citizen 2005). These largest operators, along with large food processing corporations that profit from cheap raw materials, then wield enough political power to secure enormous public subsidies, including US$165 billion going to farmers from 1995 through 2005, of which 73 per cent went to just 10 per cent of recipients (Environmental Working Group 2006). One result is that 25 000 US cotton growers receive on average US$200 000 yearly from taxpayers, allowing them to prosper even while selling cotton so cheaply that it undercuts the livelihoods of Africa's 20 million cotton growers (Rusu 2006; USDA Economic Research Service 2006). Total government subsidies paid to farmers in industrial countries come to US$279.5 billion, or almost three-quarters of a billion dollars a day (Griswold et al. 2006, pp. 42–9).

In the same vein, poor Mexican corn growers saw prices for their crops drop by almost half after their government, responding to interests of large food processors, signed a 1994 trade agreement with the USA allowing subsidised US corn to flood Mexico (King 2005, p. 115). To protest this type of unaccountable power leaving small farmers in ruins, South Korean farmer Lee Kyung Hae immolated himself in 2003. 'What would be your emotional reaction,' his suicide letter asked, 'if your salary drops suddenly to half without knowing clearly the reason' (Rosset 2006b, p. xiii).

The result is what some economists call 'immiserating trade'—as in 18 poor countries where during the 1990s exports increased while private consumption per person fell (UN Conference on Trade and Development 2004, p. 152). In coffee-export-dependent Guatemala, for example, as coffee prices skidded, undernourishment spread from 16 to 23 per cent of the population between 1990–92 and 2002–03 (UN FAO 2006a, p. 19).

Debt burden falling on the poor. In other ways as well, poverty and hunger are not static states of 'lack' but are actively generated. Poor nations are paying US$200 billion in debt repayments each year to wealthy nations, roughly four times more than they receive in foreign aid (Shah 2006). Yet most of this onerous debt was incurred not by or for the poor majorities who are suffering under the burden of repayment, but by elite-dominated governments. In many cases loans were taken by brutal dictators like Mobutu Sese Seko in the Democratic Republic of Congo (formerly Zaire) and Ferdinand Marcos in the Philippines, who used the funds to enrich themselves (Hanlon 1998). Over the last decade, citizen campaigns for debt relief have succeeded

Frances Moore Lappé

in eliminating about US$76 billion of the debt load on the 20 poorest countries, but 150 poor countries are still paying on a total US$2.8 trillion debt in 2005, at the rate of about half a trillion dollars a year (Jubilee Debt Campaign 2006).

Rules governing trade, government subsidies, debt and more are made by the economically more powerful and serve to transfer wealth and potential wealth from poor to rich. By 2006 this resulted in a net annual transfer of US$658 billion from poorer countries to wealthier countries, while a decade ago the balance was even (UN World Economics Situation and Prospects 2007). The unequal distribution of global income has been represented as a champagne glass, as in Figure 2.1, which shows a world in which the richest 20 per cent (the widest top of the glass) have 75 per cent of the world's income, while the bottom 60 per cent of people (the narrow stem) live on around 6 per cent of global income.

Figure 2.1   Unequal distribution of world income: The Champagne-glass effect

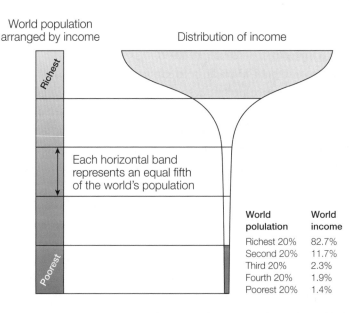

Source: Adapted from UN Development Programme (2005)

The power of beliefs

Power imbalances have always been created and maintained not by brute force alone but by belief systems that justify them and encourage their embrace even by those suffering from their consequences. In earlier societies, extreme inequalities have been justified by such notions as a chief's lineage, a caste's inherited rank, a king's or, in Islamic societies, a caliph's divine right. In many places these beliefs still hold sway. Yet today the belief system that industrial countries, especially the USA, are spreading throughout the world justifies power inequalities in the following way: to be effective, economic life must be driven by a single goal, that is, the highest return to corporate shareholders, a small fraction of humanity; and it must operate in response to supply and demand market cues operating independently, largely without accountability to democratic polities. In effect, then, the economic system's raison d'être is to return wealth to the wealthy. In this chapter, the shorthand for this ideology is 'one-rule economics'.

Through conditions on aid and trade set by international agencies, such as the World Bank, International Monetary Fund (IMF) and the World Trade Organization (WTO), the logic of one-rule economics has penetrated economies throughout the world. Beginning in the 1980s, most countries in the Global South were required, in order to receive foreign help, to cut back government's role in guiding the economy and to reduce public sector spending on education and health care while opening local markets to increased penetration by global corporations (Bello et al. 1994). Extreme imbalances in wealth and power, making hunger inevitable, flow from this belief system. Fortunately, though, alternative understandings are gaining ground.

How are people effectively uprooting hunger?

As more and more people abandon the flawed premise that hunger is about 'things'—the lack of them—and begin to see hunger as symptomatic of extreme imbalances in power in human relationships, much changes. They see possibilities for constructing new norms as well as ever-more democratic decision-making bodies; they begin to grow and distribute food and to create communities in ways more consistent with their interests and values.

Realism and hope

In order to act, however, human beings must have hope that the situation can change. So it may be helpful to note that the human qualities most needed to address power imbalances at the root of hunger are increasingly recognised as universal. The dominant economic model's assumption that human beings are motivated only by narrow self-interest is being replaced by an appreciation of common human needs for fairness, efficacy and meaning (Hauser 2006; World Bank 2006, pp. 76–88).

During the long sweep of human social evolution such extreme imbalances as those now generated by one-rule economics appear to be an aberration, at least in terms of access to food. For over two million years hominids—our precursors—evolved as hunter-gatherers; as did we *Homo sapiens*. Studying hunter-gatherer societies, anthropologist Michael Gurven concluded that humans are unique in their 'pervasive sharing' of food 'especially among unrelated individuals' (Gurven 2004, pp. 543–83). Except in times of extreme privation, when some eat, all eat. The most productive hunters, it turns out, share the most (Alvard 2004, accompanying Gurven

2004, pp. 543–83). In more recent eras, too, a norm of mutual responsibility concerning food was widespread, as suggested in the origin of the word 'lord'. It derives from *hlaf-weard* (loaf-guardian), reflecting the early Germanic tribal custom of superiors being responsible for ensuring access for all. Note also that far short of achieving truly fair participation in power, even a minor righting of the balance would result in a striking alleviation of suffering. The International Labor Organization (ILO) notes that a shift towards the world's poor of only 2 per cent of the global Gross National Income could furnish all poor people minimum income security, as well as meet basic educational and health needs (Somavia 2004, p. 38).

Towards the end of hunger

With such a realistic sense of possibility we can then ask: How are people expressing their deep needs for fairness, efficacy and meaning by gaining power over the health of their communities and our planet's future? From the village level to the level of international commerce, growing numbers of people are working effectively to end hunger and poverty by:

1 freeing their political systems from control by concentrated wealth through economic and political rules to keep power equitably shared and to expand citizen engagement in problem solving
2 creating fair and efficient economies by ensuring that access to life's essentials— food, land, health care, and education—are governed by standards that sustain life, including fairer business and financial models, not simply by supply and demand
3 building knowledge-intensive, ecologically sound agriculture sustained by the ongoing learning of farmers who increase available food as they sustain eco- systems.
These points will be examined in detail below.

1. Freeing political systems from the influence of money

In the effort to free the political process from the control of wealth, consider Bolivia, where almost a quarter of citizens, mostly among the indigenous population, are undernourished despite rich agricultural resources (UN FAO 2006a, p. 32). Thus, when the first president of indigenous-majority origin, Evo Morales, was elected in 2006, many wondered how a poor majority overcame long-entrenched minority power.

Most important are decades of community organising in which those disenfranchised began to realise their united power. Also, public financing of campaigns has at least begun to remove the grip of money on Bolivia's electoral process, as is true of other Andean countries. In an interview soon after his election,

President Morales (2006) stressed the importance of public financing of campaigns. He himself took no private money and after the election returned back to the state half of the million dollars in public funds he'd received. Not bound by expectations of wealthy donors, Morales moved forward on land reform, the hunger-fighting potential of which is enormous when considering that today the wealthiest 7 per cent of Bolivians control roughly 90 per cent of the land (Reel 2006).

Nowhere does the goal of freeing politics from the influence of money seem more distant than in the USA. Yet, even there, voluntary public financing of elections, called 'Clean Elections', is already succeeding in two states to remove the influence of wealth and to bring candidates without private wealth into the democratic process. In 2005, a third state approved the approach, and campaigns for Clean Elections are under way in about a dozen more states. With the influence of wealth removed, elected officials seem more likely to reflect the values of the majority of Americans who place ending poverty (and therefore, hunger) as a top priority (Public Agenda 2004).

Citizens use governments for ending hunger

In India, the southern, densely populated state of Kerala teaches lessons about the significance of viewing hunger through the lens of power in human relationships, not of a scarcity of things. Since the 1950s, citizens of Kerala have viewed government as a means for developing people's power to achieve greater fairness. They regularly elected progressive governments, which in 1969 instituted a distributive reform enabling 1.5 million tenants to become small farm owners (Franke & Chasin 1994, p. 58). Aware that good health and literacy also enhance one's power, Keralians made access to health care and education top government priorities (Isaac & Franke 2002, p. 16). In 1989, a massive government-sponsored literacy campaign used 50 000 volunteer trainers to virtually wipe out illiteracy. By the late 1990s, Kerala's citizens, whose incomes are about 5 per cent the size of average Americans, had achieved literacy and life expectancy rates roughly 90 per cent of those in the USA (Franke 1999).

Just a decade ago Kerala's political culture took a further huge step towards equitable participation in power. Through a People's Campaign for Decentralized Planning, control over 35 to 40 per cent of the state's development expenditures devolved to more than a thousand local governments. The People's Campaign trained hundreds of thousands of citizens in budgeting and planning, and local governments created participatory exercises in which citizens directly shaped policies and projects. Compared to previous, more centrally prepared plans, results include a greater share of resources benefiting the poorest with greater emphasis on education, sanitation, safe drinking water, improved housing and environmental protection (Isaac & Franke 2002; Brizzi et al. 2005).

Similarly, in Brazil **participatory budgeting** involves citizens in determining the use of as much as a fifth of a city's budget through multi-step, face-to-face neighbourhood deliberations. Hundreds of Brazilian cities now use the approach,

Frances Moore Lappé

which is shifting resources to those who most need them (Baiocchi 2003, pp. 47–50; Baiocchi 2005, pp. 12–13).

While in diverse cultures citizens are learning to create democratic governments accountable to their values, many people still see government's responsibility in ending hunger as, at most, the provision of things to hungry people—food, a minimal dole, homeless shelters, and so on. None of these things, however, necessarily expands citizens' power to create, over time, the lives they want. But if one reconceives government's primary roles as those of *convener* of key interests in creating solutions plus *standards-and-rules setter* to ensure fair human relationships, then government can expand power to create sustainable solutions to hunger.

Consider the experience of Belo Horizonte above. As convener, the city government's food security agency brings small local farmers together with city markets and school-food providers and other institutions. It links university researchers with citizens' groups to post weekly notices of stores offering the best food prices. As rule setter, the city requires the farm produce stands that are allowed to use prime city-owned plots, to sell food at below market prices. Here, both farmers and poor people benefit because no middlemen take a cut. Another rule requires the benefiting farmers to truck produce weekly to sell in outlying poor neighbourhoods.

Government serving as standards-and-rule setter and convener of key players in addressing hunger is not necessarily costly. In Belo Horizonte, the city-led initiatives claim roughly 1 per cent of the city's budget (Aranha 2000). Of course, in these two roles, effective government also increases wealth, augmenting government funds. The Brazilian constitution's rule that arable land serve a social function made possible new rural communities so successful that they disproportionately contribute to local taxes (Rosset 2006b, p. 11).

Government rule-setting that establishes workers' rights to form trade unions, thus gaining bargaining power, also helps lower the risk of hunger. In the USA, for example, median salaries of unionised workers are a quarter higher than non-union (Democratic Staff of the Committee on Education and the Workforce, for Miller 2004). Imagine then, on a global scale, both the reduced poverty and lighter demands on public budgets if more governments had exercised their rule-setting power and ratified and enforced ILO conventions protecting the rights of workers. Yet almost a century after the ILO's founding, the two nations with the largest economies, the USA and China, have yet to ratify two core ILO conventions protecting workers' rights to organise (ILO 2006).

It can be difficult, however, for people to see how positive interaction between government and the economy can end hunger because the dominant frame sees government and the market as enemies; in this frame the goal is to 'free' the market from government control (Friedman 1962). In fact, however, an effective market *depends on* government—on a truly democratic one answering to citizens. Without it, economies driven by highest return to shareholders end up in monopoly power, destroying an open market. In global food and farming industries, two companies—Cargill and ADM—control most (some report three-quarters) of the world's cereals trade. Four control most of the oil seed trade. Three companies—Cargill, Dreyfus, and Tate & Lyle—dominate the trading and refining of sugar (Vorley 2003, p. 11).

This concentration proves that corporate capitalism is not inherently competitive. Economist James Galbraith notes that 'corporations exist to control markets and often to replace them' (Galbraith 2006, p. 34). Continuing competition depends on enforcing anti-monopoly standards, another key rule-setting function of government with an impact on hunger.

2. Citizens creating fair and efficient economies including fairer business and economic models

What should be considered a human right, not just a commodity in the market? For increasing numbers of people one answer is food. In 2004 the UN's FAO Council adopted 'voluntary guidelines for the progressive realization of the right to adequate food' (Windfuhr & Jonsén 2005, p. 15); and today 22 countries have enshrined this right in their constitutions, either for all citizens or specifically for children (UN FAO 2001).

Brazilians are tackling this right more energetically than most. There, the Workers Party, founded in 1980 on an anti-poverty platform, made possible the election of Brazil's first working-class president, Luís Inácio ('Lula') da Silva, in 2002. Immediately, Lula declared the goal of Zero Hunger and within three years his administration had invested US$14 billion towards this end. Zero Hunger moved beyond 'one-rule economics' and established food as a basic human right. This shift in frame spurred the creation of 6000 urban farms; created over 100 public restaurants with healthy food at below-market prices; and set up a system paying 11 million poor families a monthly cash dividend as long as their children stayed in school and received regular health check-ups (Aranha 2006).

Helping to guide this national campaign has been the hunger-fighting experience of Brazil's fourth-largest city, Belo Horizonte. Declaring healthy food a right of citizenship in 1993, city officials drew together voices from labour, church and citizen organisations. Their out-of-the-box innovations, coordinated by a new municipal office of food security, include fair-price produce stands supplied by local farmers, open-air restaurants serving 12 000 subsidised meals daily, and city-sponsored radio broadcasts leading shoppers to the least expensive essentials (Aranha 2000; Chappell 2006). As a result, the city's infant death rate, a widely accepted measure of hunger, fell a striking 56 per cent over the first decade of these efforts (Andrade 2006).

Gain land, end hunger

As noted above, rural people without access to land are vulnerable to hunger. Worldwide, over 170 million landless rural people are among the world's poorest

(UN FAO 2004a, p. 25), but in Brazil they have created arguably the largest and most effective citizen movement in the western hemisphere. Founded in 1980, this is the Landless Workers Movement, known by its acronym MST.

The MST began with a commonsense argument: all suffer if fertile land lies idle while eager workers go hungry. And many non-poor agreed; so much so that they supported a 1988 constitution that requires (Article 184) the government to ensure that farmland serves a 'social function'. Using this legal underpinning as well as civil disobedience to press its case, the MST has enabled the legal transfer of land to 350 000 families, or over a million formerly landless Brazilians. Among those gaining land, infant mortality had fallen by the late 1990s to only half the national average (Rosset 2006a, pp. 312, 314). The MST has focused on organising and teaching democratic skills—such as village and business self-management, and democratic concepts—such as gender equity—that are necessary for building power. Its members' expanding power has so far birthed over 2000 settlements and 1800 schools (MST 2003).

One can see landlessness as another deficiency to be corrected; or one can, as does the MST, see lack of access to land as one aspect of powerlessness to be overcome. Where land reforms based on the first perspective have redistributed land but left beneficiaries without a political voice to secure credit and markets, farmers have gained little. But where power shifts occurred during land reform processes of the twentieth century, as happened in Japan, South Korea, Taiwan, China and Cuba, rural people saw big improvements in their lives (Rosset 2006a, p. 312).

New business models to end hunger

Hunger-ending economies also require new models of business fostering more equitable power relationships. One model merges the role of owner and worker (a distinction assumed to be essential in the dominant economic model) in worker **cooperatives** that are controlled neither by a single owner nor by outside investors but by workers who are also owners. In other cooperatives, consumers own the enterprise; in social cooperatives, such as childcare, users are often the owners. In all cooperative varieties, a core principle is the equitable sharing of responsibilities and benefits.

Membership in cooperatives has more than doubled in the last 30 years to nearly 800 million, according to the Geneva-based International Co-operative Alliance. While rarely covered by the world's press, cooperatives are not marginal. They provide 100 million jobs worldwide, one-fifth more than multinational corporations offer (International Cooperative Alliance 2007). In some African countries, the cooperative movement is surpassed only by government as the largest employer (Committee for the Promotion and Advancement of Cooperatives 1999).

Consider India. Press reports highlight India's information-technology enterprises. But as of 2004, they provided less than 1 per cent of GDP and employed fewer than one million Indians (Joshi 2004); other estimates range up to three million. Missed by the press is the power of cooperatives; they not only create many more jobs but create *hunger-ending* jobs. In only three decades, poor Indians, mostly women, have created a network of over 100 000 village-level dairy cooperatives owned by nearly 11 million members (Secretary-General of the United Nations 2005, p. 6, citing Verghese 2004, pp. 25–7). Their efforts have helped India to become the world's biggest milk producer.

Note that while roughly half of global agricultural output is marketed through cooperatives, most simply supply private corporations that then brand and sell the products, and so reap much of the profit. The Indian dairy cooperative network is different; it retains control over marketing and therefore garners a greater share of the return. In Bangladesh, the MilkVita cooperative has replicated the Indian success, enabling about 300 000 households to increase earnings tenfold (Secretary-General of the United Nations 2005, p. 6, citing Department of International Development 2006). Unlike trends extracting wealth from poor communities, leaving behind deprivation and hunger, cooperatives 'favor long-term development of their enterprise compatible with the interests of the communities in which it operates,' concluded a 1999 report (Committee for the Promotion and Advancement of Cooperatives 1999, citing Secretary-General of the United Nations 1996).

New financial models empower the poor

India's Gross Domestic Product per person is nearly a third greater than that of Bangladesh (UN FAO 2006a, p. 36), yet the latter has achieved a child death rate 23 per cent *lower* than India's (UN FAO 2004, p. 38). We can make sense of this only by shifting from a narrow focus on material resources to a mental frame centred in relationships among people.

In the early 1970s, Bangladeshi Muhammad Yunus realised that credit is a form of power. He saw that poor people who were forced to borrow from moneylenders that charged exorbitant interest rates remained poor, no matter how hard they worked. Because the low interest commercial banks would not lend to the poor, Yunus developed a new model of **microcredit** called Grameen ('Village') bank (see Box 2.4). Yunus (2006) who received the Nobel Peace Prize in 2006, calls Grameen a 'social business', a profit-making institution serving the goal of poverty alleviation.

Grameen is only one of three large microcredit networks in Bangladesh now reaching 80 per cent of the population (Yunus 2006). Microcredit is, according to the World Bank, responsible for 40 per cent of the country's entire reduction in moderate poverty in rural Bangladesh—with an even bigger impact on extreme poverty (Rosenberg 2006). Altogether these microcredit-funded, self-directed economic activities have likely freed three times as many from poverty as are employed in roughly 3000 export garment factories in Bangladesh, where insecure jobs offer wages of 8 to 18 cents an hour (Yunus 2006).

Grameen's success helped launch an international microcredit movement, now reaching nearly 100 million borrowers in more than 100 countries (Rosenberg 2006).

Frances Moore Lappé

Among the fastest growing may be those involving no 'bank' at all. Borrowers, usually groups of poor women, themselves handle the collection and borrowing decisions. To choose one example: A project called WORTH in Nepal began in 1998, where 56 000 poor women started small enterprises and generated US$3 million in new revenues during the first 18 months.

BOX 2.4

Social business creating new financial models and holistic village empowerment in Bangladesh

Microcredit

In Bangladesh over the last 30 years, networks of learning and action groups have spread to most of the country's roughly 80 000 villages (UN Economic and Social Commission for Asia and the Pacific 2006). Their intent is to remove financial, learning and health obstacles that stop poor people from realising their power.

In the Grameen ('Village') Bank small groups of poor women join together, vouch for each other's loans, and get credit on reasonable terms to advance their money-earning enterprises—such as weaving, dairy, chicken-production and small-scale retailing. As of late 2006, about US$6 billion in tiny loans from Grameen had gone to seven million poor people, mostly women, in 73 000 villages. Their repayment rate has been 99 per cent, and almost 60 per cent of the borrowers, the Bank reports, have now 'crossed the poverty line' (Yunus 2006).

Grameen is not a miniaturisation, via mini-loans, of capitalist banking as practised in the dominant economic model. The poor borrowers themselves, not outside investors, own 90 per cent of the bank; the government owns 10 per cent. Grameen is also a social movement through which borrowers commit to what they call '16 Decisions'—pledges to each other to take community-improving steps, such as keeping their families small, sending their children to school, building latrines and growing gardens (Yunus 1999).

Holistic village empowerment

In 1972, another social business was created in Bangladesh by Fazle Hasan Abed when he founded the Bangladesh Rural Advancement Committee (BRAC) to aid refugees after the war of independence from Pakistan. While still officially a 'relief agency', BRAC earns more than three-quarters of its own budget and directly employs almost 100 000 people (BRAC 2005). By taking into account the effect on all villagers where it operates, BRAC says that it 'provides and protects livelihoods of around 100 million people'; that is, two-thirds of the country's entire population (BRAC 2005).

▶

BOX 2.4

Through BRAC, almost five million poor and landless Bangladeshis, mostly women, have created over 142 000 Village Organizations. Here they meet together to address what BRAC calls the 'principal structural impediments to their development' (BRAC 2005). This wording itself suggests a frame of sufficiency, not scarcity; it assumes people have the talent and resources needed to improve their lives, if together they remove the obstacles in their paths. Through the village groups, BRAC members gain credit, open savings accounts and learn about their basic legal rights, gender equity, and how to maintain good health. BRAC uses 'popular theatre' to deepen awareness of social problems and to suggest solutions. Training and using health volunteers and paid health workers, BRAC has collaborated with the government to achieve an 80 per cent immunisation coverage. Through BRAC more than 97 million people receive curative and preventive services (BRAC 2005).

BRAC has helped to create 15 000 diverse small businesses enabling Bangladeshi producers to retain a more equitable share of the wealth they produce than do most small producers working in the dominant economic model (International Finance Corporation 2007). BRAC's craft marketing arm Aarong helps more than 300 000 rural, mostly female artisans working in small community groups to market their diverse crafts. Because 80 per cent of the crafts are sold in the organisation's eight Aarong retail stores, there are no middlemen to take a cut of the profits, leaving more for the artisans (BRAC-Aarong.com 2003; Ten Thousand Villages 2007). Participating in these initiatives, villagers also gain 'confidence', acknowledging that poor people not only need opportunity but also must make an internal shift to reject the frame of limitation placed on them.

3. Empowered farmers, ecologically sustainable solutions

Ultimately, hunger cannot be ended and remain history unless food is produced in ways that maintain healthy soils and water as well as communities. In the dominant frame, one-rule economics leads towards a particular way of producing food: a centralising, standardising system in which global corporations sell identical inputs (patented seeds and fossil-fuel based fertilisers and pesticides) to farmers worldwide who sell their crops to pay for them and to buy food. Farms become ever bigger and increasingly dependent on distant suppliers and buyers.

As alarm grows over the devastating ecological and community consequences of this model, noted early in the chapter, a very different approach is gaining ground. Often called agro-ecology or **sustainable farming**, it has both social and ecological dimensions. It promotes small farms and diversified farming to ensure decentralised power and more satisfying community relationships. Moreover, a study in 15 countries

Frances Moore Lappé

BOX 2.5

Citizens voice their values through marketplace choices

Western consumers can also support the end of world hunger through the market. What does a market look like that is ending hunger? It is driven not by the single rule of highest return to existing wealth; rather it advances several ends simultaneously: the well-being of the enterprise, including owners and all who work in it, along with the wider community—from those living near the business to purchasers of what is made and users of services rendered. A hunger-ending market also serves the well-being of our ecological home.

Where governments beholden to corporate interests are failing to protect these multiple interests, citizens are stepping in directly, by setting standards that prevent the use of dangerous chemicals and ensure a fair return to producers. One such global effort, the Fair Trade Movement, began in Europe in the 1980s. The concept is simple: a certifying body ensures that a producer has received a fair wage and attaches a label to alert consumers. Consumers determined to end hunger then selectively choose products carrying the fair trade labels. The Fair Trade Movement covers at least 20 products and operates in over 50 countries. Already, the Fair Trade Movement estimates that the higher prices secured through this certifying process have lifted over a million coffee-producing families out of destitution. Its commonsense appeal—that all workers should be paid a fair wage—means that fair trade sales jumped by over 50 per cent in just one year, 2004 (Fairtrade Labelling Organizations International 2005, p. 4). In England, roughly half the population recognises the fair trade label (O'Nions 2006, p. 18).

Through the Fair Trade Movement, purchasers, who have long imagined they had little power over an economy's fairness, directly ally with poor producers, who are also believed to have little power. Together, they create new power and further a shift towards equity in human relationships. Beyond the fairer return to specific workers affected, these efforts help to change norms that condone hunger-level wages.

In addition to groups covering agricultural products, parallel producer–citizen partnerships are tackling 'sweatshop' labour conditions. These efforts range from the United Students Against Sweatshops and the Fair Labor Association based in the USA to the Clean Clothes Campaign in the Netherlands. Other organisations, including trade unions, are working towards hunger-ending fair markets by insisting that trade agreements include provisions protecting workers' rights (Fair Labor Association 2007; Workers' Rights Consortium 2007).

in the Global South found small farms to be two to 10 times more productive than larger ones (Rosset 1999, p. 7).

In the sustainable farming approach, farmers work with flora and fauna peculiar to their place, which is the opposite of standardisation. Pest control and desired yields are achieved by understanding and managing ecological interactions and using minimal purchased inputs. Such farming is often called 'low-input' or 'low-intensity'. Actually, it is low in use of purchased inputs but is attention and knowledge intensive. Farmers do not simply follow a manufacturer's or government agent's uniform instructions; they share their experience and, often, labour and seeds. Sustainable farming works to improve output less by applying purchased products and more by developing better methods—including double-dug beds, intercropping, composting, manures, cover crops, crop sequencing, natural pest control, no-tillage and more. The approach is proving powerful (Lappé & Lappé 2002; Pretty 2002).

In this spirit, the international movement of small farmers, La Via Campesina, is pursuing policies to enable countries to achieve what it calls **food sovereignty**— producing enough domestically to be free from hunger regardless of the vagaries of the international market. And, lest one assume it is too late to reverse the globalisation of food, note that except for oils and some fruits, 85 to over 90 per cent of food is not traded (UN FAO 2007). In response to well-organised farmer pressure, the West African country of Mali became in 2006 one of the first countries in the world to make the goal of food sovereignty explicit public policy.

From agro-ecology to food sovereignty, the key is empowered people—an insight of the founder of BRAC, Fazle Abed, in Bangladesh. In 2005, reflecting on his own approach, he noted: 'We were inspired by Paolo Freire's [*Pedagogy of the Oppressed*, 1972] ... thinking about poor people and how they can become actors in history and not just passive recipients ...' Abed realised he could help poor people 'analyse their own situation, see how exploitation works in society, and see what they need to do to escape these exploitative processes' (Abed 2005, p. 14).

Conclusion

It is tempting to view hunger as a moral crisis, when it is more usefully understood as a crisis of imagination. Humanity is trapped in a failed frame, a way of seeing that underestimates both nature's potential and the potential of human nature. Exposed daily to news of deprivation alongside apparent indifference, many find it hard to hold out hope. How tragic; for mounting sociological evidence reveals that most humans have, inherently, what it takes to end hunger: deep needs for fairness, efficacy and meaning. The challenge is therefore to reframe hunger as a crisis of human relationships that is within our proven power to address, to search out and

Frances Moore Lappé

broadcast lessons of success and, most importantly, to fearlessly engage oneself—for, ultimately, can anyone believe that poor people, often facing great obstacles, can gain power to overcome hunger if one feels powerless oneself?

Acknowledgment

The author thanks Matthew Morrissey for his research assistance.

SUMMARY OF MAIN POINTS

- The question of why we have world hunger has traditionally been answered by 'scarcity', with the proposed solution being economic growth.
- The dominant belief that poverty and hunger are caused by a *lack of things*—seeds, fertile soils, irrigation and roads—ignores the real roots of hunger. These deficiencies are actually symptoms of *extreme power imbalances in human relationships* that are the inevitable result of, or made worse by, 'one-rule economics'.
- Generating more balanced, creative power to end hunger, citizens are working to remove control by wealth over the political process, taking responsibility for creating fairer markets.
- Citizens are devising more democratic business and financial models; and acting through their governments they are creating participatory decision making to establish standards and rules (including the right to healthy food) grounded in shared values of fairness, inclusion, and mutual accountability.
- Citizens are proving that empowered farmers, building on traditional land wisdom and advancing ecologically sound practices, not only increase available food and free people from dependence on an ever-more concentrated market; they also offer the best hope for future food security.

SOCIOLOGICAL REFLECTION

- What are some steps you could take to help end hunger?
- What policies could your country implement to contribute to ending world hunger?

DISCUSSION QUESTIONS

1. What is the prevailing view of world hunger, its causes and cures?
2. In searching for solutions, what does it mean to shift focus from a scarcity of 'things' to equitable relationships among people?
3. What does power mean to you and how does the author define power?

4. What are the biggest obstacles to ending hunger?
5. What are some of the new models of economic relationships citizens throughout the world are developing to end hunger?
6. What are the most important roles of government in ending hunger?

Further investigation

1. What specific changes in national and international economic policies and business structures can help to end hunger?
2. What might the realisation of a *right* to healthy food look like in your community or nation? What would be the costs and benefits?

FURTHER READING AND WEB RESOURCES

Books

Lappé, F.M. & Lappé, A. 2002, *Hope's Edge: The Next Diet for a Small Planet*, Tarcher/ Penguin, New York: Via a journey on five continents, captures diverse, democratic approaches to more effective food systems.

Lappé, F.M., Collins, J. & Rosset, P. 1998, *World Hunger: Twelve Myths*, 2nd edition, Grove Press, New York: Takes on each of the most common misunderstandings about hunger and highlights solutions.

Pretty, J. 2002, *Agri-culture: Reconnecting People, Land, and Nature*, Earthscan, London: Emphasises the great unrealised productive potential of ecological farming methods in which farmers themselves are leaders.

Rosset, P.M. 2006, *Food is Different: Why We Must Get the WTO Out of Agriculture*, Palgrave Macmillan, New York: Argues that food should be treated as a right and protected to ensure sustainability. It demystifies policies of the World Trade Organization and introduces small farmers' movements working for national policies of food sovereignty.

Sen, A. 1999, *Development as Freedom*, Knopf, New York: Nobel-winning economist, Amartya Sen, argues that democratic rights are essential to ending hunger, and that access to life's essentials is as important to freedom as political rights.

Shiva, V. 2005, *Earth Democracy: Justice, Sustainability and Peace*, New Society Books, Boston: Defines a reconceptualisation of democracy to include economic life and our relationship to the natural world.

Websites

FIAN International, Defending the Right to Food: www.fian.org
Focus on the Global South: www.focusweb.org
Food First/Institute for Food and Development Policy: www.foodfirst.org

Frances Moore Lappé

International Forum on Globalization: www.ifg.org
New Economics Foundation: www.neweconomics.org
Oakland Institute: www.oaklandinstitute.org
Small Planet Institute: www.smallplanetinstitute.org
UN Human Development Reports: http://hdr.undp.org/english/

Documentaries

The Future of Food, Lily Films 2004, www.thefutureoffood.com.
The Global Banquet: Politics of Food, Old Dog Documentaries, Inc., 2000, www.
    olddogdocumentaries.com/vid_gb.html.
The Roots of Change: The Journey of Wangari Maathai, Marlboro Productions and the
    Hartly Film Foundation, 2007, www.marlboroproductions.com/.
Seeds of Change: Farmers, Biotechnology, & the New Face of Agriculture, Dead Crow
    Productions, www.seedsofchangefilm.org.

REFERENCES

Abed, F. 2005, 'Social Entrepreneurship—Its Promise and its Challenges, Fazle Hasan
    Abed Interview', *Alliance*, Allavida, London, vol. 10, no. 1, March 2005, www.
    allavida.org/alliance/mar05e.html.
Alvard, M. 2004, 'Good Hunters Keep Smaller Shares of Larger Pies', Open Peer
    Commentary, accompanying Gurven, M. 2004, 'To Give or Not to Give: The
    Behavioral Ecology of Food Transfers', *Behavioral and Brain Sciences*, vol. 27,
    Cambridge University Press, Cambridge, 2005, pp. 543–83.
Andrade, F. 2006 (pers. comm.), University of Wisconsin, citing Brazilian government
    <www.datasus.org.br>; also http://cs.server2.textor.com/alldocs/Lansky%202.
    pdf.
Aranha, A. 2000 (pers. comm.). Then Director of Program for the Defense and
    Promotion of Nutritional Consumption, Secretariat of Municipal Supply
    Policy, Belo Horizonte, Brazil. Now Special Consultant, Brazilian Ministry of
    Social Development and the Fight Against Hunger.
—— 2006, 'FOME Zero/CFSC/Bridging Borders Toward Food Security Conference',
    Vancouver, www.smallplanetinstitute.org/worldhunger/fomezero.pdf.
Baiocchi, G. 2003, 'Participation, Activism, and Politics: The Porto Alegre Experiment',
    in A. Fung & E.O. Wright (eds), *Deepening Democracy*, Verso, New York, pp.
    47–50.
—— 2005, *Militants and Citizens: The Politics of Participation in Porto Alegre*, Stanford
    University Press, Stanford, Ca.
BBC 2005, 'SA Proposes Quicker Land Reform', *BBC*, July 25, http://news.bbc.co.uk/2/
    hi/africa/4720023.stm.

—— 2007, 'India Rising,' BBC World Service.com, www.bbc.co.uk/worldservice/ specials/1620_india/page2.shtml.

Bello, W. et al. 1994, *Dark Victory: The United States and Global Poverty*, Food First Books, Oakland.

BRAC 2005, 'BRAC History', BRAC website, www.brac.net/history.htm.

—— 2006, 'BRAC At a Glance: As of June 2006', www.brac.net/downloads_files/ June_06_AAG_BW.pdf.

BRAC-Aarong.com 2003, 'Aarong-Terms and Conditions', www.brac-aarong.com/ exportservices.asp.

Brizzi, A., Chaudhuri, S., Shah, A. & Shah, P. 2005, 'Building Democracy: The People's Campaign for Decentralized Planning in Kerala', World Bank, PowerPoint presentation, http://info.worldbank.org/etools/BSPAN/PresentationView.asp? PID=1380&EID=676

Chappell, M. 2006 (pers. comm.), University of Michigan. Specifics of 40 farmers and 12,000 meals daily.

China Daily 2006, 'China's Poverty Line Too Low', *China Daily*, Quoting Wu Zhong, official, State Council Leading Group Office of Poverty Alleviation and Development, China, www.chinadaily.com.cn/china/2006-08/23/content_ 672510.htm.

Committee for the Promotion and Advancement of Cooperatives 1999, *The Contribution of Cooperatives to the Implementation of the World Summit for Social Development Declaration and Programme of Action*, New York, 17–28 May 1999, www.copacgva.org/wssd99.htm.

De Long, Bradford J. 1998, *World GDP, One Million B.C.—Present*, University of California at Berkeley, San Francisco, pp. 1–12, http://delong.typepad.com/ print/20061012_LRWGDP.pdf.

Democratic Staff of the Committee on Education and the Workforce, for Rep. George Miller (D-Calif.), Senior Democrat 2004, 'Everyday Low Wages: The Hidden Price We All Pay for Wal-Mart', US House of Representatives, http:// edworkforce.house.gov/publications/WALMARTREPORT.pdf.

Department of International Development 2006, 'Can Cooperatives Save the World?', in *Developments: The International Development Magazine*, Department of International Development, United Kingdom of Great Britain and Northern Ireland.

Environmental Working Group 2006, Farm Subsidy Database, 'United States', www. ewg.org/farm/region.php?fips=00000.

ETC Group 2005, 'Global Seed Industry Concentration—2005', *Communiqué* iss. 90, www.mindfully.org/Farm/2005/Global-Seed-Industry6sep05.htm.

Fair Labor Association 2007, http://fairlabor.org/index.html.

Fairtrade Labelling Organizations International 2005, *Annual Report 2004/2005: Delivering Opportunities*, Fairtrade Labelling Organizations International: Bonn, Germany, www.fairtrade.net/uploads/media/FLO_AR_2004_05.pdf.

Franke, R.W., Professor of Anthropology, 1999, 'Lessons in Democracy from Kerala State, India', University Lecture, March 25, 1999, http://chss2.montclair.edu/anthropology/frankekeralastate.htm.

—— & Chasin, B. 1994, *Kerala: Radical Reform as Development in an Indian State*, Food First Books, Oakland.

Friedman, M. 1962, *Capitalism and Freedom*, University of Chicago Press, Chicago.

Galbraith, J.K. 2006, 'Mission Control', *Mother Jones*, November/December.

Gardner, G. & Halweil, B. 2000, 'Overfed and Underfed: The Global Epidemic of Malnutrition', *WorldWatch Institute, WorldWatch Paper 150*, March.

Grameen Bank 2006, 'Grameen Bank', www.grameen-info.org/.

Griswold, D., Slivinski, S. & Preble, C. 2006, 'Six Reasons to Kill Farm Subsidies and Trade Barriers', *Reason*, February, pp. 42–9.

Gurven, M. 2004, 'To Give or Not to Give: The Behavioral Ecology of Food Transfers', *Behavioral and Brain Sciences*, vol. 27, Cambridge University Press, Cambridge, pp. 543–83.

Hanlon, J. 1998, 'Dictators and Debt', Jubilee Research, London, www.jubileeresearch.org/analysis/reports/dictatorsreport.htm.

Hauser, M.D. 2006, *Moral Minds*, HarperCollins, New York.

Hirvonen, P. 2005, 'Stingy Samaritans: Why Recent Increases in Development Aid Fail to Help the Poor', *Global Policy Forum*, Global Policy Forum, New York, www.globalpolicy.org/socecon/develop/oda/2005/08stingysamaritans.htm.

International Cooperative Alliance 2007, 'Statistical Information on Cooperatives', International Cooperative Alliance: Geneva, www.ica.coop/coop/statistics.html.

International Finance Corporation 2007, 'New Markets for Local Banks: The Case of Bangladesh', www.ifc.org/ifcext/media.nsf/Content/Feature_New_Markets_Bangladesh.

International Labor Organization 2006, 'Ratifications of the Fundamental Human Rights Conventions by Country', Database of International Labor Standards, www.ilo.org/ilolex/english/docs/declworld.htm.

International Textile, Garment and Leather Workers' Federation 2002, 'Future of Bangladesh Clothing industry in the Hands of Employers and Government', ITGLWF website, www.itglwf.org/DisplayDocument.aspx?idarticle=467&langue=2.

——2006, 'Bangladesh Employers Told to Stop Destroying Garment Industry', ITGLWF website, www.itglwf.org/DisplayDocument.aspx?idarticle=15042&langue=2.

Isaac, T.M.T. & Franke, R.W. 2002, *Local Democracy and Development: The Kerala People's Campaign for Decentralized Planning*, Rowman & Littlefield, Lanham.

Joshi, V. 2004, 'The Myth of India's Outsourcing Boom', *The Financial Times*, London, 16 November.

Jubilee Debt Campaign 2006, 'Hasn't All the Debt Been Cancelled?', Jubilee Debt Campaign Website, www.jubileedebtcampaign.org.uk/?id=98.

King, A. 2005, 'Trade and Totomoxtle: Coping with NAFTA in the Totanacan Region of Veracruz', *Strengthening Rural Communities: Bread for the World Institute's 15th Annual Report on the State of World Hunger*, BFWI, Washington DC.

Kingstone, S. 2004, 'Brazil's Land Wars Hit New Height', BBC, 17 April, http://news.bbc.co.uk/2/hi/americas/3634107.stm.

Krznaric, R. 2005, 'The Limits on Pro-Poor Agricultural Trade in Guatemala: Land, Labour and Political Power', *Human Development Report 2005*, UN Development Programme, New York, http://hdr.undp.org/docs/publications/background_papers/2005/HDR2005_Krznaric_Roman_17.pdf.

Lappé, F.M., Collins, J. & Rosset, P. 1998, *World Hunger: Twelve Myths*, 2nd edition, Grove Press, New York.

Lappé, F.M. & Lappé, A. 2002, *Hope's Edge, The Next Diet for a Small Planet*, Tarcher/Penguin, New York.

Mgbeoji, I. 2006, *Global Biopiracy—Patents, Plants, and Indigenous Knowledge*, Cornell University Press, Ithaca.

Morales, E. 2006, 'Bolivian President Evo Morales on Latin America, U.S. Foreign Policy and Rights of Indigenous People of Bolivia', *Democracy Now*, 22 September 2006, www.democracynow.org/article.pl?sid=06/09/22/1323211&mode=thread&tid=25.

MST 2003, 'History of the MST', 'About the MST', www.mstbrazil.org.

National Agricultural Statistics Service 2005, 'Number of Farms, Average Size of Farm, and Land in Farms, United States, 1974–2003', National Agricultural Statistics Service, www.nass.usda.gov/ky/B2004/p010.pdf.

National Research Council 1996, *Lost Crops of Africa Volume 1: Grains*, Board on Science and Technology and International Development, National Academy Press, Washington, DC.

NetAid.Org 2007, 'U.S. Leadership', www.netaid.org/global_poverty/united-states/.

Nord, M., Andrews, M. & Carlson, S. 2005, 'Household Food Security in the United States, 2004', Economic Research Report No. (ERR11), United States Department of Agriculture, October 2005, pp. 5–6, www.ers.usda.gov/publications/err11/.

Nowels, L. & Tarnoff, C. 2004, 'Foreign Aid: An Introductory Overview of U.S. Programs and Policy', *CRS Report for Congress*, Congressional Research Service, Library of Congress, www.fas.org/man/crs/98-916.pdf.

O'Nions, J. 2006, 'Fairtrade and Global Justice', *Seedling Magazine*, July, p. 18, www.grain.org/seedling/?type=64.

Oxfam America 2006, 'Grounds For Change: Creating a Voice for Small Coffee Farmers and Farmworkers with the Next International Coffee Agreement', www.oxfamamerica.org/newsandpublications/publications/research_reports/research_paper.2006-05-10.1341802122/Grounds_for_Change.pdf.

Oxfam Great Britain 1999, 'Loaded Against the Poor: World Trade Organization', p. i.

Oxfam International 2002, *Rigged Rules and Double Standards: Trade, Globalization and the Fight Against Poverty*, London.

Pretty, J. 2002. *Agri-Culture*, Earthscan, London.

Public Agenda 2004, 'Poverty and Welfare: People's Chief Concerns', www.publicagenda.org/issues/pcc_detail.cfm?issue_type=welfare&list=1.

Public Citizen 2005, 'The Ten Year Track Record of the North American Free Trade Agreement: U.S., Mexican and Canadian Farmers and Agriculture', www.citizen.org/documents/NAFTA_10_ag.pdf.

Reel, M. 2006, 'Two Views of Justice Fuel Bolivian Land Battle', *The Washington Post*, www.washingtonpost.com/wp-dyn/content/article/2006/06/19/AR200606 1901221.html?nav=rss_world/southamerica.

Rockefeller Foundation, The, Bill and Melinda Gates Foundation 2006, 'Press Release: Bill and Melinda Gates, Rockefeller Foundations Form Alliance to Help Spur "Green revolution" in Africa', www.rockfound.org/initiatives/agra/ agra1.pdf.

Rodney, W. 1973, *How Europe Underdeveloped Africa*, Bogle-L'Ouverture Publications, London; Tanzanian Publishing House, Dar-Es-Salaam.

Rosenberg, T. 2006, 'Talking Points, How to Fight Poverty: 8 Programs That Work', *The New York Times*, 16 November, New York, http://select.nytimes.com/2006/11/16/ opinion/15talkingpoints.html?_r=1&pagewanted=print.

Rosset, P. 1999, 'The Multiple Functions and Benefits of Small Farm Agriculture in the Context of Global Trade Negotiations', *Food First Policy Brief* no. 4, Food First, Oakland; Transnational Institute, Amsterdam, p. 7.

—— 2006a, 'Moving Forward: Agrarian Reform as Part of Food Sovereignty', in P. Rosset, R. Patel and M. Courville, *Promised Land: Competing Visions of Agrarian Reform*, Food First Books, Oakland.

—— 2006b, *Food is Different: Why We Must Get the WTO Out of Agriculture*, Palgrave Macmillan, New York.

Rostow, W.W. 1960, *The Stages of Economic Growth: A Non-Communist Manifesto*, Cambridge University Press, Cambridge.

Rusu, L. 2006, 'US Must Reform Agricultural Subsidy Program', Oxfam America, www. oxfamamerica.org/newsandpublications/press_releases/press_release.2006- 09-01.3724151415/?searchterm=farm%20subsidies.

Sachs, J. 2005, *The End of Poverty: Economic Possibilities for Our Time*, The Penguin Press, New York, pp. 36, 73, 204, 208, 329–46. For Sachs' current work: Millennial Promise, www.milennialpromise.org.

Schell, O. 2004, 'A Lonely Voice in China Is Critical on Rights and Reform', *The New York Times Books*.

Secretary-General of the United Nations 1996, 'Status and role of cooperatives in the light of new economic and social trends', United Nations General Assembly (A/51/267).

—— 2005, 'Cooperatives in Social Development', United Nations General Assembly (A/60/138).

Shah, A. 2006, 'The US and Foreign Aid Assistance', *Global Issues*, www.globalissues. org/TradeRelated/Debt/USAid.asp#MoreMoneyIsTransferredFromPoorCount riestoRichThanFromRichToPoor.

Sharma, D. 2005, 'Bhagawati, Globalization and Hunger', Global Policy Forum, www. globalpolicy.org/socecon/trade/subsidies/2005/0329bhagwati.htm.

Shiva, V. 1991, *The Violence of the Green Revolution*, Zed Books, London, UK.

—— 1993, *Monocultures of the Mind*, Zed Books and Third World Network, London, UK.

—— et al. 2002, *Corporate Hijack of Food*, Navdanya, New Delhi, India.

Smith, J. 2007, *Genetic Roulette: The Documented Health Risks of Genetically Engineered Foods*, Chelsea Green Publishing, White River Junction, Vermont.

Somavia, J. 2004, 'A Fair Globalization, the Role of the ILO', *International Labour Conference, 92nd Session*, World Commission on the Social Dimension of Globalization, International Labour Office, Geneva, www.ilo.org/public/ english/standards/relm/ilc/ilc92/pdf/adhoc.pdf.

Ten Thousand Villages 2007, 'Brac-Aarong', www.tenthousandvillages.ca/cgi-bin/ category.cgi?item=art_6615&type=store&template=fullpage-en.

UN Millennium Development Goals 2007, *UN Millennium Development Goals*, www. un.org/millenniumgoals/, [accessed 06.07.07].

UN Conference on Trade and Development 2004, *The Least Developed Countries Report 2004: Linking International Trade with Poverty Reduction*, United Nations, New York and Geneva, p. 152.

——2007, *World Economic Situation and Prospects 2007*, United Nations, New York and Geneva, p. 57.

UN Development Programme 1999, *Human Development Report 1999*, United Nations Development Programme, New York.

—— 2003, *Human Development Report 2003*, Oxford University Press, New York.

—— 2005, *Human Development Report 2005*, United Nations Development Programme, New York.

UN Economic and Social Commission for Asia and the Pacific: Human Settlements 2006, 'Country Paper: Bangladesh', United Nations Economic and Social Commission for Asia and the Pacific, Human Settlements, www.unescap.org/ lgstudy/country/Bangladesh/Bangladesh/html.

UN Food and Agriculture Organization 2001, 'The Right to Food', United Nations, Rome, www.fao.org/worldfoodsummit/english/fsheets/food.pdf.

—— 2002, 'World Agriculture 2030: Main Findings', United Nations, Rome, www. fao.org/english/newsroom/news/2002/7833-en.html.

—— 2004a, *The State of Food Insecurity in the World 2004*, Rome, www.fao.org/ docrep/007/y5650e/y5650e00.htm.

—— 2004b, 'The State of Agricultural Commodity Markets 2004', Rome, p. 10, www.fao.org/docrep/007/y5419e/y5419e00.htm.

—— 2006a, *The State of Food Insecurity in the World 2006*, Rome, www.fao.org/docrep/009/a0750e/a0750e00.htm.

—— 2006b, Statistics Division, 'China', United Nations, www.fao.org/faostat/foodsecurity/MDG/EN/China_e.pdf.

—— 2006c, 'Food and Agriculture Statistics Global Outlook', Statistics Division, June 2006, p. 1, http://faostat.fao.org/Portals/_Faostat/documents/pdf/world.pdf.

—— 2006d, 'World Hunger Increasing: FAO Head Calls on World Leaders to Honour Pledges, Food and Agriculture Organization of the United Nations', www.fao.org/newsroom/en/news/2006/1000433/index.html.

—— 2007, (pers. comm.).

UN Department of Economic and Social Affairs, United Nations Conference on Trade and Development 2007, 'World Economics Situation and Prospects', New York, www.un.org/esa/policy/wess/wesp2007files/wesp2007.pdf.

USDA Economic Research Service 2006, 'Farm Income and Costs: 2005 Farm Sector Income Estimates', www.ers.usda.gov/Briefing/FarmIncome/2005incomeaccounts.htm.

Verghese, K. 2004, 'India's Milk Revolution: Investing in Rural Producer Organizations', paper presented at the World Bank conference, *Scaling Up Poverty Reduction: A Global Learning Process and Conference*, Shanghai, pp. 25–7.

Vorley, B. 2003, *Food, Inc.: Corporate Concentration from Farm to Consumer*, U.K. Food Group, London, pp. 11, 24, 25, www.ukfg.org.uk/docs/UKFG-Foodinc-Nov03.pdf.

Windfuhr, M. & Jonsén, J. 2005, *Food Sovereignty: Towards Democracy in Localized Food Systems*, www.ukabc.org/foodsovpaper.htm.

Woodward, D. & Simms, A. 2006, *Growth Isn't Working: The Unbalanced Distribution of Benefits and Costs from Economic Growth*, New Economics Foundation, London, UK, www.neweconomics.org/gen/z_sys_publicationdetail.aspx?pid=219.

Workers' Rights Consortium 2007, www.workersrights.org.

World Bank 2005, *World Development Report 2005*, Washington D.C., p. 30.

—— 2006, 'Equity and Development', Ch. 4', *World Development Report 2006*, pp. 76–88.

World Food Summit 1996, 'World Food Summit: 13–17 November 1996 Rome Italy', World Food Summit, www.fao.org/wfs/index_en.htm.

Worldwatch Institute 2007, *The State of the World: Our Urban Future*, Worldwatch Institute, Washington, D.C.

Yunus, M. 1999, *Banker to the Poor: Micro-Lending and the Battle Against World Poverty*, Public Affairs, New York.

—— 2006, *Nobel Lecture*, Oslo, http://nobelprize.org/nobel_prizes/peace/laureates/2006/yunus-lecture-en.html.

Ziegler, J. 2004, 'The Right to Food: Report Submitted by the Special Rapporteur on the Right to Food, Jean Ziegler', Commission on Human Rights, United Nations Economic and Social Council, 9 February.

CHAPTER 3

Unsustainable Food Production: Its Social Origins and Alternatives

Terry Leahy

OVERVIEW

- What are the environmental problems of agriculture today?
- What agricultural technologies are available to deal with these problems?
- What are the social causes of these problems and what are the social alternatives?

As we humans of the planet earth go about producing and consuming our food we set in train a long list of environmental problems. The process is unsustainable because the environmental damage we are causing will make it increasingly harder for us to live well. We are also drastically reducing the opportunities for other forms of life. These problems arise from specific social structures. It is not 'us' as a mass of individuals, or even 'us' meaning the whole of society, who create environmental problems. These problems come from our relationships with each other, relationships of class, economy, work and power. It is possible to set out some of the ways in which current practices of food production damage the environment and also to look at some of the alternatives. Agricultural strategies designed to achieve commercial success are inevitably constrained by the market. Often the more satisfactory environmental solution is impossible in the marketplace. This chapter will also look at the kinds of social structures that might deal with this crisis of environmental damage. While capitalism may be considered to be part of the problem, alternative social structures seem unlikely to gain popular support soon, whether we are talking about more nationalised ownership of the economy, an anarchist gift economy or a deconstruction of industrial civilisation.

Key terms

agroforestry	food forest	ruralisation
alienated labour	monoculture	salinity/salinisation
capitalism	oil crunch	social structure
cash crops	organics	sustainable agriculture
gift economy	permaculture	transnational corporations
global warming	polyculture	

Environmental problems and food production

As we go about producing and consuming food, we set in train a long series of environmental problems. Current agricultural methods, while highly efficient, are unsustainable because the environmental damage they cause reduces the productivity of the land for future agricultural use. Major environmental problems are caused by **monoculture**, fertilisers, pesticides, overgrazing, overfishing, tree clearing, irrigation and the use of fossil fuels. What sociology can offer is the insight that these problems develop as a consequence of specific **social structures**.

Monocultures, fertilisers, pests and weeds

In rich countries with high labour costs, technologies designed to save labour costs cause environmental problems. With the farming industry based on large pieces of land serviced by machinery and cheap fuel, monocultural (single crop) production is cheaper than growing a variety of crops together. However, a single crop is the perfect environment for a pest or disease—both spread easily and can destroy all the produce (Lawrence & Vanclay 1992, p. 53; Watson 1992). Toxic chemical pesticides are used to prevent these problems, but they cause some damage to human health and also kill off microbes, earthworms, insects and animals that could actually aid food production (Leu 2006). After time, pests develop resistance to pesticides, and as a consequence the crop may be unable to be grown at all or even more toxic pesticides could be called in (Lawrence & Vanclay 1992; Mannion 1995).

Monocultural production also makes considerable use of artificial fertilisers such as super-phosphates. These destroy micro-organisms that normally create soil fertility, and acidify soils. The result is reduced agricultural productivity. Up to 60 million hectares of Australian agricultural land will become too acidic for plant growth in the next 10 years (Cullen et al. 2003, p. 3). Soluble fertiliser is washed into waterways and causes a problem of nutrient overload, stimulating algal growth. The algae use up oxygen, and as result water weeds, fish and insects die. The algae can itself be poisonous, like the blue green algae of the Darling River (Lawrence & Vanclay 1992; Thomas & Kevan 1993; Vanclay & Lawrence 1995). We can look at two kinds of solutions to these problems: **food forest** solutions and **organics**.

Food forest solutions

As an alternative to monoculture, some **permaculture** writers recommend systems that mimic natural woodland environments (Mollison & Holmgren 1978; Soule & Piper 1992; French 1993; Fern 1997; Whitefield 1998). For example, a **polyculture** or food forest is where a mixed variety of foods are grown together. 'Forest gardening' is a strategy in which carbohydrates are provided by trees or bushes—a food forest of nuts and fruits with an understorey of low vines and shrubs. If pest species do cause a problem it is then confined to some crops, while the rest flourish. Pests do not easily move between small pockets of the same crop. In companion planting a specific plant is grown that helps control the pests of the second species. Animals are also part of the food forest, providing fertiliser and eating many pest species (Mollison 1988; French 1993; Morrow 1993). Crops chosen for a particular location are those that flourish and resist pests (Mollison & Holmgren 1978; Mollison 1988; Watson 1992; Morrow 1993).

Methods of polycultural production could work very well if we did not have a **capitalist** system. If people grew food for their local neighbourhood and had plenty of time to plant, maintain and harvest by hand, a mixture of species that had to be cared for individually would take time but could sustain the soil and be fun to grow. However, for farmers who are saving on labour costs by using harvesting machinery, the polyculture solution seems unrealistic (Lawrence & Vanclay 1992, pp. 52–3).

Organic solutions

Another kind of solution to these problems is 'organic' agriculture. In organics, inputs come from organic plant or animal resources, such as animal manure for fertiliser and plant species used to deter pests. No artificial fertilisers or synthetic pesticides are used (Kristiansen & Merfield 2006; Leu 2006). Originally, this kind of agriculture was developed to be healthy for people. There is no danger of long-lasting chemical toxicity that can lead to cancers and diseases of the nervous system. This system of agriculture also protects the environment.

Methods such as crop rotation, growing living mulch and slashing it to lie on the ground, the use of animal manures, the planting of legumes that fix nitrogen in the soil, or the building of earthworks to increase water retention are all techniques used in organic agriculture to create soil fertility. In organic agriculture, there are no artificial fertilisers to destroy soil organisms, acidify soils and wreck aquatic environments with nutrient overloads, and no long-lasting pesticide or weed-killing chemicals to harm wild species and the micro-organisms in soils (Kasperczyk & Knickel 2006).

While crop yields per hectare are generally lower in organic agriculture, costs of inputs are less and farmers can end up better off if they get higher prices for organic produce (Pretty 1999). Reductions in crop yields after conversion to organics were as high as 40 per cent in some European countries but only 10 to 20 per cent in Australia, Canada and the USA (Wynen 2006). While organic yields can be low immediately after conversion, they improve over the next five years and can be as high as in conventional agriculture (Leu 2006).

The market for organic produce has been growing at a phenomenal rate in the rich countries of the world—at rates of between 8 per cent and 20 per cent per year

(Lockie et al. 2006, p. 245). In 2004 the total value of the organics market was US$23 billion (Kristiansen & Merfield 2006, p. 10). On the other hand, organic food is still up to 80 per cent more expensive—usually more than the 15 per cent to 20 per cent extra that most buyers will be prepared to pay (Lockie et al. 2006, p. 247; Wynen 2006, p. 234). The basic reason for the added expense is the extra labour that goes into organics, in producing composts, spreading manure, weeding by hand, companion planting, and resting fields to grow cover crops (Lawrence & Vanclay 1992; Thomas & Kevan 1993).

Existing farmers attempting to transfer to organic methods face considerable challenges. If their farms are near others that use chemicals, it is unlikely they could get certification as an 'organic' farmer because of the drift from chemical sprays from neighbouring farms. It takes approximately five years to reach the same level of production as conventional approaches using organic methods—the time needed for soils and beneficial organisms to build up after toxic chemicals have been removed (Wynen 2006). This five-year window can be financially crippling. Grain producers have the added expense of installing their own mill to keep their crop separate and market their organic product. Organic farming also involves a considerable investment in skills and knowledge, which in itself is expensive (Campbell 1991; Vanclay & Lawrence 1995; Pretty 1999). It is hard to imagine that the organics market is going to grow year by year until it dominates 90 per cent of the market. It is still only 1 to 2 per cent of the food market in rich countries and growth is levelling off where it has been most successful (Lockie et al. 2006, p. 245).

Ploughing, cultivation and weed control

Ploughing with machinery creates a seedbed and controls weeds. It saves on labour costs and favours monocultural production. When soil is ploughed the top layer is turned over completely. This destroys micro-organisms that create soil fertility. The use of heavy machinery packs the soil down and creates an infertile hard pan (Thomas & Kevan 1993). Ploughed fields are very susceptible to erosion. Rain washes away the topsoil—a non-renewable resource for agriculture. The removed topsoil silts waterways, polluting them with excessive nutrients (Land & Water Australia 2002). For these reasons, monocultural production of cereals and potatoes is unsustainable. For example, in Australia's top wheat growing areas 13 tonnes of soil is lost through erosion for every tonne of wheat produced (Lawrence & Vanclay 1992, p. 40). A 30-year study has revealed that 8 tonnes of soil per hectare are lost in summer cropping of annual cereals, compared with 0.01 tonnes lost from undisturbed native forests (Turner et al. 2004). In the world as a whole, soil is being lost to erosion at the rate of 5 tonnes per person per year (Trainer 1995, p. 18; see also Watson 1992, p. 21).

Clearly, a food forest strategy is one kind of solution—tree crops produce carbohydrates without the soil being constantly disturbed and ploughing is abandoned. Within the organics framework, cereal monocultures are achieved by rotating different crops in different seasons, using hand weeding and some ploughing to reduce weeds. Living mulch, legume crops and fallowing fields are used to keep organic matter in the soil and retain moisture—soils are less frequently exposed to rain and suffer less erosion. In this way, organics protects soils from the effects of ploughing, while retaining a cereal as the basic carbohydrate crop (Morse 2006).

Minimum tillage

Within typical commercial farming one approach that has been used is 'minimum tillage', or 'no-till' or 'conservation farming' as it is variously called. After the grain is harvested, the stubble and crop residue is left on the field to add organic matter to the soil. The fields are regularly sprayed with herbicides to kill weeds. This technology has been widely adopted in the last few decades. By 1996, up to 80 per cent of Australia's cropping farms were using some or all aspects of this technique (Cullen et al. 2003, p. 11). Importantly, the method comes without the labour costs associated with organic agriculture.

Minimum tillage technology acts to improve soils, and the amount of carbon in the soil is higher in conservation farming systems than on conventional farms. There is less ploughing to control weeds and soil is not turned over by the plough (a procedure that kills soil organisms). Instead, to prepare for sowing, tractors are fitted with machinery that chisels a thin furrow deep into the soil. Crop residues and dead weeds rot down to improve soil, protect the ground from sunlight and retain moisture.

Nevertheless, this technology has certain pitfalls. Most of these weed-killing chemicals have a damaging effect on wildlife. For example, 'Roundup', the most common weed killer, washes into waterways where it kills frogs. It is acutely toxic to beneficial insects, fish, birds, earthworms and soil micro-organisms. It is also a danger to the health of farm workers (Sundquist 2004, p. 7; Leu 2006, p. 2). Other weed-killing chemicals are as bad or worse (Sundquist 2004, p. 7). Atrazine is one of the world's most commonly used herbicides, and has been found in rain samples from 30 to 90 per cent of sites tested in Greece and the USA. It interferes with the endocrine system, causing cancers in humans and animals (Leu 2006, p. 2).

The most problematic aspect of no-till technology for farmers is that weeds are developing resistance to all these chemicals. The result is a complicated schedule of different chemical sprays in different months and years to kill different kinds of weeds. The end result of this is that farmers rarely avoid ploughing for weeds at least once a season—with the attendant problems of diminishing soil quality and soil erosion. In other words, the problems of soil erosion that permaculture or organics can actually solve are not addressed in the long term by 'conservation farming'. The toxic effects associated with these chemicals intensify as weed species develop resistance and more chemicals are sprayed.

Large grazing animals

Large animals grown for meat generally cause environmental problems. Overgrazing is a common response to competitive pressures on prices (Watson 1992). Yet too many sheep or cattle pack the soil down hard, destroying soil aeration and killing soil micro-organisms, leaving a hard crust that grows little fodder and does not admit rain. Without cover, the soil easily washes away. These problems are rampant in grazing around the world (Crosby 1986; Thomas & Kevan 1993).

Grazing solutions adapt permaculture to commercial production. Deep-rooted perennial pasture species reduce the risks of **salinity** and soil erosion. Properties are fenced so paddocks can be rested. In 'rotational grazing', livestock are moved regularly between paddocks. Nevertheless, these systems do not necessarily have much impact on how many animals can be grazed (the 'stocking rate'). The solution to grazing pressure is always to reduce herds and farmers worry that profitability will be reduced. The time required to run a careful grazing management is also relevant (Hutchings 2004; Sundquist 2004).

Agroforestry

Another common technique is to combine grazing with timber crops—**agroforestry**. The farm benefits from the biodiversity of species in a woodland environment (Holmgren 1994). This can be profitable—for example, in improving the quality of milk, the numbers of stock and reproduction rates improves even though up to 8 per cent of the pasture has been removed to grow trees (Cullen et al. 2003, pp. 10, 14). Nevertheless, agroforestry costs money in fencing and planting trees, and returns on the timber take decades to eventuate. So innovative farmers pioneer agroforestry but most others ignore it. While it is advised that 30 per cent of native vegetation cover may be necessary to prevent ecological damage, figures between 2 and 4 per cent are most common (Cullen et al. 2003, pp. 13, 14).

Salinity

The National Land and Water Resources audit of 1997–2002 showed that 6 million hectares of agricultural and pastoral land in Australia is suffering from dryland salinity problems, and predicted that 17 million hectares would be affected by 2050 unless drastic measures were taken (National Dryland Salinity Program 2004, p. 10). There are also salinity problems with irrigated agriculture—2.5 million hectares in Australia at present (Murray-Darling Basin Commission 2004). With irrigation, a constant supply of water causes the water table to rise. Salts lower down dissolve and rise to the surface. A salt pan inhibits the growth of plants. This effect is extremely hard to reverse and the irrigated area becomes a useless desert (Lawrence & Vanclay 1992; Thomas & Kevan 1993).

Where land has been cleared, a similar problem arises known as dryland salinity. Rainfall on higher areas travels down the slope, where it causes the water table to rise, bringing salt to the surface. This salty area of low ground becomes poisonous to most plant life. Prior to land clearing, this salinisation process was prevented by deep-rooted tree species. These trees brought water up from their roots, released it as vapour into the air and stored it in their foliage. Water did not move down the slope, causing problems of salinity further down (Lawrence & Vanclay 1992).

There is a commercial angle to these issues. Irrigated land is very profitable before problems of salinity develop. Clearing slopes for pasture or cereal crops is also profitable. Once salinity develops it is expensive or impossible to reverse. A common finding is that almost all the area of land upslope from the salting problem has to be replanted with trees and shrubs—80 per cent is a typical requirement. Then, it is likely to take between 50 and 100 years for the salting to be reduced (Stirzaker et al. 2002, p. 35; National Dryland Salinity Program 2004, p. 39).

The unfortunate reality is that in most areas where salinity is a problem there are no tree or shrub alternatives that can return a profit. 'The conclusion of recent studies is that no profitable system of farming, even applying "current best practice" could control salinity' (National Dryland Salinity Program 2004, pp. 73, 79, 83). Large amounts of public money would have to be spent. An estimated 17 million hectares of trees would need to be planted in areas with low rainfall, and farmers compensated for the area taken out of grazing or cropping.

Deep drainage

A quick-fix engineering solution to salinity is to dig channels that are deeper than the water table. The rising saline water is drained away from the zone where plant roots grow. About 10,000 kilometres of these deep drains have been constructed (National Dryland Salinity Program 2004, p. 87). There are various drawbacks to this scheme. The raised edges of channels have to be maintained to prevent surface water from draining into the channels and filling them when rainfall is heavy. If the channels become blocked, they will also fill up, spilling salty water onto fields. What can be done with the salty water from these drains? It is all too common for farmers to channel their drains to a big pond on the edge of their farm. After heavy rain, the pond spills onto the neighbouring farm. Salt leaks out to destroy roads and buildings. Grand visions of channels all the way to the coast become a rationale for ignoring these negative effects.

Costs of salinity

The long-term 'costs' of Australia's salinity problem are difficult to assess. The annual cost in lost production and destroyed infrastructure is estimated at A\$230 million, which is only a small fraction of the value of Australia's A\$35 billion agricultural industry (Stirzaker et al. 2002, p. 4). So, while these up-front costs of salinity are low, the costs of stalling salinity are prohibitive. Yet other large costs are looming. The

Murray River is becoming too salty to supply Adelaide with drinking water—by 2020 it will be too salty 40 per cent of the time (Stirzaker et al. 2002, p. 5).

Environmental problems beyond the farm gate

Ecological problems are not confined to the paddock. Farming, food transport and storage use fossil fuels, an irreplaceable resource. Today, many more calories of energy are used to produce fertilisers, run farm machinery, and transport and store food than are present in the food itself. In the USA, three units of energy are used in farming for every unit of food energy consumed. Adding the energy costs of transporting and processing food, there are 10 units of energy needed. As a result, 17 per cent of energy use goes into food production and distribution. If every country in the world was using energy at this rate to produce food, all fossil fuel reserves would have been exhausted by 1996 (Soule & Piper 1992; Mannion 1995). So modern agriculture is dependent on cheap fossil fuel energy—especially oil.

One reason that this poses a problem is **global warming**. The Intergovernmental Panel on Climate Change maintains that we need to cut carbon dioxide emissions (and fossil fuel use) by between 60 and 80 per cent. To allow for economic growth in developing countries, rich countries would have to cut emissions to about 5 per cent of what they now use (Trainer 1995). Unless this is done, the most likely result is a devastating climate change that would seriously increase the costs of agriculture (Maslin 2002; Flannery 2005). This is just the beginning of the problems of global warming. The likely results are catastrophic.

We are also likely to run out of accessible oil reserves. The peak of oil discoveries was in 1960 and since then less and less oil has been discovered. Yet the world consumption of oil is rapidly increasing. An estimate can be made of when oil is going to become much more expensive—the **oil crunch**. Most forecasts suggest this will occur by 2020 (Campbell 1997; Heinberg 2003). What would make most sense is to begin setting up the physical and social structures that are going to be necessary in an agricultural economy without cheap oil (Gunther 2002; Holmgren 2002).

Without cheap energy for transport and refrigeration, we would have to produce almost all food in the local neighbourhood, within walking distance (Trainer 1995). However, today the average distance food has travelled to reach the plate of a US resident is 2000 kilometres (Durning 1991, p. 159). This far-flung distribution of food makes perfect economic sense. Consumers spend more buying exotic foods. For a large supermarket chain, producing a uniform product and distributing it over a large area is cheaper than marketing a variety, which is different in each locality. This is why bananas from Coffs Harbour are sent to Sydney to be bought by big food conglomerates and redistributed back to Coffs Harbour to be sold.

Packaging of food also causes environmental problems. The two factors producing excessive packaging are long-distance transport of food and competition between

Terry Leahy

businesses to attract consumers. The consumer merely chooses the most attractive packet on the shelf. Consumers become part of a system in which unnecessary mountains of plastic, aluminium and paper are manufactured and distributed.

Food production and environmental problems in developing countries

In developing countries, peasant and tribal subsistence has been replaced by food production for the international market (Bennett & George 1987; Trainer 1994). A wealthy landlord or business class monopolises land. Ted Trainer estimates that 80 per cent of land in developing countries is owned by 3 per cent of the population (Trainer 1989, p. 17; see also George 1988; Trainer 1995). Africa, a continent where many starve, actually has more farming land per person than the USA but much of it is used for export crops (Trainer 1995, p. 155). On the land used to produce **cash crops** for the international market, environmental problems are similar to those in developed countries—erosion, toxic pollution, overgrazing and so on. As in developed countries, these problems are caused by competition on the international market.

Displaced subsistence farmers either starve, try to find some employment in towns or remain in rural areas. They may be unemployed and driven to eke out a subsistence by clearing less productive and previously forested land. The environmental effect is that areas of high biodiversity are destroyed by farming. Often soil erosion or leaching of nutrients makes these effects virtually irreversible (George 1988; Fargher & Cadaweng 1990; Pearce et al. 1990; Trainer 1994).

Produce such as rubber, sugar, tea, coffee and meat are all grown in areas where wild animals and plants were dominant. Sixteen million hectares in developing countries are planted for export crops of coffee, tea and cocoa (Trainer 1995, p. 155). Annually, 100 million kilograms of meat is exported to the USA from Central America, mostly from land that was recently tropical rainforest (Trainer 1995, p. 34; see also Pearce et al. 1990; Revkin 1990; Trainer 1994). Recently, the World Wide Fund for Nature has found that 20 per cent of a national park in Sumatra, Indonesia has been occupied by illegal coffee plantations exporting their product and selling it to companies including Nestlé, Kraft, Lavazza and Starbucks—this is a park that is home to endangered Sumatran tigers, elephants and rhinoceroses (Shahab 2007).

As Jules Pretty (1999) points out, **sustainable agriculture** solutions can work well in developing countries if the training and government infrastructure are in place to support them. With labour costs very low in these countries it makes sense to use more labour and fewer industrial inputs of chemical fertilisers and pesticides.

Nevertheless, solutions to environmental problems in developing countries require time, effort and money. In a world where wealth is very unevenly distributed there is little left to deal with these problems (Trainer 1994; 1995). For those of us in the rich countries, our affluence is bought at the expense of environmental destruction, not only in the countries in which we live, but also in the rest of the world.

How are environmental problems linked to global capitalism?

As the above material shows, the ecological problems of food production are related to economic and political structures. There are three basic classes in today's world. First, there is the global capitalist class. The richest 2 per cent of adults own more than half the global household wealth, with the richest 1 per cent alone owning 40 per cent (UNU-Wider 2006). For example, 25 million rich Americans receive as much income as 57 per cent of the world's people (New Internationalist 2004, p. 21). Second is the affluent middle class of all countries and the relatively affluent working class of the developed world. These people are the global consuming class. They are probably between 10 and 20 per cent of the world's population—no more than 1 billion people (UNU-Wider 2006). Twenty per cent of the world's people in the high-income countries account for 86 per cent of total private consumption expenditures (UNDP 1998, p. 2). Third, the rest of the world's population are the global poor—the unemployed of developed countries and the subsistence peasants, low-wage workers and unemployed urbanites of developing countries. A large fraction of these people—840 million—do not get adequate energy and protein in their diet and at least another billion are anaemic and suffer food shortages (UNDP 1998, pp. 49, 50; Sachs 2005). Each of these three groups has a role in the ecological problems of food production. It is their interaction that creates the problems.

Prior to the colonial period, most land in developing countries was used for subsistence production either by peasants or by tribal owners—horticulturalists or hunters and gatherers. Now, most land is being used to produce food for the commodity economy, for sale for cash.

In developing countries today, larger landowners produce food for a global market. Much land is controlled by the global rich and is used for cash crops. These are exported for sale to the affluent consumer class in developed countries. Ecological problems come about because this land is farmed unsustainably or because the land has been converted from forests or woodlands to its present use. The transport and packaging of cash crops exported from developing countries is itself an ecological problem. For the shareholders in the **transnational corporations** that manage this farming, environmental controls are seen to interfere with profits. If profits fall, they move their shares to another company or another country. So farmers in poor countries compete to reduce prices. Often those prices crash—cotton prices dropped by 47 per cent between 1998 and 2001 and coffee by 69 per cent in the same years (New Internationalist 2004, p. 18).

Large food companies dominate markets internationally. In 2003, four companies based in the USA and linked in two alliances controlled 80 per cent of the world's seed market and 75 per cent of the agrochemical market. Six corporations handled 85 per cent of the world market in grain and 15 controlled 85 to 90 per cent of coffee

Terry Leahy

sales (New Internationalist 2003, p. 20; Garcia 2004). Multinationals also dominate the market in other commodities such as tobacco, tea, cocoa and sugar (Trainer 1995). International competition squeezes small farmers and large companies alike.

In the developed world with high wages, the effect is to reduce human labour in farming, through high input agriculture and heavy machinery. For investors, spending money on more sustainable farming would just reduce profits, and managers know they cannot afford such risks. For small owner-operated farms, the price of environmental repair is too high given that farm income is minimal. In many industrialised countries government subsidies prop up farm incomes while supermarket chains make the profits (Garcia 2004; Crosthwaite et al. 2006).

The basic problem of capitalism and the environment is a mismatch between profit and sustainability. It costs money to halt soil erosion, so in any given year profits remain high if nothing is done (McLaughlin 1993, p. 32). The economic system makes it difficult for owners and managers to choose a more expensive strategy. Along with this, a capitalist system makes it very hard to regulate markets. Owners are assumed to have full rights to use their property for maximum profit. Any impediment has to be fought for as a special case, usually after environmental damage has become too obvious to ignore. The wealth of owners makes them a powerful lobby group (McLaughlin 1993).

For a government in the developed world, a serious investment in environmental repair could be achieved in one of two ways. Regulations could force changes on the agricultural industry. The profitability of farming would drop as farm owners had to pay to conform to the regulations. Export earnings would fall and food prices rise. Alternatively, taxpayers could fund this restructuring. Then, the money paid by consumers in higher taxes would be diverted from other industries that supply the consumer goods taxpayers now buy. There would be a damping down of consumer demand. Either way, this investment in rural restructuring would be at the expense of the profitability of the economy.

Governments are of course aware that agriculture is gradually destroying farm-land, and that this is ultimately disastrous for both the farming industry and the economy alike (Lawrence & Vanclay 1992). Caught between these pressures, governments make some effort to support sustainable land use, but it is far from adequate. In Australia, former Prime Minister John Howard introduced a plan for the major waterway upon which much agriculture relies—the Murray-Darling River system. The plan focuses on forestalling the salting up of the water supply to maintain an agricultural industry facing prolonged drought. The basic idea is to use less irrigation water, with open channels replaced by pipes. Some irrigators will sell their water licences back to the government. This is a 10-year program with an average funding of A$1 billion per year (Farr 2007). This is just scratching the surface of the problems in agriculture and yet it is worth about 3 per cent of the annual value of Australia's agricultural industry (ABS 2006). What this reveals is, first, that commercial agriculture has not been able to run in a sustainable way. This failure has ended up costing Australians a lot of government money. Second, the costs of actually fixing the problems are so large as to call into question the future of agriculture in Australia.

A fundamental group to be considered are the affluent consumers of the global market. Capitalism has depended on sales of mass-produced consumer goods to the employed populations of industrial countries. With increases in productivity, the provision of consumer goods has continually increased. Consumers choose food that is either the cheapest or fits their desire for luxury goods. They are reluctant to pay more or restrict their choices—by buying only organic produce, only free range meat, less meat, only food that is locally produced, only food supplied in bulk in reusable jars or paper bags without labels and so on. One approach would be to castigate these consumers for their wasteful consumption and their environmental ignorance.

But why does this consumption appear necessary and attractive? Affluent consumers are also **alienated labour** (Cardan 1974; Marx 1978a,b; Willis 1990). Using this term from Karl Marx, I want to indicate that affluent consumers have to get a paid job to live. As employees they have no control of what they produce, no control over who gets the products, and no control over their conditions at work. Work is perceived as a burden, not as a creative and sociable pleasure. It is in consumption and leisure that affluent workers exercise free choice and their creative and social capacities.

All this ties into the way affluent consumers look at food. Expensive, well-packaged and luxurious food seems the appropriate moral reward for a life of thankless labour. Within a puritanical culture, food is one of the few morally legitimate pleasures (Pont 1997). In fact, the foods that are transported from developing countries—at great cost to the environment—are the epitome of luxury and morality. Meat and dairy products are an appropriate reward for hard masculine labour and necessary for healthy growth; sugar a sweet pleasure and an apt reward for appropriate femininity; coffee, tea and chocolate—all stimulating but legitimate drugs—an aid to concentration at work or a reward after work. These factors make it difficult to get consumers to reform their food purchasing habits environmentally. It becomes unlikely that consumers would embrace tough environmental regulations if this meant they would pay more for food or have less choice of foods.

Ruralisation and suburban farming

It may be considered that urbanisation is a factor that distances urban consumers from the environmental consequences of food production in far distant farms and other countries. Within capitalism, it makes sense economically to separate farms from affluent cities, so that cheap labour or large machinery can be readily used. It makes sense culturally for alienated workers to want luxuries from far off places, as compensation for their forced labour. This separation is not necessary.

People could be reorganised to grow their own food locally (Trainer 1995). Frederick Gunther, a Swedish writer, suggests relocation of urbanites and **ruralisation**. We have

Terry Leahy

to stop transporting food long distances and start composting our sewage. Agricultural products would be produced close to consumers, with villages of 200 people supplied by farms of 40 hectares. Villages would end up being a kilometre apart. Food would be produced by, rather than imported into, the village. The energy used in redistributing and recycling soil nutrients would be 1 per cent of that used just to treat sewage now. No energy would be needed to make synthetic fertilisers, as these would be replaced by waste recycling and legume crops (Gunther 2002, p. 266).

Writers such as David Holmgren and Ted Trainer think local farming can be achieved without relocation out of the cities. They argue that it would be more practical to make use of the land available in our suburbs to produce most food in the cities where people now live (Trainer 1995; Holmgren 2005).

Social alternatives to capitalism

Nationalisation

The aspects of capitalism that lie behind environmental damage are unlikely to disappear without a radically different social organisation. Yet Soviet-style nationalisation seems no better at dealing with environmental problems than capitalism. Despite the fact that the government is in a position to control environmental damage—through its ownership of firms—there are other problems. One is the inefficiency of allocation of resources that goes with government bureaucratic structures (Feher et al. 1983). Another problem is that labour is alienated—people do not have any control in their jobs. As in capitalist societies, people expect an increasing affluence to justify their compliance. The environment comes last for a government attempting to increase consumer satisfaction despite the inefficiencies of the bureaucratic command economy. The sense that good work is not rewarded by opportunities for private consumption erodes dedication and undermines efficiency. Waste is endemic.

The gift economy

The **gift economy** is another kind of alternative to capitalism that may be considered to be more benign environmentally. There would be no money and no wage labour. Instead people would produce things for their own consumption or as gifts. It would be a vast extension of the kinds of voluntary work now done by citizen groups. Clubs and associations would produce technologically complex goods and services. People would be motivated to work by desires for status and the pleasure of giving, as well as by the knowledge that their work was necessary for the whole community. The standard of living would be the effect of multiple gift networks (Vaneigem 1983; Coates & Leahy 2006). Coordination would be by links between collectives of producers and consumers, and by collectives of researchers, media and administrative workers.

This social alternative could help the environment. Farmers would conserve their agricultural and environmental resources, to live well in the future and to be able to continue gaining social recognition by giving farm produce to the community. Status would come from work that looked after the natural environment. Because 'income' would depend on gifts, no amount of hard work would lead to wealth. There would be no point in producing useless items.

Creativity and choice would be here turned to creating a productive process that was also environmentally benign. People would not depend on increasing material well-being for their creative outlet. An organic agriculture with an emphasis on tree crops would work well—which would provide enjoyable and creative work as well as sustainable production (Mollison & Holmgren 1978; see also Mollison 1988; Soule & Piper 1992; French 1993; Fern 1997). The gift economy would depend on generosity and egalitarianism. Pleasure would come from giving to those in need. Other species would also be regarded as appreciating gifts of care and concern. This is a somewhat rosy view. Where would the political will come from?

Conclusion: An end to civilisation?

Given the environmental problems discussed in this chapter, and the lack of political effort to address them, some commentators predict we will end up like civilisations in the past that have undermined their agricultural base, resulting in an inevitable collapse in food production, a major decline of the population, and finally the collapse of government and the literal massacre of the ruling class (Diamond 2005). A scenario one would not wish on anyone's grandchildren! The success of sustainable forms of agriculture ultimately depends not only upon the actions of concerned individuals and communities, but also on state regulation in the form of incentives, subsidies and planning. The experiments in sustainable agriculture discussed in this chapter show that viable social alternatives are available and feasible.

SUMMARY OF MAIN POINTS

- The problems of modern agriculture come from technologies that maximise profits by cutting costs.
- Technological solutions to these problems are only accepted if they promise to compete on profits.
- Environmentally adequate solutions are unable to dominate the market.
- Environmental problems in agriculture also go beyond the farm gate.
- In developing countries, cash crops displace poor farmers and take up the habitat of wild species.

Terry Leahy

- Global capitalism can be seen as a major social cause of the environmental damage produced by agriculture.
- Social alternatives to capitalism might work but do not have much popular appeal at present.

SOCIOLOGICAL REFLECTION

Go to your local large supermarket and examine the origin of the foods you usually eat.

- For all the foods you usually buy, is there an organic alternative available? What is the price difference compared with your usual product? Where is the organic food grown? How many of the foods that you usually eat could be grown in your own neighbourhood? How would you cope emotionally if your diet was restricted to foods that could be grown in your local area and fresh foods that would be available only when harvested?
- Look at the pesticides and herbicides sold in the supermarket. Do a web search and find out if the chemicals contained in these products could be harmful to your health

DISCUSSION QUESTIONS

1. What environmental problems are addressed by minimum tillage, agroforestry and deep drainage?
2. What are the problems with these solutions?
3. What are the economic disincentives for food forests, organic agriculture and localised agriculture?
4. Why is it so hard to get effective environmental reform of agriculture?
5. Would nationalisation or a gift economy work better than capitalism to solve the environmental problems of farming?
6. Is a collapse of civilisation the most likely outcome of our current environmental crisis?

Further investigation

1. Capitalist agricultural practices are the prime cause of environmental degradation. Discuss.
2. Sustainable agriculture makes social and economic sense. Discuss.

FURTHER READING AND WEB RESOURCES

Books

Diamond, J. 2005, *Collapse: How Societies Choose to Fail or Survive*, Penguin, Camberwell, Victoria. An excellent historical and cross-cultural comparison of societies facing environmental problems.

Flannery, T. 2005, *The Weather Makers: The History and Future Impact of Climate Change*, Text Publishing, Melbourne. Readable and authoritative.

Heinberg, R. 2003, *The Party's Over—Oil, War and the Fate of Industrial Societies*, Clairview, New York. Well written, a good critique of some of the more optimistic scenarios for replacement energy sources.

Holmgren Design Services 2005. *Melliodora, Hepburn Permaculture Gardens: A Case Study in Cool Climate Permaculture Design 1985–2005*. A detailed account of the planning and setting up of a sustainable house and agricultural system based on tree crops. Pictures of the property at different stages from all angles. eBook from www.holmgren.com.au.

Mollison, B. 1988, *Permaculture: A Designers' Manual*, Tagari Publications, Tyalgum, Australia. A comprehensive how-to manual for sustainable agriculture in different climate zones.

Pretty, J. 1999, *Regenerating Agriculture: Policies and Practice for Sustainability and Self-Reliance*, Earthscan, London. Global in scope, a thorough introduction to the problems of industrial agriculture and the kinds of alternatives that are working.

Trainer, T. 1995, *The Conserver Society*, Zed Books, London. Shows why capitalism cannot solve environmental problems and the kind of society that could.

Websites

David Holmgren: www.holmgren.com.au. Founder of permaculture and a leading permaculture designer.

Gift Economy: http://gifteconomy.octapod.org. Website of Terry Leahy (author of this chapter) with much detailed discussion of agriculture and other topics.

The Simpler Way: http://socialwork.arts.unsw.edu.au/tsw/. Ted Trainer's website, with detailed information on many environmental and social issues.

United Nations Development Programme: www.undp.org/reports/global/. Annual reports on everything to do with developing countries.

Documentaries

Garcia, D.K. 2004, *The Future of Food*, Lily Films. Covers the problems of GM foods and multinational control over agriculture, as well as sustainable alternatives.

The Community Solution 2006, *The Power of Community: How Cuba Survived Peak Oil*, Community Service Inc. A fascinating documentary. After the fall of the Soviet Union, Cuba's cheap oil vanished and it had to reconstruct its agriculture.

Post Carbon Institute 2004. *The End of Suburbia: Oil Depletion and the Collapse of the American Dream*, Electric Wallpaper, Canada. A documentary that proposed solutions somewhat different to those proposed by Australian permaculture writers.

Terry Leahy

REFERENCES

ABS 2006, *7503.0 Value of Agricultural Commodities Produced, Australia, 2004–05*, Australian Bureau of Statistics, www.abs.gov.au [accessed 26 February 2007].

Bennett, J. & George, S. 1987, *The Hunger Machine: The Politics of Food*, Polity Press, London.

Campbell, A. 1991, *Planning for Sustainable Farming: The Potter Farmland Plan Story*, Lothian Books, Melbourne.

Campbell, J.Z. 1997, *The Coming Oil Crisis*, Multiscience and Petroconsultants, Brentwood, UK.

Cardan, P. 1974, *Modern Capitalism and Revolution*, Solidarity, London.

Coates, J. & Leahy, T. 2006, 'Ideology and Politics: Essential Factors in the Path Towards Sustainability', *Electronic Green Journal*, Spring, Issue 23, http://egj.lib.uidaho.edu/egj23/index.htm/ [accessed 28 February 2007].

Crosby, A.W. 1986, *Ecological Imperialism: The Biological Expansion of Europe, 900–1900*, Cambridge University Press, Cambridge.

Crosthwaite, J., Malcolm, B., Moll, J. & Dorough, J. 2006, 'Future Investment in Landscape Change', in *Conference Proceedings: International Landcare Conference*, State of Victoria Department of Sustainability and the Environment, Melbourne.

Cullen, P., Williams, J. & Curtis, A. 2003, *Landcare Farming: Securing the Future for Australian Agriculture*, Landcare Australia, Chatswood.

Diamond, J. 2005, *Collapse: How Societies Choose to Fail or Survive*, Penguin, Camberwell, Victoria.

Durning, A. 1991, 'Asking How Much is Enough', in L. Brown et al., *State of the World 1991: A World Watch Institute Report on Progress Toward a Sustainable Society*, Allen & Unwin, Sydney.

Fargher, J. & Cadaweng E. 1990, 'Grassland Management for Reforestation in Tropical Uplands', *Permaculture International Journal*, no. 37, pp. 33–4.

Farr, M. 2007, 'Drought Proof: Howard's $10 bn Plan to Safeguard Australia', *Daily Telegraph*, 26 January, p. 1.

Feher, F., Heller A. & Markus, G. 1983, *Dictatorship Over Needs: An Analysis of Soviet Societies*, Basil Blackwell, Oxford.

Fern, K. 1997, *Plants for a Future: Edible & Useful Plants for a Healthier World*, Permanent Publications, Hampshire.

Flannery, T. 2005, *The Weather Makers: The History and Future Impact of Climate Change*, Text Publishing, Melbourne.

French, J. 1993, *The Wilderness Garden: Beyond Organic Gardening*, Aird Books, Melbourne.

Garcia, D.K. 2004, *The Future of Food*, Lily Films.

George, S. 1988, *A Fate Worse than Debt*, Penguin, Harmondsworth.

Gunther, F. 2002, 'Fossil Energy and Food Security', *Energy and Environment*, vol. 12, no. 4, pp. 253–275.

Heinberg, R. 2003, *The Party's Over: Oil, War and the Fate of Industrial Societies*, Clairview, New York.

Holmgren, D. 1994, *Trees on the Treeless Plains*, Holmgren Design Services, Hepburn, Victoria.

—— 2002, *Permaculture: Principles & Pathways Beyond Sustainability*, Holmgren Design Services, Hepburn, Victoria.

—— 2005, *Retrofitting the Suburbs for Sustainability*, Holmgren Design Services, www.holmgren.com.au.

Hutchings, P. 2004, 'Grazing Management', in K. Kent, G. Earl, B. Mullins, I. Lunt and R. Webster (eds), *Native Vegetation Guide for the Riverina*, Charles Sturt University, Murray Catchment Authority, Deniliquin, NSW, www.csu.edu.au/herbarium/riverina/ [accessed 27 October 2004].

Jensen, D. 2006, *Endgame: The Problem of Civilization*, Vols 1 & 2, Seven Stories Press, New York.

Kasperczyk, N. & Knickel, K. 2006, 'Environmental Impacts of Organic Farming', in P. Kristiansen, A. Taji & J. Reganold (eds), *Organic Agriculture: A Global Perspective*, Comstock, New York, pp. 259–94.

Kristiansen, P. & Merfield, C. 2006, 'Overview of Organic Agriculture', in P. Kristiansen, A. Taji & J. Reganold (eds), *Organic Agriculture: A Global Perspective*, Comstock, New York, pp. 1–23.

Land & Water Australia 2002, *Managing Phosphorus in Catchments*, Fact Sheet 11, River Landscapes, Australian Government, Canberra, ACT.

Lawrence, G. & Vanclay, F. 1992, 'Agricultural Production and Environmental Degradation in the Murray-Darling Basin', in G. Lawrence, F. Vanclay & B. Furze, *Agriculture, Environment and Society: Contemporary Issues for Australians*, Macmillan, Melbourne.

Leu, A. 2006, 'Beyond Silent Spring: Organic Agriculture as a Model for Environmental Sustainability', in *Conference Proceedings: International Landcare Conference*, State of Victoria Department of Sustainability and the Environment, Melbourne.

Lockie, S., Halpin, D. & Pearson, D. 2006, 'Understanding the Market for Organic Food', in P. Kristiansen, A. Taji & J. Reganold (eds), *Organic Agriculture: A Global Perspective*, Comstock, New York, pp. 245–58.

Mannion, A.M. 1995, *Agriculture and Environmental Change: Temporal and Spatial Dimensions*, John Wiley & Sons, Chichester, UK.

Maslin, M. 2002, *The Coming Storm: The True Causes of Freak Weather*, ABC Books, Sydney.

Marx, K. 1978a, 'Economic and Philosophic Manuscripts of 1844', in R.C. Tucker, *The Marx-Engels Reader*, W.W. Norton, New York.

—— 1978b, 'Wage Labour and Capital', in R.C. Tucker, *The Marx-Engels Reader*, W.W. Norton, New York.

McLaughlin, A. 1993, *Regarding Nature: Industrialism and Deep Ecology*, State of NY Press, Albany.

Mollison, B. 1988, *Permaculture: A Designer's Manual*, Tagari Publications, Tyalgum, Australia.

—— & Holmgren, D. 1978, *Permaculture One*, Corgi Books, Uxbridge.

Morrow, R. 1993, *Earth User's Guide to Permaculture*, Kangaroo Press, Kenthurst, Australia.

Morse, R. 2006, 'Developing No-tillage Systems Without Chemicals: The Best of Both Worlds?', in P. Kristiansen, A. Taji & J. Reganold (eds), *Organic Agriculture: A Global Perspective*, Comstock, New York, pp. 83–91.

Murray-Darling Basin Commission 2004, *The Murray-Darling Basin*, Canberra, ACT.

National Dryland Salinity Program 2004, *Dryland Salinity and Catchment Management*, Land & Water Australia, Canberra, ACT.

New Internationalist 2003, 'Food and Farming: The Facts', *The Politics of Food and Farming*, January/February vol. 353, pp. 20–1.

—— 2004, 'Free Trade', *The Free Trade Game*, December vol. 374, pp. 18–19.

Pearce, D., Barbier, E. & Markandya, A. 1990, *Sustainable Development: Economics and Environment in the Third World*, Earthscan, London.

Pont, J.J. 1997, *Heart Health Promotion in a Respectable Community: An inside view of the Culture of the Coalfields of Northern New South Wales*, PhD thesis, University of Newcastle.

Pretty, J. 1999, *Regenerating Agriculture: Policies and Practice for Sustainability and Self-Reliance*, Earthscan, London.

Revkin, A. 1990, *The Burning Season: The Murder of Chico Mendes and the Fight for the Amazon Rain Forest*, William Collins Sons, London.

Sachs, J. 2005, *The End of Poverty: How We Can Make it Happen in Our Lifetime*, Penguin, London.

Shahab, N. 2007, 'Firms Told to Clean up Illegal Coffee Act', *Sydney Morning Herald*, 18 January, p. 10.

Soule, J.D. & Piper, J.K. 1992, *Farming in Nature's Image: An Ecological Approach to Agriculture*, Island Press, Washington, D.C.

Stirzaker, R., Vertessy, R. & Sarre, A. 2002, *Trees, Water and Salt*, Joint Venture Agroforestry Program, Australian Government Publications, Canberra, ACT.

Sundquist, B. 2004, *Grazing Lands Degradation: A Global Perspective*, http://home.alltel. net/bsundquist1/og2 [accessed 27 October 2004].

Thomas, V.G. & Kevan, P.G. 1993, 'Basic Principles of Agroecology and Sustainable Agriculture', *Journal of Agricultural and Environmental Ethics*, vol. 6, no. 1, pp. 1–19.

Trainer, T. 1989, *Developed to Death: Rethinking Third World Development*, Green Print, Merlin, London.

Trainer, T. 1995, *The Conserver Society: Alternatives for Sustainability*, Zed Books, London.

Turner, J., Wareing, K., Flinn, D. & Lambert, M. 2004, *Forestry in the Agricultural Landscape*, Department of Primary Industries, Melbourne.

UNDP 1998, *Consumption for Human Development*, United Nations Development Programme, www.undp.org/reports/global/ [accessed 26 February 2006].

UNU-Wider 2006, *Pioneering Study Shows Richest Two Percent Own Half World Wealth*, United Nations University, World Institute for Development Economics Research, www.wider.unu.edu [accessed 26 February 2006].

Vanclay, F. & Lawrence, G. 1995, *The Environmental Imperative: Ecosocial Concerns for Australian Agriculture*, Central Queensland University Press, Rockhampton.

Vaneigem, R. 1983, *The Revolution of Everyday Life*, Left Bank Books and Rebel Press, London.

Watson P. 1992, 'An Ecologically Unsustainable Agriculture', in G. Lawrence, F. Vanclay and B. Furze, *Agriculture, Environment and Society: Contemporary Issues for Australians*, Macmillan, Melbourne.

Whitefield, P. 1998, *How to Make a Forest Garden*, Permanent Publications, Hampshire.

Willis, P. 1990, *Common Culture: Symbolic Work at Play in the Everyday Cultures of the Young*, Westview Press, Boulder, Colorado.

Wynen, E. 2006, 'Economic Management in Organic Agriculture', in P. Kristiansen, A. Taji & J. Reganold (eds), *Organic Agriculture: A Global Perspective*, Comstock, New York, pp. 231–44.

CHAPTER 4

Agribusiness, Genetic Engineering and the Corporatisation of Food

Geoffrey Lawrence and Janet Grice

OVERVIEW

- What is 'agribusiness' and what role does it play in food production?
- What types of biotechnologies are used in the food and agricultural industries and what do consumers think of them?
- What is the future of genetically modified foods?

This chapter deals with the connections between agriculture and food production, highlighting, in particular, the global nature of the agri-food sector and its commitment to biotechnology. It examines consumer attitudes to food biotechnologies and argues that the growing consumer wariness about genetically engineered foods (together with a surge in interest in organic foods) may alter the current pro-biotechnology trajectory of the agri-food sector.

Key concepts

agribusiness	food safety	neo-liberalism
agri-food	genetic engineering	substitutionism
appropriationism	genetically modified	transgenic organisms
biotechnology	organisms (GMOs)	vertical integration
capitalism	globalisation	
DNA	horizontal integration	

Introduction

Why would scientists wish to take a gene from a fish (the flounder) and insert it into a tomato? Why would they select a gene from a chicken and put it in a potato? The answers, according to food industry scientists, are that, in the first case, the tomato will have a better flavour and longer shelf life, and in the second case, the potato will be able to develop increased resistance to disease. Geneticists are also attempting to produce a variety of wheat that is resistant to pests: it will need fewer, if any, chemical sprayings to control insect infestations. How would this work? A gene from the soil bacterium *Bacillus thuringiensis* produces a substance toxic to insects but not to humans. If inserted and expressed in the plant it provides continuous pest control. In another experiment, scientists have developed a pig with the capacity to grow more quickly on less food and produce leaner pork. The pig has been genetically altered so that it contains extra hormone genes derived from human **DNA**.

For science and industry, the benefits that will be derived from the **genetic engineering** of plants and animals outweigh the risks and concerns. The food processing industry, in particular, will benefit financially if foods can be processed more easily, have a longer shelf life, travel without damage, and exhibit characteristics desired by consumers.

However, according to studies undertaken in Australia and abroad, there appears to be growing consumer resistance to genetically modified foods (GM foods). Why, then, would major segments of the **agri-food** industry be so convinced of the desirability of going down a 'biotech' path in the production of foods? Answers to this question can be found in an understanding of **agribusiness** and its role in farming and food production.

Corporate agribusiness

'Agriculture' is often conceived as the on-farm production of foods and fibres. Farmers grow the products necessary to sustain life, which are then distributed and marketed locally, nationally and globally. Farmers in this sense are viewed as largely independent producers, making on-farm decisions with a very firm understanding of the marketplace and deciding, individually, what to produce and when and how to produce it. In one of the earliest formulations of the term 'agribusiness', American John Davis—writing in the 1950s—believed this view of farming was flawed and antiquated. Farming must be seen as part of a wider network of production relations. Agribusiness is 'the sum of all farming operations, plus the manufacture and distribution of all farm production supplies, plus the total of all operations performed in connection with the handling, storage, processing and distribution of farm commodities' (Davis 1956, p. 109).

What Davis was highlighting was the full integration of farming into wider circuits of **capitalist** production—a process that accelerated in the United States of America and other Western nations after World War II as the corporate sector began to horizontally and vertically integrate its activities. **Horizontal integration** is the purchasing of like companies (for example, a flour mill purchasing other flour mills), while **vertical integration** is the purchase of unlike companies that can form strategic production linkages (for example, a flour mill purchasing a biscuit or bread manufacturer or a supermarket chain). Both are strategies to increase the size of operations, to draw closer connections between affiliates, to increase the level and efficiency of production, and to raise profits. Both lead, in the agri-food industries, to the progressive integration of farming into corporate business operations. How is this achieved?

On the upstream side, the corporate sector, including companies such as John Deere, ConAgra, Syngenta, DuPont (Pioneer), Aventis and Dow, and firms in the finance industry, supply the inputs used by farmers—the tractors, headers, ploughs, fertilisers, seeds, insecticides and irrigation pipes—and the credit to purchase them. On the downstream side of farming, companies such as Goodman Fielder, Kraft, Bunge, Simplot, Kelloggs, McDonald's, Tesco, Wal-Mart, Woolworths and Coles take agricultural produce and store it, process it, package it, transport it, and sell it through a host of outlets, including supermarkets. The influence of firms involved in upstream and downstream activities has had a significant impact on farming. In entering contract relations with firms in the corporate sector, farmers find they must conform to corporate demands. The food corporations can specify that certain seeds be used, that certain varieties of potato or tomato or pineapple be grown instead of others, that crops be harvested at specific times, that particular chemicals be sprayed, that company-determined pay rates for employees be enforced, and that certain standards be reached before produce is accepted by the company (Burch & Lawrence 2007). Not all of this is 'negative': it does appear that supermarkets are enforcing higher standards on suppliers—standards that might foster more sustainable practices in farming as well as along the entire agri-food supply chain (see Campbell, Lawrence & Smith 2006). But what we can be certain of is that a combination of economic power and **globalisation** gives the corporate sector ultimate control over food production in the developed world (Jansen & Vellema 2004; Rama 2005).

Globalisation and agribusiness

The 'seedling to supermarket' arrangements described above not only allow control throughout the marketing of foods and fibres, but also ensure profits are made along the production chain. In the USA, the agribusiness/food sector is the second-most-profitable industry after pharmaceuticals (Magdoff et al. 2000, p. 2). Cargill, a privately owned company based in the USA, is one of the world's largest agribusiness corporations employing some 149 000 workers in over 60 countries. It recorded sales of US$75 billion in 2006 (see Cargill 2007). ConAgra, also based in the USA, owns 56 companies operating in 26 countries with a workforce of 58 000. It recorded sales of US$14.6 billion in 2005, with the company boasting that 96 per cent of all households in the USA stock ConAgra products (ConAgra 2007; see also McMichael 2000, p. 103). Both these companies are vertically integrated and are examples of corporations that have used their market positioning to secure transnational advantage. Another company of interest is Tyson Foods. According to McMichael (2000, p. 103), Tyson sends US chicken meat to Mexico for processing, taking advantage of cheap labour (one-tenth the cost of labour in the USA) to prepare chicken for the Japanese market.

Other firms have been accused of exploiting unprotected child labour in their profit-making endeavours (McMichael 2000, p. 99), some have 'bargained' for lower payments for contract production (with the threat of withdrawal if the growers refused the offer) (Burch & Rickson 2001), and others have taken advantage of lower environmental standards in certain countries to produce foods more cheaply (Constance et al. 2003). For an export country like Argentina, the presence of the agri-food transnational corporations has contributed to relative food price increases, the removal of farmers, and increased unemployment and income loss among the lower-income sectors of society (Teubal & Rodriquez 2003). Agri-food change in the wine industry in South Africa has brought workers 'little improvement, either in the form of wages, or living conditions' (Ewert 2003, p. 167). Finally, itinerant female agri-food workers in developing countries such as Mexico and Kenya are among the most exploited of all workers worldwide (Dolan 2004; McMichael & Friedmann 2007).

There are many other examples of the transformative pressures placed upon food commodity chains by agribusiness. Both directly and through agro-political organisations, agribusiness has pressured governments in places such as Australia and New Zealand to deregulate the agricultural sector, allowing corporate takeovers of what were once state-controlled or cooperative ventures (Le Heron & Roche 1999; Pritchard 2005a, 2005b). Hand-in-hand with deregulation of the agricultural sector and **neo-liberal** policies that foster corporate financial advantage have come mergers, takeovers, partnerships and joint ventures, leading to the concentration of the activities of particular agri-food industries in a small number of firms. In the latest and most comprehensive account of the US agri-food sector, Heffernan (1999) reports that four companies in the beef-packing industry are responsible for some 79 per cent of US output. Similarly, the top four companies are responsible for 62 per cent of flour milling, 57 per cent of pork production and 49 per cent of chicken production. Such market concentration gives these top four firms enormous economic and political clout (Tozanli 2005).

Trade in undifferentiated commodities (raw sugar, unprocessed wheat, generic beef, wool and so forth) has previously been undertaken through statutory authorities

Geoffrey Lawrence and Janet Grice

and producer boards—particularly in places such as New Zealand, Canada and Australia. However, as deregulation has occurred, agribusinesses have taken over much of this trade, converting raw materials into 'durable' foods so as to add value to exports. There is obviously financial benefit in global trading, but there is a growing realisation that consumers—particularly in the West—are demanding not more food, but better food, or so-called high-value foods (HVFs). These foods include poultry meat, fruits and vegetables, and fish, dairy and organic products that can be shifted around the world to meet consumer demand (Lang & Heasman 2004). HVFs are not standardised bulk commodities but 'quality' products that serve niche markets (Nestle 2003; Lockie et al. 2006). In their aptly titled book *From Columbus to ConAgra*, Bonanno and colleagues (1994) describe the changes that have occurred in the USA. Their argument is that flexibility is the major driving force in corporate expansionism. By exercising Just-in-Time principles (delivery-on-demand of agricultural products, rather than the need to store) many firms have moved away from the 'durable' manufactured, processed, canned and frozen foods to fresh foods and other HVFs. These foods are sourced globally so as to save on labour costs as well as to guarantee year-round supply—largely for consumers interested in purchasing 'clean and green' foods that are identified with health and good living (Watts & Goodman 1997; Burch & Lawrence 2005).

It is the global organisation of production that is the defining characteristic of both forms of trade—in durable and fresh foods. The so-called 'world steer' is now understood to be the agricultural equivalent of the 'world car'. As the fast-food industry has grown, beef has become a world commodity, with 'components' manufactured (grown) and assembled (in the case of the beef animal, disassembled) in various locations around the globe. Cattle ranching takes place in locations such as Central America, Australia, Argentina and South Africa. Semen is sent from the USA to 'enhance' breeding. This is supplemented by antibiotics and other veterinary medicines manufactured by transnational pharmaceutical companies—with origins in places like Switzerland and Germany. Beef is fattened with grains often imported from the USA, and the meat is sent to the USA, Russia, the Philippines, Mexico—and indeed to any country proud to display the Golden Arches—as a generic product to be 'ground' for hamburger meat (see descriptions in Rifkin 1992, pp. 192–3; McMichael 2000, pp. 101–2).

The two processes that have underpinned—and help us explain—agribusiness expansion are **appropriationism** and **substitutionism** (Goodman et al. 1987; Goodman & Redclift 1991). Appropriationism is the progressive use of manufactured inputs in agriculture. What were once farm-derived inputs (seeds kept from the year before, silage stored from the past season, 'natural' fertilisation of the soil via crop rotation and the use of horses to haul machinery) have been appropriated by off-farm industries that now supply the seeds, fertilisers and machinery as farm inputs. In so doing, agribusiness makes money from these sales, while providing farmers with the technical means to increase output. A contemporary example is the 'redesigning' of plants and animals so that they conform to the corporate agenda of having farmers purchase seeds that will only respond to the company's proprietary chemicals (discussed below). Another is the development of tomato varieties specifically suited to particular mechanical harvesting equipment (Pritchard & Burch 2003, p. 34).

The second process—substitutionism—is the replacement of costly and/or unreliably supplied inputs with 'generic ingredients' in the food processing industry. As Friedmann (1991, p. 74) explained over a decade ago, what food processors want 'is not sugar, but sweeteners; not flour or cornstarch, but thickeners; not palm oil or butter, but fats; not beef or cod, but proteins. Interchangeable inputs, natural or chemically synthesized, augment control and reduce costs better than older mercantile strategies for diversifying sources of supply…'. Substitutionism allows for greater corporate control over agriculture because of the ability of firms to substitute components in food production. Firms can use 'sugar' made from the cornstarch, for example, rather than that derived from cane or beet—particularly if it is cheaper, more readily available and has other positive characteristics, such as being easy to manufacture (see discussion below). The firms have the capacity to bypass particular farmers, particular commodities and particular regions in sourcing generic food ingredients, again placing more control in the hands of agribusiness.

Agri-food biotechnologies

Why might biotechnologies be so desired by agribusiness? Biotechnologies have been employed for centuries to make cheeses, bake breads and brew beers. Traditional **biotechnology** is the harnessing of natural biological processes to produce foods, beverages and medicines. One example is the use of micro-organisms to ferment substances (such as grapes into wine). In more recent times, through the application of advanced cell-biology techniques, other processes have been made possible. Biotechnologies applied in the agri-food sector today include large-scale fermentation, cell culture and fusion, cloning, gene marker technology, DNA sequencing, diagnostic probes and genetic engineering (Norton 2002, p.4). It is this last component of biotechnology—genetic engineering—that is proving both profoundly transformative and controversial. Genetic engineering involves the manipulation of genes, and components of genes, to alter the characteristics of bacteria, plants, and animals.

Entirely new **transgenic organisms** can be created by the cross-species insertion of genetic material. As well as the examples given at the beginning of the chapter, there are others of considerable interest to agri-food industries:

- Scientists are experimenting with placing a gene from a waxmoth into a potato (to increase resistance to bruising) and a gene from a trout into a catfish (to encourage faster growth of the catfish). They have already been successful in placing a gene from a pea plant into rice (to add new protein to rice grains – the so-called 'golden rice'). These are but a few examples; there are thousands of other transgenic foods being developed throughout the world.

- In the area of animal production, the natural hormone bovine somatotropin has been extracted from cattle, synthesised biogenetically, and injected into cows, increasing milk production by 30 per cent.
- Scientists hope to be able to insert a gene responsible for root-nodule formation in legumes into non-leguminous crop plants such as wheat and barley. If successful, this process would enable those crops to 'fix' their own nitrogen, potentially reducing the amount of fertiliser that farmers need to apply.
- Experiments have been successfully performed to make commercial crops resistant to herbicides. Chemicals can be sprayed to rid the soil of weeds, while still allowing the crops to grow without damage or loss of vigour.
- Enzymes from bacteria, yeast, fungi and plants are being extracted and biogenetically engineered and 'grown' in fermentation tanks to provide the food industry with substances that speed up food-manufacturing processes and impart new characteristics to food (Lawrence et al. 2001; Norton 2002; Hindmarsh & Lawrence 2004).

While some of these innovations would seem, at face value, to be desirable in a world of food scarcity, there are many critics who argue that these sorts of experiments will have negative animal-welfare implications, have the potential to create health problems and will not help feed the world's poor (Ho 1998; Hindmarsh & Lawrence 2001; McMichael 2003). So why persist? By looking a little more closely at the last two examples listed above, the advantages of genetic engineering for agribusiness will become obvious.

Appropriationism

Herbicide resistance provides an excellent case of appropriationism. Agribusiness companies have genetically engineered seeds that will tolerate spraying with particular herbicides. The most well-known case is that of Monsanto and its proprietary herbicide, Roundup. This herbicide is toxic to most herbaceous plants, including soybeans. Scientists have engineered a soybean plant that will not only resist Roundup, but will actually need to be sprayed with it in order to reach peak production. The company is developing a total seed-and-herbicide package that it can sell to farmers. The plant is a productive one, weeds can be removed more readily and the farmer could potentially increase profits by growing the Roundup Ready seeds. However, the farmer cannot keep the seed and grow it the next year. If that occurs, the farmer can be sued by the company for breaching intellectual property laws that protect the seed's genetic make-up. When contracts are signed with Monsanto, farmers are forbidden from cultivating other varieties, using herbicides other than those produced by Monsanto, or exchanging the seeds with neighbours. The farmer must also allow Monsanto officials to inspect paddocks and fields for three years (de la Perriere & Seuret 2000, p. 16; see also Hindmarsh & Lawrence 2004).

By 1998, only four years after the first authorisations allowing the sowing of genetically modified (GM) crops, some 30 million hectares of GM cotton, soybeans, tomatoes, potatoes and canola had been planted. By 2001 there were 50 million hectares planted with GM crops—mostly in the USA, Canada, Argentina and China (Pretty 2002, p. 128). In 2006, the area planted with GM crops had grown to 102 million hectares in over 22 countries (ISAAA 2006). A new crop—herbicide resistant alfalfa (Lucerne)—was launched in the USA in 2006 (ISAAA 2006). The global market for GM crops in 2006 was estimated at US$6.15 billion and is expected to rise to approximately US$6.8 billion in 2007 (ISAAA 2006).

In the case of herbicide-resistant canola, it is now acknowledged that there are serious risks of cross-pollination, with spontaneous hybridisation occurring between the genetically engineered crop and its close relatives—including wild radish and hoary mustard. This might result in the growth of 'superweeds' that can resist herbicide treatment, as well as other impacts. For example, given that canola pollen can travel up to 2 kilometres from the crop, neighbouring farmers wanting to grow and sell 'non-GM' canola will find it virtually impossible to protect their crop. Organic honey producers will not know whether bees have taken pollen from the GM crop—thus preventing the honey from being labelled 'organic' (and, hence, taking away the opportunity of obtaining premium prices for the product) (Allen 2000, p. 65; Fitzsimons 2000, pp. 192–3). There are other major concerns about genetic engineering of crops and animals:

- **Genetically modified organisms (GMOs)** are complex and 'unstable' and have the potential to affect the environment in ways not able to be predicted by science. Even GM advocates are urging caution in the release of GM fish, for fear that these fish will invade the habitats of native species and eliminate them (see report in Associated Press 2003, p. 1).
- Insect resistance will inevitably occur, reducing the ability of GM crops to survive infestations. Scientists will then look for alternative insect-resisting genes to insert into crops and insects will eventually become resistant to them. The problem is linked to large-scale monocropping (planting vast areas exclusively or almost exclusively with one variety), yet monocropping is likely to accelerate as agriculture becomes increasingly industrialised (de la Perriere & Seuret 2000, pp. 43–4; Magdoff et al. 2000).
- Organic producers who have relied on natural biological controls, such as the soil bacterium *Bacillus thuringiensis* (Bt), will face major problems as insects become

Geoffrey Lawrence and Janet Grice

resistant to plants genetically engineered with Bt (de la Perriere & Seuret 2000, pp. 43–4).

- GM products could seriously compromise the treatment of human and animal diseases. Some GM crops have antibiotic-resistant genes that, if they transferred to bacteria, could make those bacteria immune to drugs, thus undermining current treatments.

- Science has yet to understand the extent of the allergic reactions that people and animals may experience from ingesting GM foods. Allergies relate to particular proteins produced by plants. The recombination of plant genetic material can lead to allergic reactions that have the potential to harm or kill those eating the novel foods (Conner 2000). In Australia, under current **food safety** regulations, GM foods are tested to ensure they are not allergenic by considering if new proteins come from organisms containing significant allergens, or if new proteins are similar to known allergens, or if new proteins have other characteristics similar to allergens. If a GM food were shown to be allergenic, approval would not be given (FSANZ 2005).

Despite these and other concerns, the vertical integration of firms in the seed and chemical industries has provided enormous potential for appropriationist strategies. In the end, the farmers are dependent upon the corporations for virtually all of the inputs for farming—apart, of course, from their own labour power.

Substitutionism

Substitutionism occurs as the food industry seeks to use biotechnology to produce generic inputs rather than rely upon specific crops. The best example is that of sugar. Historically, sugar has been extracted from cane and from beet. Today, the reaction of a genetically engineered enzyme upon cornstarch forms what is called *high-fructose corn syrup* (HFCS). Corn is wet-milled to extract starch, and an enzyme is added to extract glucose—with enzymatic isomerisation turning glucose into fructose. The liquid fructose becomes an input into the industrial food process, where it is used in soft drink and other food manufacturing processes. It is highly regarded by the food industry because it provides an excellent substrate for yeast; blends easily with acids, flavourings and other sweeteners; retains moisture; and allows for greater all-round control in food processing (*Food Resources* 2003, p. 1). It was first used in the 1960s, but consumption soared when raw-sugar prices rose in 1974–75. By 1986, HFCS accounted for over half the caloric-sweetener market in the USA (Llambi 1994, p. 200) but, today, it is used in 'virtually all the sodas and most of the fruit drinks sold in the supermarket' (Pollan 2006, p. 18). The concern, here, is that HFCS has been strongly implicated in the growth of obesity in the USA. Not only does HFCS add hundreds of calories per day to the food intake of the average US consumer, but it also appears to be implicated in stimulating the appetite, thereby increasing food consumption (Boyles 2004; Pollan 2006).

Yet, according to Goodman and Redclift (1991, p. 190), because sweeteners can now be made from corn, wheat, sorghum and potatoes, and can be used interchangeably in food production, corporate firms have more flexibility than they used to. They can literally pick which field crops they will use to make not only industrial sugars, but also proteins, starches and oils. Their prediction, at the beginning of the 1990s, that 'agri-food systems gradually will merge with the chemical and pharmaceutical industries to form a 'bio-industrial processing complex'' (Goodman & Redclift 1991, p. 109) has become a reality at the beginning of the twenty-first century (see Lang & Heasman 2004).

This does not mean there are not 'spaces' for actors to protest, or for alternative food regimes (such as organics) to emerge (Hendrickson & Heffernan 2003; Nestle 2003; Lang & Heasman 2004). In fact, there is evidence that as a result of the contradictory forces that are part of global industrial expansion, homogenisation is being accompanied by differentiation, centralisation is being matched by decentralisation, and integration is occurring alongside fragmentation (Pritchard & Burch 2003). Nevertheless, what is argued above is that biotechnology is being used to enhance both appropriationism and substitutionism in the agri-food industries. Despite some public opposition, biotechnologies continue to be applied widely in agriculture, and are now found in, or are used to produce, over 30 000 varieties of food (AfroCentric News 2003, p. 3). And yet, at the same time, it can be argued that '... Agricultural biotechnology has been, so far, a massive pyramid scheme financed by hopes of great wealth down the road. Few, if any, companies that invested heavily in biotechnology have recovered that investment through sales of a genetically-engineered product' (Charles 2001, p. 295). Monsanto profited from the sales of its herbicide, Roundup, but has since become a subsidiary of the Swedish-owned firm Pharmacia. Others have profited by selling their holdings 'at a good price when the next wave of speculative money came along' (see Charles 2001, p. 296).

Public perceptions of GMOs and GM foods

A number of studies around the world (but largely confined to Western nations) confirm that there is growing public suspicion of GMOs. While people seem to be quite at ease with the application of biotechnologies in the pharmaceuticals industry (to manufacture synthetic chemicals for human and animal health), or to help clean up the environment (bio-remediation) or grow novel plants for export (for example, developing a 'blue rose' for the international marketplace) they are much less convinced of the benefits of eating GM food. Public surveys in Australia, Brazil, Canada, Japan, the United Kingdom and the USA indicate that consumers have a generally negative

Geoffrey Lawrence and Janet Grice

view of GM foods, with respondents considering that the risks of such foods outweigh any benefits (see Norton 1999). Consumers appear to be concerned about the health and safety aspects of food production and manufacture. There is growing suspicion that artificial chemicals in foods (preservatives, flavour enhancers and so forth) are responsible for ill-health, and the public appears to view genetic manipulation as yet another form of 'interference' that compromises naturalness. GM foods are products that consumers believe they and their families could well do without (INRA 2000, p. 50). The 2005 Eurobarometer survey demonstrated support for medical and industrial applications but opposition to agricultural applications. Without positive benefits of GM foods to consumers, the public remains sceptical, although Gaskell et al. (2006) have claimed that 'resistance to GM food is the exception rather than the rule' where biotechnologies are concerned.

In Australia, researchers have established that there is no 'blanket' dislike for genetic engineering—it all depends on the sort of manipulation taking place. Genetic engineering of plants gains more acceptance than for animals, and for animals more than for humans (Norton et al. 1998). While one Australian survey received quite positive responses to questions about genetic engineering (Kelley 1995), a close analysis of the questions indicated they were worded so as to elicit favourable responses (Hindmarsh et al. 1995). The majority of respondents to another Australian survey believed it was morally wrong to insert human genetic material in other species (for example, pigs) and they believed there would be long-term health problems associated with the ingestion of GMOs. The public believed that accidental releases would result in environmental damage, and that, on the whole, the benefits of genetic engineering were outweighed by the risks (Norton et al. 1998). There was over 95 per cent agreement that particular transgenic foods should be labelled, 93 per cent agreement that consumers should be consulted before the release of GM foods, and 92 per cent support for government control of GM foods (Norton et al. 1998). In Europe, people have argued for the right to choose whether or not they would eat GM foods (in other words, that all GM foods be labelled as such) and have called for their banning until they are proven to be harmless (European Commission 2001).

Furthermore, it appears that it is not—as some scientists suggest—only a matter of 'educating' the public about the benefits of GM foods: consumer acceptance is premised on concern for food safety. And it seems that the more people are learning about GM foods (and worrying about food safety), the less confident they are becoming about those foods (Norton 1999; Nestle 2003). Importantly, women are more wary than men of GM foods—and it is women, by and large, who purchase the family's food supplies (Norton 1999). As well, in Australia, the public is largely unaware of the regulatory processes that are in place to govern the introduction of GM crops and foods (Grice & Lawrence 2004). Busch and colleagues (1991) have argued that three issues are of importance when consumers purchase food commodities—consent, knowledge and fairness. With GM foods, consent and knowledge are linked to labelling, which allows people to make informed decisions about food purchases. In Australia, foods that contain less than 1 per cent of GM ingredients do not need to be labelled. Further, foods such as cotton oil or corn oil that contain no DNA also do not require labelling even if they are sourced from GM crops. In relation to the third criterion—fairness—people are coming to see that it is big business that will benefit from the sale of GM products, not consumers (Norton & Lawrence 1996; Grice et al. 2003). In other words, consumers have reason to be wary of ingesting foods that are developed to fulfil the profit-making needs of corporations rather than the desires of consumers for healthy and nutritious foods. Nutritionists Young and Lewis (1995, p. 930) have argued that advances in genetic engineering:

> have been based on relatively little knowledge of basic human nutritional needs. More importantly, these advances have been predicated with no understanding of dietary nutrient interactions. Changing nutrient composition of foods through biotechnology may alter nutrient interactions, nutrient-gene interactions, nutrient availability, nutrient potency, and nutrient metabolism. Biotechnology has the potential to produce changes in our foods and in our diet at a pace far greater than our ability to predict the significance of those changes ...

The point is that scientists, food industry officials and the public simply do not know what problems will be caused by the genetic manipulation of foods. The scientists and food industry seem to believe that the benefits of experimentation with and releasing of GMOs will outweigh any risks. The public is beginning to question this assessment.

Conclusion: The future of GM foods

Any critical assessment of agribusiness must start with recognition of the fact that there has been, since the 1950s, a strong technological push in commercial agriculture and food production. Within the commercial agriculture sector, producers have found it necessary to purchase the latest seeds, fertilisers, tractors and management techniques to stay economically viable. Farmers have sought virtually any new inputs that would help to boost productivity or efficiency or both. Genetically engineered inputs promise a continuation of this trend. The agribusiness sector has found a receptive market among farmers for its latest GM seed/pesticide/fertiliser packages. For many farmers, and for the agribusiness-input industries, the use of GM seeds is simply a continuation of the productive, 'high-tech' approach to farming that has increased food production enormously over the past 20 years. For the food industry, the use of genetically engineered enzymes, bacteria, plants and animals promises to speed up production, create novel products of great benefit to society, and literally 'feed the world' with genetically enhanced plants and animals.

Geoffrey Lawrence and Janet Grice

So why would there be any opposition to such a glowing future? There are basically six reasons why there has been, and we might expect there to be, strong challenges from throughout the world:

1. GM foods do not seem to provide obvious benefits to consumers. Rather, they seem to benefit the companies selling GM seed/fertiliser/insecticide packages to farmers, and the companies using GMOs to catalyse chemical reactions in foods that are part of the food processing industry. What advantage will the 'end users' (consumers) of the new foods and fibres derive? This has not been well explained by proponents of biotechnology.

2. Genetic engineering has not been proven safe and beneficial. There are major concerns about the unknown health effects of genetic interactions when GM foods are ingested, and when the release of genetically engineered plants and animals allows novel genes to become widespread in the environment.

3. Some important industries, both traditional and new (such as 'commercial organics'), may be compromised by the release of GMOs. Will farmers growing non-GM cotton, canola, corn and soybeans be able to segregate their crops? Will those wanting to label their products as 'non-GMO' be able to do so when the extent of 'genetic pollution' from GMO crops is unable to be monitored?

4. There is evidence that, throughout the world, large supermarket chains are banning GMOs and stacking their shelves with organic produce—a certain sign that consumer resistance to GMO is not going away, and a reflection of people's desire for natural 'clean and green' foods (Lockie et al. 2006; Burch & Lawrence 2007).

5. The release of GMOs will make it harder for countries to claim that they are producing food in a sustainable manner. There are likely to be arguments (some decades hence) that a GMO-based agricultural production system is not sustainable, particularly when GMO products are perceived to corrupt 'natural' products and natural production systems (see Campbell & Coombes 1999; McKenna & Campbell 2002). If this occurs, foods from a GMO-based agri-food regime might be deemed unacceptable as imports, thereby severely limiting the exportation of foods from those nations that have gone down the GMO path.

6. The idea that GMOs will 'feed the world' is viewed as nothing more than a cynical justification for the perpetuation of corporate control of food (Crouch 2001). The 'green revolution' technologies of the 1960s and 1970s were going to feed the world but failed. Why? Because the world food problem has less to do with the volume of production than with the patterns of distribution. We have enough food now to feed the world, but there is little political will to ensure that it is available to those in need. Biotechnology cannot address what is essentially a global geopolitical problem, even if the rhetoric of 'food for all' can be used as an ideological device to promote corporate involvement in food production (McMichael 2000, 2003).

It is important to understand the intensity of the opposition to GMOs. There are literally thousands of organisations around the world opposed to the introduction of GM inputs to agriculture and to the further development and commercialisation of GM foods (Phelps 2001; Tokar 2001, pp. 420–42). A genetically engineered future for foods should not, therefore, be taken as a given.

What has been argued in this chapter is that two dominant processes—appropriationism and substitutionism—are helping to fashion agri-food industries in a manner that increases the profits, and level of control, of the corporate sector in relation to food production. There is no conspiracy here. Companies are attempting to meet demand for particular products, satisfy shareholders' desires for strong returns on invested capital, and employ the latest technologies in an effort to save costs and increase productivity. This logic is entirely consistent with the behaviour of most firms within the system of capitalism. The problem for the agri-food firms is that the powerful techniques that they are now harnessing—biotechnologies in general, and genetic engineering in particular—are different from older forms of food production and processing and have uncertain (and potentially harmful) outcomes. Not surprisingly, there is growing consumer resistance to their application in the food sector.

What is the future of GM foods? Writers are divided on this question. For some, agribusiness will use its power to 'enforce' the adoption of GM foods. This, they argue, will be achieved through the World Trade Organization (WTO), a body that has the power to overrule what are considered to be unfair barriers to trade. If the WTO decides that the consumers in WTO-affiliated nations must accept genetically modified foods (and that banning them would be an unacceptable trade block), then it is clear that a major hurdle will have been overcome by the corporate food sector (McMichael 2003).

For other writers, the level of protest against GM foods will be such that those dealing with GMOs at point of sale (that is, the supermarkets) will determine that it is in their own interest to remove GM foods from their shelves. As stricter (mandatory) labelling is put in place, consumers will be able to gauge immediately which foods are GM and which are not. If, as many expect, there is a strong rejection of GM foods, it will not take the supermarkets long to remove these products and replace them with alternatives that are in higher demand. Evidence is growing that this is currently occurring (Burch & Lawrence 2007). Many people are predicting a very rosy future for organic products as consumer rejection of GM food grows, and as the organics industry becomes better organised and more market savvy (Lockie et al. 2002; Lockie et al. 2006).

There is, of course, a third possibility—that the two trajectories (growth in the application of GMOs and growth in organics and other 'clean and green' options) will occur, simultaneously. Indeed, this option appears the most likely to come to pass. If it does, we can be certain that there will be a heightened battle (or, in Lang

Geoffrey Lawrence and Janet Grice

and Heasman's words, 'food wars') between the agri-food corporations and the organic and other'clean and green' producers for the hearts, minds and stomachs of consumers.

SUMMARY OF MAIN POINTS

- The term 'agribusiness' refers to corporate involvement in the 'upstream' provision of farm inputs and the 'downstream' processing and sale of farm products.
- Aided by biotechnologies, agribusinesses in the 'upstream' sector are developing chemical and seed 'packages' to sell to farmers; on the 'downstream' side, they are contracting farmers to provide both generic inputs into the food processing industry and fresh foods for the supermarkets.
- The two key processes driving agribusiness penetration into the farming and food industry sectors are appropriationism and substitutionism. Both allow for increased profit making, as well as higher levels of control, for the agribusiness sector.
- There is substantial public resistance to genetically engineered foods.
- Recent evidence suggests that while agribusiness as a whole remains enchanted with GMO technology, some major players in the food industry—in particular the supermarkets—are seeking to minimise the presence of GMO-derived products in their stores.
- There is little doubt that there will be significant battles between consumer/non-GMO farmer groups and the agribusiness sector over the next decade.

SOCIOLOGICAL REFLECTION

The essential proposition in this chapter is that capitalism is—as Karl Marx claimed over 150 years ago—a dynamic system that is based upon continual profit making by firms that are obliged to become larger, more capital intensive and more global in their focus. For Marx this would occur through what he termed the concentration and centralisation of capital. Agri-food industries—the large input suppliers, the banks providing finance, the food manufacturers, transport firms and the supermarkets—have all exhibited strong tendencies to increase in size, shrink in number, and grow in power and influence. Marx praised capitalism for the economic vitality of such a system, but he also saw the 'dark' side of such change including the exploitation of workers, the collapse of small businesses, and the social and environmental problems that arose from unfettered growth.

- Are we witnessing the inevitable 'corporatisation' of food, and if so, what might this mean for farmers and consumers in the developed, and developing, worlds?
- Is there any good reason to 'resist' a strong corporate presence in the food industry, or are we so reliant upon that industry that any opposition would be counterproductive?

- Finally, what might another sociological approach to the study of food (for example, functionalist, feminist, Weberian or postmodernist) tell us about the dynamics of change in the food industry and its implications?

DISCUSSION QUESTIONS

1. Is agribusiness really a 'juggernaut', or can its GMO trajectory be altered or stopped?
2. Why would people in the Third World oppose genetic engineering when the new technology promises a more abundant food supply?
3. Appropriationism and substitutionism are seen to be two key processes driving agribusiness expansion. Are there any others?
4. Of the following genetic engineering procedures, which would you approve and why?
    a) Placing a gene from a cornflower plant into a rose so that the rose flower is deep blue.
    b) Placing a hormone of human origin into a pig so that the pig demands less feed, matures quickly and produces lean meat.
    c) Adding a fish gene to a tomato so that the tomato has more flavour and colour and can be harvested without bruising.
    d) Placing a gene from a soil bacterium into a wheat plant so that the wheat plant requires less chemical pesticide sprays.
5. As a consumer, will you purchase genetically modified foods?
6. Can we count upon the supermarkets to provide safer and more wholesome (clean and green) foods to consumers?

Further investigation

1. Choose a specific genetically modified food available in your community and investigate its advantages and disadvantages for agribusiness and consumers.
2. Genetically modified food is the new 'green revolution' with advantages for agribusiness and consumers alike. Discuss.
3. Is genetically modified food really 'franken-food' as some critics suggest?

FURTHER READING AND WEB RESOURCES

Books

Burch, D. & Lawrence, G. (eds) 2007, *Supermarkets and Agri-food Supply Chains: Transformations in the Production and Consumption of Foods*, Edward Elgar, Cheltenham, UK.

Geoffrey Lawrence and Janet Grice

Dixon, J. 2002, *The Changing Chicken: Chooks, Cooks and Culinary Culture*, University of New South Wales Press, Sydney.

Hindmarsh, R. & Lawrence, G. (eds) 2004, *Recoding Nature: Critical Perspectives on Genetic Engineering*, University of New South Wales Press, Sydney.

Lang, T. & Heasman, M. 2004, *Food Wars: The Global Battle for Mouths, Minds and Markets*, Earthscan, London.

Lockie, S., Lyons, K., Lawrence, G. & Halpin, D. 2006, *Going Organic: Mobilising Networks for Environmentally Responsible Food Production*, CABI, Wallingford.

Pollan, M. 2006, *The Omnivore's Dilemma: The Search for a Perfect Meal in a Fast-food World*, Bloomsbury, London.

Websites

Agribusiness Accountability Network: www.coc.org/focus/private/aai.html

Australasian Agri-food Research Network: www.csafe.org.nz/afrn/index.htm

Food Standards Australia New Zealand: www.foodstandards.gov.au

International Federation of Organic Agriculture Movements: www.ifoam.org/

International Journal of Sociology of Agriculture and Food: www.csafe.org.nz/ijsaf/

Office of the Gene Technology Regulator: www.ogtr.gov.au/

Films and Documentaries

Fast Food Nation (2006): Movie about the health risks of fast food (116 minutes).

Fed Up! Genetic Engineering, Industrial Agriculture and Sustainable Alternatives (2002): Documentary examining agribusiness and GM food (57 minutes).

Food Wars (2004): TV series.

Peaceable Kingdom (2004): Documentary examining inhumane practices in the meat industry (70 minutes).

Super Size Me (2004): An amusing documentary that examines the connections between the fast-food industry and obesity, notable for filmmaker Morgan Spurlock's 30 days of consuming only McDonald's food (100 minutes).

REFERENCES

AfroCentric News, 16 January 2003, pp. 1–4, www.afrocentricnews.com/html/food.html.

Allen, T. 2000, 'The Environmental Costs of Genetic Engineering', in R. Prebble (ed.), *Designer Genes: The New Zealand Guide to the Issues, Facts and Theories about Genetic Engineering*, Dark Horse, Wellington, pp. 61–8.

Bonanno, A., Busch, L., Friedland, W., Gouveia, L. & Mingione, E. (eds) 1994, *From Columbus to ConAgra*, University Press of Kansas, Kansas.

Boyles, S. 2004, 'Soft Drink Sweetener Blamed for Obesity', WebMD, http://onhealth. webmd.com/script/main/art.asp?articlekey=56856 [accessed 7 February 2007].

Burch, D. & Lawrence, G. 2005, 'Supermarket Own Brands, Supply Chains and the Transformation of the Agri-food System', *International Journal of Sociology of Agriculture and Food*, vol. 13, no. 1, pp. 1–18.

—— (eds) 2007, *Supermarkets and Agri-food Supply Chains: Transformations in the Production and Consumption of Foods*, Edward Elgar, Cheltenham, UK.

Burch, D. & Rickson, R. 2001, 'Industrialised Agriculture: Agribusiness, Input-dependency and Vertical Integration', in S. Lockie & L. Bourke (eds), *Rurality Bites: The Social and Environmental Transformation of Rural Australia*, Pluto Press, Sydney, pp. 165–77.

Busch, L., Lacy, B., Burkhardt, J. & Lacy, L. 1991, *Plants, Power and Profit: Social, Economic and Ethical Consequences of the New Biotechnologies*, Basil Blackwell, London.

Campbell, H. & Coombes, B. 1999, 'Green Protectionism and Organic Food Exporting from New Zealand: Crisis Experiments in the Breakdown of Fordist Trade and Agricultural Policies', *Rural Sociology*, vol. 64, no. 2, pp. 302–19.

Campbell, H., Lawrence, G. & Smith, K. 2006, 'Audit Cultures and the Antipodes: The Implications of EurepGAP for New Zealand and Australian Agri-food Industries', in T. Marsden & J. Murdoch (eds), *Between the Local and the Global: Confronting Complexity in the Contemporary Agri-food Sector*, Elsevier, Amsterdam, pp. 69–93.

Cargill 2007, Cargill Home Page, www.cargill.com/worldwide/index.htm [accessed 5 February 2007].

Charles, D. 2001, *Lords of the Harvest: Biotech, Big Money and the Future of Food*, Perseus Publishing, Cambridge, Massachusetts.

ConAgra 2007, ConAgra Home Page, http://company.conagrafoods.com/phoenix. zhtml?c=202310&p=irol-history [accessed 5 February 2007].

Conner, T. 2000, 'Crops: Food, Environment and Ethics', in R. Prebble (ed.), *Designer Genes: The New Zealand Guide to the Issues, Facts and Theories About Genetic Engineering*, Dark Horse, Wellington, pp. 141–52.

Constance, D., Bonanno, A., Cates, C., Argo, D. & Harris, M. 2003, 'Resisting Integration in the Global Agro-food System: Corporate Chickens and Community Controversy in Texas', in R. Almas & G. Lawrence (eds), *Globalization, Localization, and Sustainable Livelihoods*, Ashgate, Aldershot, UK, pp. 103–18.

Crouch, M. 2001, 'From Golden Rice to Terminator Technology: Agricultural Biotechnology will not Feed the World or Save the Environment', in B. Tokar (ed.), *Redesigning Life: The Worldwide Challenge to Genetic Engineering*, McGill-Queen's University Press, Montreal, pp. 22–39.

Davis, J. 1956, 'From Agriculture to Agribusiness', *Harvard Business Review*, vol. 34, pp. 107–15.

de la Perriere, R. & Seuret, F. 2000, *Brave New Seeds: The Threat of GM Crops to Farmers*, Zed Books, London.

Dolan, C. 2004, 'On Farm and Packhouse: Employment at the Bottom of a Global Value Chain', *Rural Sociology*, vol. 69, no. 1, pp. 99–126.

European Commission 2001, *Eurobarometer 55.2, Europeans, Science and Technology*, European Opinion Research Group, Brussels.

Ewert, J. 2003, 'Co-operatives to Companies: The South African Wine Industry in the Face of Globalization', in R. Almas & G. Lawrence (eds), *Globalization, Localization, and Sustainable Livelihoods*, Ashgate, Aldershot, UK, pp. 153–69.

Fitzsimons, J. 2000, 'The Nuclear-free Issue of the 21st Century', in R. Prebble (ed.), *Designer Genes: The New Zealand Guide to the Issues, Facts and Theories About Genetic Engineering*, Dark Horse, Wellington, pp. 187–96.

Food Resources, 16 January 2003, p. 1.

Friedmann, H. 1991, 'Changes in the International Division of Labor: Agrifood Complexes and Export Agriculture', in W. Friedland, L. Busch, F. Buttel & A. Rudy (eds), *Towards a New Political Economy of Agriculture*, Westview, Boulder, pp. 65–93.

FSANZ 2005, *GM Foods: Safety Assessment of Genetically Modified Foods*, www. foodstandards.gov.au [accessed 25 January 2007].

Gaskell et al. 2006, *Europeans and Biotechnology in 2005: Patterns and Trends*, www. ec.europa.eu/research/press/2006/pdf/pr1906_eb_64_3_final_report-may2006_en.pdf [accessed 20 January 2007].

Goodman, D. & Redclift, M. 1991, *Refashioning Nature: Food, Ecology and Culture*, Routledge, New York.

Goodman, D., Sorj, B. & Wilkinson, J. 1987, *From Farming to Biotechnology*, Basil Blackwell, Oxford.

Grice, J., Wegener, M., Romanach, L., Paton, S., Bonaventura, P. & Garrad, S. 2003, 'Genetically-Engineered Sugar Cane: A Case for Alternate Products', *Agbioforum*, vol. 6, no. 4, pp. 162–8.

Grice, J. & Lawrence, G. 2004, 'Consumer Surveys of Biotechnology: Asking the Questions Until We Get the Answers We Want OR Empowering the Public to Express Their Opinion?', *Revista Iberoamericana de Ciencia, Tecnología y Sociedad*, Centro Redes, Buenos Aires.

Heffernan, W. 1999, *Consolidation in the Food and Agriculture System* (report to the National Farmers' Union), University of Missouri Department of Rural Sociology and the National Farmers Union, Colorado.

Hendrickson, M. & Heffernan, W. 2003, 'Opening Spaces through Relocalization: Locating Potential Resistance in the Weaknesses of the Global Food System', *Sociologia Ruralis*, vol. 42, no. 4, pp. 347–69.

Hindmarsh, R. & Lawrence, G. (eds) 2001, *Altered Genes II: The Future?*, Scribe, Melbourne.

—— (eds) 2004, *Recoding Nature: Critical Perspectives on Genetic Engineering*, UNSW Press, Sydney.

Hindmarsh, R., Lawrence, G. & Norton, J. 1995, 'Manipulating Genes or Public Opinion?', *Search*, no. 26, pp. 117–21.

Ho, M-W. 1998, *Genetic Engineering: Dream or Nightmare? The Brave New World of Bad Science and Big Business*, Gateway Books, UK.

INRA (Europe) & European Consumer Safety Organisation 2000, 'Eurobarometer 52.1: The Europeans and Biotechnology', www.europa.eu.int/comm/research/eurobarometer-en.pdf [accessed November 2003].

ISAAA 2006, ISAAA Brief 35-2006: Executive Summary, www.isaaa.org/Resources/Publications/briefs/35/executivesummary/default.html [accessed 20 January 2007].

Jansen, K. & Vellema, S. (eds) 2004, *Agribusiness and Society: Corporate Responses to Environmentalism, Market Opportunities and Public Regulation*, Zed Books, London.

Kelley, J. 1995, *Public Perceptions of Genetic Engineering: Australia, 1994*, Department of Industry, Science and Technology, Canberra.

Lang, T. & Heasman, M. 2004, *Food Wars: The Global Battle for Mouths, Minds and Markets*, Earthscan, London.

Lawrence, G., Norton, J. & Vanclay, F. 2001, 'Gene Technology, Agri-food Industries and Consumers', in R. Hindmarsh & G. Lawrence (eds), *Altered Genes II: The Future?*, Scribe, Melbourne, pp. 143–59.

Le Heron, R. & Roche, M. 1999, 'Rapid Regulation, Agricultural Restructuring, and the Reimaging of Agriculture in New Zealand', *Rural Sociology*, vol. 64, no. 2, June, pp. 203–18.

Llambi, L. 1994, 'Opening Economies and Closing Markets: Latin American Agriculture's Difficult Search for a Place in the Emerging Global Order', in A. Bonanno, L. Busch, W. Friedland, L. Gouveia & E. Mingione (eds), *From Columbus to ConAgra: The Globalization of Agriculture and Food*, University of Kansas Press, pp. 184–209.

Lockie, S., Lyons, K., Lawrence, G. & Halpin, D. 2006, *Going Organic: Mobilising Networks for Environmentally Responsible Food Production*, CABI, Wallingford.

Lockie, S., Lyons, K., Lawrence, G. & Mummery, K. 2002, 'Eating "Green": Motivations Behind Organic Food Consumption in Australia', *Sociologia Ruralis*, vol. 42, no. 1, April, pp. 20–37.

Magdoff, F., Foster, J. & Buttel, F. (eds) 2000, *Hungry for Profit: The Agribusiness Threat to Farmers, Food and the Environment*, Monthly Review Press, New York, www.monthlyreview.org/hungry.html.

McKenna, M. & Campbell, H. 2002, 'It's Not Easy Being Green: The Development of "Food Safety"Practices in New Zealand's Apple Industry', *International Journal of Sociology of Food and Agriculture*, vol. 10, no. 2, pp. 110–41.

McMichael, P. 2000, *Development and Social Change: A Global Perspective*, 2nd edition, Pine Forge, Boston.

—— 2003, 'The Power of Food', in R. Almas & G. Lawrence (eds), *Globalization, Localization, and Sustainable Livelihoods*, Ashgate, Aldershot, UK, pp. 69–85.

—— & Friedmann, H. 2007, 'Situating the "Retail Revolution"', in D. Burch & G. Lawrence (eds), *Supermarkets and Agri-food Supply Chains: Transformations in the Production and Consumption of Foods*, Edward Elgar, Cheltenham, UK, pp. 293–323.

Nestle, M. 2003, *Safe Food: Bacteria, Biotechnology and Terrorism*, University of California Press, Berkeley.

Norton, J. 1999, *Science, Technology and the Risk Society: Australian Consumers' Attitudes to Genetically-Engineered Foods*, unpublished PhD thesis, Central Queensland University, Rockhampton.

—— 2002, *Potential of Biotechnologies to Enhance Sustainable Development of the Central Queensland Region* (Occasional Paper 3/2002), Institute for Sustainable Regional Development, Central Queensland University, Rockhampton.

—— & Lawrence, G. 1996, 'Consumer Attitudes to Genetically-engineered Food Products: Focus Group Research in Rockhampton, Queensland', in G. Lawrence, K. Lyons & S. Momtaz (eds), *Social Change in Rural Australia*, Rural Social and Economic Research Centre, Central Queensland University, Rockhampton, pp. 290–311.

—— , Lawrence, G. & Wood, G. 1998, 'The Australian Public's Perceptions of Genetically-Engineered Foods', *Australasian Biotechnology*, vol. 8, no. 3, pp. 172–81.

Phelps, B. 2001, 'Opposing Genetic Manipulation: The GenEthics Campaign', in R. Hindmarsh & G. Lawrence (eds), *Altered Genes II: The Future?*, Scribe, Melbourne, pp. 187–202.

Pollan, M. 2006, *The Omnivore's Dilemma: The Search for a Perfect Meal in a Fast-food World*, Bloomsbury, London.

Pretty, J. 2002, *Agri-Culture: Reconnecting People, Land and Nature*, Earthscan, London.

Pritchard, B. 2005a, 'Implementing and Maintaining Neoliberal Agriculture in Australia – Part 1. Constructing Neoliberalism as a Vision for Agricultural Policy', *International Journal of Sociology of Agriculture and Food*, vol. 13, no. 1, pp. 1–12.

—— 2005b, 'Implementing and Maintaining Neoliberal Agriculture in Australia – Part 11, *International Journal of Sociology of Agriculture and Food*, vol. 13, no. 2, pp. 1–14.

—— & Burch, D. 2003, *Agri-food Globalization in Perspective: International Restructuring in the Processing Tomato Industry*, Ashgate, Aldershot, UK.

Rama, R. (ed.) 2005, *Multinational Agribusinesses*, Haworth Press, New York.

Reichardt, T. 2000, 'Will souped up salmon sink or swim?' *Nature*, 406, 6 July, pp. 10–12.

Rifkin, J. 1992, *Beyond Beef: The Rise and Fall of the Cattle Culture*, Penguin, New York.

Teubal, M. & Rodriguez, J. 2003, 'Globalization and Agro-food Systems in Argentina', in R. Almas & G. Lawrence (eds), *Globalization, Localization, and Sustainable Livelihoods*, Ashgate, Aldershot, UK, pp. 119–34.

Tokar, B. 2001, *Redesigning Life: The Worldwide Challenge to Genetic Engineering*, McGill-Queen's University Press, Montreal, Canada.

Tozanli, S. 2005, 'The Rise of Global Enterprises in the World's Food Chain', in R. Rama (ed.), *Multinational Agribusinesses*, Haworth Press, New York, pp. 1–72.

Watts, M. & Goodman, D. 1997, *Globalising Food*, Routledge, London.

Young, A. & Lewis, G. 1995, 'Biotechnology and Potential Nutritional Implications for Children', *Pediatric Nutrition*, vol. 42, no. 4, pp. 917–30.

CHAPTER 5

Operating Upstream and Downstream: How Supermarkets Exercise Power in the Food System

Jane Dixon

OVERVIEW

- What activities comprise the sphere of food distribution and exchange?
- How have retail traders wrested power from primary producers and food processors (secondary producers and manufacturers) in the Australian food system?
- How can a cultural economy approach illuminate the balance of power in commodity and food systems?

This chapter focuses on a relatively neglected part of the food system, the distribution and exchange of food commodities and food-related services. The dynamics of this sphere are explored through a case study of the role that supermarkets have played in building the popularity of chicken meat. The power of these highly profitable retail traders is explained using the concept of cultural economy activities. The influence of supermarket chains over many aspects of Australia's food system and culinary culture sheds light on the changing nature of expertise and values underpinning household food-consumption patterns.

Key terms

agri-food

Commodity
Systems Analysis (CSA)

cultural capital

cultural economy

flexible accumulation

food system

just-in-time (JIT)

monopsonic power

time famines

Introduction

In the late 1960s, Australians ate 40 kilograms of red meat and only 8 kilograms of chicken per year. Thirty years later, the figures were 36 and 31 kilograms, respectively (DAFF 2005a, p. 68), with chicken and beef projected for equal consumption by 2010 (Bailey 2005, p. 73). This trend can be partly attributed to the changing demographic mix: since the 1960s, different ethnic groups have arrived in Australia with culinary cultures that either do not use much meat (Italians), or use mostly pork and chicken (many Asian and Pacific Islander subgroups). (See Michael Symons' (1993) treatment of the influence of migrants to Australia's culinary culture.) The other significant influence on meat consumption has been the way a large proportion of the population has come to justify their consumption patterns using a mixture of values that coalesce in the idea of 'healthy convenience' (Gofton & Ness 1991). Largely promoted by Australia's two major supermarket chains, 'healthy convenience' reflects the twin concerns of food that does not contribute to heart disease and other diseases (often associated with red meat and full-fat dairy products) with a desire for food that allows the household manager, most often the family cook, to use time and money wisely.

One explanation for the rapid shift from red to white meat is that consumers have displaced producers in exercising the balance of power in the **food system**. Whereas housewives used to uncritically buy what was provided by beef and sheep meat producers, their expressed concerns for their family's health and demands for 'shortcuts' and more flexible meal options signalled the growing influence of the consumer. While studies of post-1950s changes to national food systems and shopping practices generally conclude that the newly reflexive consumer is powerful (Gabriel & Lang 1995; Miller 1995; Falk & Campbell 1997), research that is based on interviews with consumers often challenges this argument. Accounts by consumers of their mundane routines and decision-making considerations portray consumption as an endless series of compromises: poorer families are forced to rely on relatively expensive foods of dubious nutritional value (Charles & Kerr 1986); women are concerned about the nutritional goodness of foods (Murcott 1993; CSIRO 1994); and working mothers are concerned that lack of time to cook during the week forces them to rely on processed and convenience foods (Dixon 2002).

The pressures of money and the perception of **time famines**, a term used by Gofton (1990), combine with the constant promotion of new products and media coverage of the latest evidence from nutrition science to unsettle shoppers and undermine confident shopping—the behaviour that most challenges marketplace authority (Douglas 1997). Lack of confidence among shoppers and the constant need to be flexible fuel volatile consumption patterns that producers have trouble interpreting. Translating consumer demands into products has become a highly specialised and expensive facet of food enterprises and supermarkets have assumed leadership in

Jane Dixon

communicating consumer wants to producers. However, supplying the latest market intelligence is only one of the ways in which supermarket chains influence what is happening in the food system. Their promotional activities—for example, categorising and advertising certain foods as 'fresh produce' and 'home-meal replacement'— influence the way that consumers think about food commodities far more effectively than the marketing campaigns of commodity producers, who are often distrusted as sources of product endorsement (Tansey & Worsley 1995; Dixon 2003).

Until recently, most research on food systems has ignored the dynamics between production and consumption. While consumer scientists (see Marshall 1995) consistently insist on the importance of the supply chain—delivering goods to market (availability)—and the value chain—the cultural norms surrounding the goods (acceptability)—systematic analyses of what happens between the two chains, that is, between production and consumption, are rare. How availability and acceptability align with one another, so that the goods on offer are sufficiently desirable to lead to their transfer from one owner to another, lies at the heart of the sphere of distribution and exchange. In this sphere, cultural processes are enlisted to facilitate economic exchange and, in turn, economic processes influence the value sets and practices that make up cultural systems. ('Value sets' are also referred to as 'regimes of value', a term coined by Appadurai (1986).)

The employment figures of the component parts of the Australian food system alone are sufficient to justify increased scrutiny of the sphere of distribution and exchange. In 2005, there were 375 000 people employed in agriculture and fisheries, 171 000 people in food processing and one million people had jobs in the food wholesaling, retailing and service sectors (Delforce et al. 2005, p. 382).

This chapter explores the interdependence of production and consumption by following the commodity path of chicken meat between the farm and the dinner table. For 30 years, supermarkets have been instrumental in fostering the everyday availability and acceptability of a meat that was traditionally associated with special occasions. The chapter begins by laying out the methodological approach adopted for data collection and in so doing outlines the elements that comprise the sphere of distribution and exchange.

The study of distribution and exchange: The case of chicken meat

One of the most influential approaches to the study of power in food systems emerged in the mid 1980s. **Commodity Systems Analysis (CSA)** encouraged researchers to explore a wide range of processes that contribute to the final form of a commodity, including production practices, science application, the labour process on the farm and in the factory, and marketing and distribution networks (Friedland

1984). William Friedland, who developed CSA, has since added further foci for study, including what he calls 'the commodity culture', which refers to the cultural forms found among commodity producers and consumers (Friedland 2001). While CSA acknowledges that primary producers are significantly influenced by distributors— including marketing boards and wholesale traders—the activities of marketing and distribution networks have remained a minor part of the overall schema.

Between 1996 and 1998, influenced by Warde (1994), I adapted the CSA approach by adding the distinctive sphere of consumption. Data were collected on the post– World War II history of chicken meat production and consumption in Australia, with a view to answering the question: have consumers displaced producers as the driving force behind the chicken meat commodity complex? (A full account of the study can be found in *The Changing Chicken* (Dixon 2002).) Chicken meat was chosen because, along with margarine, it showed the most marked increase in consumption of any food between 1970 and 1990 (Skurray & Newell 1993).

The Australian chicken meat industry has grown spectacularly over the last quarter of a century, with approximately eight million chickens coming to market each week (DAFF 2005b, p. 53). These chickens are being produced by a relatively small number of chicken farmers (about 850) and processing plants (about 90), the majority of which are owned and operated by three privately owned firms: Inghams, Bartter and Baiada. Annual turnover in the industry, which employs 40 000 employees, is A$3.6 billion (RIRDC n.d.), and the three top firms control 80 per cent of the industry (ACMF n.d.).

State governments regulate farmer pay rates and conditions, and hence provide a measure of stability for the industry. As a consequence, contract farmers have an incentive to invest in the latest technology, and developments in bird breeding have made today's birds convert feed into flesh more rapidly. Some claim this to be Australia's most successful **agri-food** industry (Fairbrother 1988; Cain 1990). Furthermore, there has never been an intermediary marketing board (as there is for eggs and red meat); farmers are contracted directly to processors, enhancing even further the smooth flow of product onto the market.

The efficiency of the production side of the complex has helped to keep wholesale prices low, and some credit chicken's cheapness relative to other meats with its success (SACMC n.d., p. 3; DAFF 2005b, p. 54). However, my focus group research showed that the esteem with which chicken is held by consumers is more complex. Among the explanations provided were a personal liking of chicken meals; the perception that chicken is healthier than red meat; the fact that it is easy to prepare and easy to chew, which was a particularly important attribute with children; and, above all, the versatility of chicken, which extended to its acceptance by vegetarian family members. It was a particularly 'family friendly' food. Interestingly, chicken also emerged from the group discussions with several negative features: removing chicken fat was viewed with disgust and the use of growth hormones and the conditions under which chickens

Jane Dixon

were raised caused anxiety. Despite these misgivings, chicken was purchased because it helped ease the pressures on the family cook. This finding makes sense in the context of the general concerns shared by family food providers in an era when so many women are part of the labour force. Social and market research indicates that, at the end of a busy day, women look for opportunities for casual eating (Mackay 1992), relief from the burden of cooking (Santich 1995) and assistance in making food-related decisions (De Vault 1991; Fischler 1993). As is often remarked upon, food is associated with both physical and metaphysical risks, and the anthropological conundrum that food must be 'good to think' before it is 'good to eat' (Harris 1986) provides employment for thousands of consumer scientists, marketers and advertisers.

Given consumer misgivings about this most popular of foods, it seemed imperative to understand how chicken was made 'good to think', and this entailed examining the operations of actors in the middle of the chicken commodity system. It was not sufficient to understand the exchange of material goods—money and meals and; the processes and effects of the trade in cultural goods, such as time, 'quality', rituals and authority, appeared to be equally important.

Applying a cultural economy approach

For insights into the distribution and exchange of foods and food-related services, anthropology is particularly helpful. Anthropologists teach us that merchants have long provided a dual function: they deliver goods to the market and they deliver stories about the goods—they imbue them with both mystery and relevance. As Appadurai has noted, 'over the span of human history, the critical agents for the articulation of the supply and demand of commodities have been not rulers but of course, traders' (Appadurai 1986, p. 33).

Economic and retail geographers have led the study of the actors responsible for mediating the relationship between producers and consumers (Wrigley & Lowe 1996; Freidberg 2003), and they have dubbed retailers 'the new masters of the food system' (Flynn & Marsden 1992). Alongside a more traditional political economy approach, with its emphasis on capital and labour relations, these diverse disciplinary influences have coalesced in a transdiscipline, called **cultural economy**.

The field of cultural economy is devoted to analyses of the many ways in which cultural and economic processes interact to influence the way in which markets and organisations operate. Cultural economists point out the twin dangers of denying the relative autonomy of cultural and economic processes and of privileging one set of processes over the other. To do cultural economy is to acknowledge that 'economic and organizational life is built up, or assembled from, a range of disparate, but inherently cultural, parts [and is concerned with] the extent to which economic and organizational relations in the present are more thoroughly "culturalized" than their historical predecessors' (du Gay & Pryke 2002, pp. 11–12).

Many inspirational works are referred to in two edited collections devoted to exploring the cultural economy approach: *Cultural Economy* by du Gay and Pryke (2002) and *The Blackwell Cultural Economy Reader* by Amin and Thrift (2004). They include Lash and Urry's *Economies of Signs & Space*, Featherstone's 1987 article 'Lifestyle and Consumer Culture' and Appadurai's (1986) edited book *The Social Life of Things*. Not mentioned is Halperin's (1994) *Cultural Economies: Past and Present*, which builds on the work of Karl Polanyi (in the 1940s) to develop a model for charting the contributions of cultural and political systems to the allocation of productive resources. Pierre Bourdieu's work is also underplayed, although elsewhere Scott Lash (1990, p. 240) credits Bourdieu (1979/1984) with being the foremost exponent of cultural economy, because much of his work interprets society and culture in the light of the interaction between symbolic and financial capital.

My appreciation of the value of 'doing' cultural economy came from an understanding of the inadequacies of assuming that the production sphere involved economic activities only and that the consumption sphere was the sole province of cultural practices (this is explained more fully in Dixon 1999). What was needed was an approach that was broad enough to account for value-adding processes that apply to more than material production. In practical terms, I required a theoretical framework that would allow me to collect and analyse data on the reasons why the desirability of particular practices, like home cooking and backyard food production, wax and wane and differ among subpopulations. My study of the chicken meat commodity complex made me aware that the cultural adding of value by both producers and consumers was too often hidden by the promotion of the economic value of goods and services.

Using in-depth interviews, ethnographic techniques, and syntheses of secondary sources, my research revealed that supermarkets, fast-food chains, nutrition educators, and other producers of food knowledge all contribute to making chicken meat desirable. It also showed how large retailers blur the boundaries between production and distribution through their direct and indirect influence over product development. The next two sections explore how, in relation to chicken meat, 'retail capital is increasingly mediating the producer-consumer relation' (Lowe & Wrigley 1996).

Supermarkets and chicken meat

An overview of the Australian supermarket sector

Australian supermarkets are by far the largest segment of Australia's food retail sector, claiming 62 per cent of the A$88 billion in total food and alcohol retailing activity in 2003–04 (Jacenko & Gunasekera 2005, p. 2). Their dominance is not surprising, considering that three factors drive the food and beverage market:

health and freshness, convenience and value (ACNielsen 2006a): all qualities that supermarkets have socially constructed through their economic and cultural activities over many years.

Supermarkets are most profitable at two ends of the value chain: in the production of what are called 'high-value foods' (HVFs), including chicken meat products; and generic house branded products like milk.

HVFs are generally fresh, minimally processed foods, such as fruit and vegetables, dairy products, shellfish and poultry. They are characterised by heterogeneity, associations with 'quality', and niche markets (Watts & Goodman 1997, p. 11). Displacing more traditional HVF providers—the greengrocer, butcher, 'continental deli' and fishmonger—has required applying vast amounts of retail capital to the restructuring of supermarket operations, and this multifaceted process is described below.

The emergence over the past decade of house branded products, 'home brands' or 'private brands', has been at the expense of food processors with their nationally recognised brands. Even though home brands sell for less than national brands, the margin on the former is estimated to be about 2 percentage points higher (Jacenko & Gunasekera 2005, p. 5). House branding of products is complemented by the house branding of a product line, and this too is described below.

Concentration and operation of retail capital

In 1999, a Parliamentary Joint Select Committee on the Retailing Sector (JSCRS) noted that Australia has one of the most concentrated supermarket sectors of any country. At that stage, the three major chains, Woolworths/Safeway, Coles and Franklins, accounted for 80 per cent of grocery sales and 60 per cent of the fresh food market (JSCRS 1999). With the sale of Franklins stores to the South African firm Metcash and the two majors, the share of the market controlled by Woolworths and Coles has grown to 76 per cent (Jacenko & Gunasekera 2005, p. 2).

When retail capital is concentrated in so few firms, the industry is characterised as a duopoly/oligopoly, which means that new firms face significant entry barriers (Jacenko & Gunasekera 2005; Smith 2006). In other countries, governments regulate the extent to which major chains can dominate food retailing, but despite lobbying from farmers' organisations and the National Association of Retail Grocers of Australia for this kind of regulation in Australia, the JSCRS refused to cap retail-firm concentration, arguing that this would be to the detriment of thousands of small shareholders, including families. The relaxed attitude by governments towards retailers is not unique to Australia: Hughes (1996) identified benign regulatory environments in the United States of America and the United Kingdom as well. Even so, Australia has a much higher degree of retail concentration than these two countries: in the UK, the top three firms hold 52 per cent market share while in the USA it takes the top five firms to reach 34 per cent market share (Jacenko & Gunasekera 2005, p. 3).

The Australian ruling was significant for chicken meat producers for two reasons. First, it consolidated the **monopsonic** conditions of the market, where there are few product buyers and many sellers. In contrast, red meat producers, while increasingly beholden to supermarkets, still sell a majority of their products through the thousands of independent butchers. They can walk away from the supermarkets when offered too little for their products, whereas the biggest customers for the major chicken meat producers are the supermarkets, and chicken meat producers could not survive by selling only to butchers and fast-food chains.

Second, supermarkets are no longer content to make profits by moving goods between the factory and wholesale operation and from the wholesale point to retail operation. They are increasingly reinvesting their own capital in food processing and value-adding activities, thus directly competing with traditional food processors. In the case of chicken meat, the major chains have set up specialist poultry sections. Supermarkets employ staff to perform the labour previously undertaken by the staff of the chicken processor: they cut up the raw meat and add the herbs, spices and sauces. On the basis of this enhanced capacity to compete directly with processors, supermarkets dictate terms to the dependent processor. Through labour substitution, the supermarkets have increased their bargaining power: if the processor cannot or will not produce the cuts the supermarket orders, the supermarket turns to its own operation. For these reasons it is not surprising that the South Australian Chicken Meat Council (SACMC) has identified retail sector influence over the structure and dynamics of the value chain as one of the top 13 factors influencing the nation's poultry industry (SACMC n.d., p. 3).

Retail concentration provides a few actors with large cash flows ready for investment in restructuring how the retail sector operates. 'Retail restructuring' is the term given to a wide range of activities designed to position retailers at the forefront of commercial and social life. The most notable activities over the last three decades include organisational and technological transformations in retail distribution, reconfiguring of labour practices within retailing, and redesigning of the retail–supply interface.

Supermarkets at the forefront of technological transformations

In terms of technological innovation, the introduction by supermarkets of the cool chain cannot be underestimated. The cool chain, developed by the UK supermarket firm Marks & Spencer, involves getting produce to stores in an unfrozen but chilled state, ready for storage in the supermarkets' refrigerated cabinets. This particular food technology was fundamental in the 1970s to encouraging housewives to buy a chicken more often than just for the weekend roast. Market research had revealed to Marks & Spencer that while chilled birds were more expensive than frozen ones, housewives preferred them for their 'convenience'. Chilled birds did not have to thawed and they tasted better, and the'flood of water released by frozen birds during thawing made them seem a poor buy in comparison with chilled birds' (Senker 1988, p. 167). Since then, there has been continuous product innovation: another factor contributing to chicken's popularity (DAFF 2005b, p. 54).

The cool chain is by no means the sole revolutionary technology that has been introduced by the supermarkets. Improved stock ordering has been made possible through computerised technologies and the bar-coding of products. For over a decade, supermarket checkout tills have supplied a central computer with a continual flow of data on what products are leaving every store. Their EPOS (electronic point of sale) systems have in turn allowed supermarkets to make the most of **just-in-time** (JIT) systems, whereby the goods producer has to anticipate the amount of stock that will be demanded by the retail customer and have the warehousing facilities to hold the stock until it is ordered. This shifting of the risk of holding stock that may or may not be sold has further consolidated the power of the retailer over the secondary producer (Foord et al. 1996).

Reconfiguring labour processes

As to changing labour practices, supermarkets and other parts of the food service sector prefigured what has since become known as **flexible accumulation**, based on having a labour force and processes that allow for both flexible production and flexible specialisation (Mathews 1989). The food service sector was among the first to dispense with a full-time male workforce in favour of a part-time and causal workforce of women and young people (Murray 1989). The adoption of a flexible workforce had a twin effect: it lowered wages bills, thus boosting the profits of the large retailers, and it allowed retailers to introduce employee multi-skilling. Unlike the butcher, whose skills are acquired in an apprentice-like relationship with a master butcher over several years, the women employed in the delicatessen and specialist poultry sections of supermarkets can be sent away for two days of training in meat preparation or a three-day course in safe food handling, and can have similarly short exposures to marketing, budgeting and staff training. Because they possess generic skills, employees with specialist talents can be deployed to different sections of the supermarket at different times.

Supermarkets have an advantage over small family-run businesses because of the large volumes in which they trade, their technological sophistication and trained staff (albeit relatively inexpensively trained). They can charge lower prices on items produced in-house, they can afford to open for longer hours and, because of the precarious nature of casual employment, employees desperate to keep their jobs are willing to accept new job demands with minimal training (Ryan & Burgess 1996).

These are exactly the same factors operating in favour of fast-food chains like KFC, another significant purveyor of chicken meat products (Lyons 1996). Furthermore, the labour practices of the retail sector have to be adopted by food processing firms so that they can maintain the 24 hours a day, seven days a week delivery schedule demanded by the retailers (Delforce et al. 2005, p. 388).

As Goodman and Redclift (1991) note, a circular logic operates between the food sector's dependence on women's employment and women's demand for convenience foods. With a majority of mothers doing two jobs—one as a paid employee and the other as the family food provider—the food service sector has effectively engineered demand for its products. The evolving 'home meal replacement' category of heat-and-serve and ready-to-eat meals being championed by the supermarkets is the logical outcome of family meal providers experiencing 'time famine'.

With their economies of scale, cheap labour and large amounts of investment capital, supermarkets have been able to develop their fresh food operations to a point where in-store bakeries and fruit-and-vegetable, meat and fish sections compete directly with small, owner-operated specialist food businesses. In many locales, these smaller shops are losing customers because they appear to be lacking in variety, convenience and specials—a feature loved by the postwar generation, which was brought up to value thrift in food purchasing. Furthermore, the Australian experiment with deregulation of shopping hours has made family owner-operated stores even less competitive, thus further diminishing competition between different retail forms. Unsurprisingly, a less competitive food sector has not delivered lower food prices (Baker & Marshall 1998).

Redesigning the retail–supply chain interface

The chicken meat complex is an exemplar of changes being experienced by other commodity complexes. At the heart of the control of retail-supplier chains lie three conditions: the designation of 'preferred suppliers', improved stock-handling proced-ures and retailer knowledge of the manufacturing process (Burch & Goss 1999).

The first factor has long been integral to Australia's chicken meat commodity complex (Dixon 2002). For over 30 years, Woolworths was supplied by Inghams, the nation's largest poultry processor, and Coles had a preferential supply arrangement with Steggles, the second-largest processor (which was previously owned by Goodman Fielder and is now owned by Barrter Enterprises). These preferential supply arrangements, which have never been subject to a formal inquiry by the nation's competition regulatory authority, created what is known in the chicken meat industry as a three-tier system. The first tier consists of the two suppliers to the two major supermarket chains; the second tier of medium-sized processors also supplies supermarkets, but is as dependent for survival on their contracts with fast-food chains and specialist poulterers; and the third tier of small processors ekes out a

Jane Dixon

precarious existence trying to supply butchers, food caterers and the shortfall created by the other two tiers.

The adoption of EPOS systems to facilitate improvements in stock handling have already been mentioned. This retailer-controlled stocktaking system has been accompanied by a form of organisational interdependence called 'relational contracting'. Relational contracts are based on interactive, flexible and stable supply networks. They rarely involve formal written documents; regular face-to-face and telephone exchanges are used to negotiate price, quality standards and ingredients. Usually the contact originates with the product manufacturer, who rings stores and tells them what product is available.

However, a few years ago the chicken meat industry became a test site for eliminating the part of the process that involved negotiation. In what was called the 'cross-docking' of poultry, the Coles supermarket chain began to fax its daily orders through to its preferred processors, and it was incumbent on the latter to meet the order, whether they had the stock or not. The rationale of the new ordering system was to achieve a marketing system that stressed economies of coordination, achieved 'through minimising stock holding and transport costs, reducing paperwork … reducing the need for market searching by the retailer etc' (Dawson 1995, p. 80). While the larger chicken meat processors were content with the new arrangements (they no longer had to employ telephone sales staff or truck drivers to deliver to scores of outlets), this form of supply disadvantages smaller processors, whose plants are not geared to deliver a range of products with just 24 hours' notice. If the business media is correct, the relentless pursuit of cost savings in supply chains is set to intensify. By adopting integrated information technology (IT) systems that directly link cash registers with product suppliers, Woolworths anticipated saving A\$4.5 billion over a five-year period (Kohler 2003, p. 14).

Dawson (1995) points out that the ability to drive these forms of marketing systems creates new kinds of channel power, which reinforces retailer power relative to the power of suppliers and consumers. Those firms that profit from the new supply arrangements grow bigger and other firms are forced out, which in turn decreases the choice of firms for producers to sell to and the spiral of size, profitability and concentration increases.

Retail power is further illustrated by other events that have affected the chicken meat commodity complex. During the years when the new supply chain arrangements were being put into place, chicken meat producers were fighting government plans to force chicken meat imports on the industry and to deregulate the arrangements that allowed chicken farmers to collectively bargain over the amounts they were paid for growing birds (Dixon 2002). While chicken farmers and processors were successfully repelling government 'reforms' justified by global free-trade pressures and national competition policy, they were succumbing without protest to retailer-led restructuring of their industry.

Redesigning the retail-consumer demand chain interface

Just as supermarkets exert considerable influence over the production sphere of the chicken meat commodity complex, they are also extremely active in shaping the practices of food consumption. Here the general strategy is one of selling 'a way of life' that provides a supportive context to the exchange of goods and services. Selling a way of life involves using particular language, images and practices in anticipation that consumers will accept and adopt them. Australian supermarkets' efforts to influence shopping and consumption practices are best explained in two social histories of Australian supermarkets, *Shelf Life* (Humphery 1998) and *Basket, Bag and Trolley* (Kingston 1994). Together they show how supermarket chains have for 80 years been proactive in shaping the consumer experience so as to maximise their profits. As supermarkets moved beyond their variety-store heritage during the 1960s, they became purveyors not simply of groceries but of three Cs: 'convenience, cleanliness and consumer choice' (Humphery 1998, p. 105). Clearly, they hoped that Mrs Housewife, an identity they helped to forge from the 1920s onwards, would forego and forget the super-convenient practice of boys delivering the weekly grocery order on bicycle or (in later years) buying her fish and vegetables from the back of a truck that meandered through suburban streets. In place of having her consumables bagged and delivered, Mrs Housewife had to learn how to participate in the consumer culture of self-service. This required a dedicated promotional effort by the supermarkets, which had to associate the shift in labour with the march of economic progress (Humphery 1998, p. 105).

In what follows, I describe how the table chicken has assisted supermarket chains to acquire the requisite **cultural capital** to continue to amass financial capital. Whereas the previous section showed how producer–retailer relations are being refashioned, this section analyses the constant reworking of the consumer–retailer interface.

Supermarkets as the heart of the household: Providing 'healthy convenience'

The humble chicken has played a significant role in the fortunes of supermarket chains. This most acceptable food has allowed supermarkets to constantly rework their identity as a family-friendly institution whose mission is to help consumers negotiate their busy lives. Nowhere is this better illustrated than in the logo that the Franklins chain adopted in the mid 1990s when trying to recruit staff to the 'Franklins Family': a giant rooster bestriding the space rocket of progress.

The cool chain, described earlier, brought benefits over and above bringing new products onto the market. The sale of chilled as opposed to frozen chickens allowed supermarkets to portray themselves as being at the cutting edge of progress, a position reached through their foresight with new technologies. As Hollander (2003)

Jane Dixon

argued, cool chains enhanced the legitimacy of supermarkets, which had become increasingly reliant on produce from far-flung reaches, to metaphorically 'freshen' the meaning of a first-world food system.

The introduction of this particular technology coincided with the advent in the 1970s of social movements concerned with health and the environment, which together encouraged consumers to desire goods that had had minimal contact with the industrial process and were 'close to nature'. What could be more natural than unfrozen and, by dint of marketing prowess, 'fresh' products? Arguably, it was their success with chicken that provided supermarkets with an opportunity to actively promote themselves as offering opportunities for a fresh and healthy life. Company annual reports reveal that, in the mid 1990s, the three major chains all promoted themselves through the discourse of 'fresh produce'. And it seems that the symbolic importance of 'freshness' has not diminished, with Woolworths codenaming its recent restructuring efforts Project Refresh (Kohler 2003, p. 14).

While supermarkets were establishing fresh-produce sections, they were also competing with small suburban takeaway and fast-food shops to supply the traditional Friday night meal. Rather than attempt the more labour-intensive fish and chips or hamburger, supermarkets introduced rotisserie chicken counters. Whole cooked chickens, with potatoes and coleslaw, consolidated their reputation for offering not only healthy convenience but meal solutions to families at the end of a busy week. Furthermore, by lowering the price of these chickens, or giving two-for-the-price-of-one deals just prior to store closing time, they communicated to Mrs Housewife that if she valued thrift then here was the place to get it. The supermarket practice of loss leading—whereby selected items are sold for less than they cost the retailer, to entice consumers to visit the store and then buy more profitable items—is an important vehicle for communicating the value-for-money ethos so esteemed by many consumers. Over the years, the range of goods used as loss leaders has been quite consistent (Coca-Cola, margarine and bacon, for example) and, from the time of the frozen chicken onwards, chicken has featured prominently.

Fashioning the discourse around home-meal replacement (HMR)

Many food retailers offer to solve a nation's problems of not having enough time, being confused about nutrition and lacking food-preparation skills by providing what the food service sector calls 'meal solutions'. The Friday night 'roto bird' described above was preceded by frozen TV dinners in the 1960s, which were a forerunner to cook-chilled meals that require minimal effort from the household cook. Not only was the first TV dinner in the USA a chicken dish (Swanson TV Brand dinners), but chicken Kiev and chicken cordon bleu ushered in the heat-and-serve cook-chill revolution. Apparently, cook-chilled meals were viewed as 'a pleasure, a relief, a welcome technical fix for the working woman's double burden: feeding the family as well as the bank balance' (Raven et al. 1995, p. 5).

Meal-replacement strategies do not simply mean product innovation; they also involve redefining what is meant by the terms 'home', 'meal' and 'replacement'. And consumer acceptance has been contingent upon a subtle effort to alleviate the guilty feeling of housewives that they were failing in their primary job by not feeding their families with foods prepared at home (Strickland 1996). The supply by the food service sector—including supermarkets, fast-food chains, takeaway shops, cafes and restaurants—of the close-to-ready main meal of the day, several days of the week, is a market niche that is being vigorously fought over (Strickland 1996). Supermarkets currently have the edge over fast-food chains in this niche because they have a longer association with offering healthy choices, thanks to their early appropriation of the 'fresh food' title.

Product differentiation to foster chain differentiation

There is plenty of evidence that supermarkets do not act purely in response to consumer demand, but that their product offerings influence those demands. For example, specialist sections selling HVFs are an integral part of supermarkets' strategy to use product differentiation to foster different communities of consumption. Product-differentiated retail systems emerge when a single chain segments its stores on the basis of store layout and services and the mix of distinctive product ranges (Harvey 1998). To determine the best ambience and product mix, supermarkets use psychographic mapping techniques, which allow market researchers to determine the lifestyles and attitudes of consumers in the catchment areas surrounding stores. The information gleaned from these techniques complements the scanner data acquired when shoppers use their store loyalty cards. As a result, supermarkets know how to micro-market their offerings: which stores should promote themselves as catering to older Australians of a conservative outlook who still like 'meat and three veg'; which should cater to young urban professionals for whom cooking is down-time; and where to introduce novel products for shoppers attracted to multicultural food experimentation, encouraged by celebrity chefs.

Each of the chains is particularly keen to attract consumers who are time-poor and who are willing to spend more on value-added foods, where the biggest profits are to be made. Coles and Woolworths are locked in a battle to assemble product and service portfolios that will appeal to the consumer market segment for whom quality is more important than price. They want this group to identify with their firm and to dismiss the other as not complementary to their social status.

As part of the market segmentation strategy, Australian supermarkets have been following their UK counterparts with the production and sale of private label foods. There are sound economic reasons for this strategy: profits are higher and, globally,

Jane Dixon

the growth of private label goods relative to manufacturer brands has been getting stronger (ACNielsen 2006a, p. 45).

By the end of 2007, Coles aims to make its house brands comprise one-third of packaged goods sales. Importantly, Coles will use its private labels to further segment the market: its three-tier strategy will involve an 'entry point' brand 'Coles $mart Buy', a mid price-quality brand 'You'll Love Coles', and the 'exceptional quality' brand 'George J. Coles', which it claims will lead innovation in that product line (Webb 2005). One business columnist reported that even the largest producers of packaged goods, including Nestlé and Coca-Cola, were alarmed at the supermarket's strategy (McMahon 2005). Further, the market analysis firm ACNielsen noted in its Grocery Report 2006 that, 'Private label clearly presents some strategic challenges for manufacturers … small to medium-sized manufacturers run a higher risk of being squeezed off shelves to make room for more profitable private label items. In response, they may embrace the idea of producing private label goods as an opportunity … Alternatively, they may focus on penetrating alternative channels outside grocery' (ACNielsen 2006b, p. 3).

Adding to the debate, Australia's high-profile consumer watchdog the Australian Consumers Association compiled a review of consumers' views regarding private labels. On the positive side, consumers believe that private labels offer 'value for money'; are 'quality assured' by a reputable retailer; and offer choice of better products through their premium tiers, 'ultimately providing an alternative to shopping in niche stores, such as delicatessens'. On the flipside consumers raised concerns about a lessening of choice as supermarkets cut out brands to accommodate their own brands on limited shelf space. Furthermore, while the two major chains have given assurances about sourcing local ingredients as long as they meet their specifications, consumers fear that Australian owned and made products may be jeopardised (Choice 2006).

Elaborating the sphere of distribution and exchange

In his study of fast food in France, Fantasia (1995, p. 201) notes that '[t]here is a vantage point situated at the intersection of economic and cultural sociology from which we can discern ever more clearly the material dimensions of culture and the non-material dimensions of goods'. That point is the sphere of distribution and exchange. Within this sphere are numerous actors, including those who work in what Sassen (1991) calls the 'producer services'—accountants, lawyers, IT specialists, psychographic researchers, market analysts, advertisers and public relations experts. Corporations are dependent on these services to make money. Other experts, including nutritionists, health educators, home economists and celebrity chefs, constitute what can be called a 'consumer services' sector (Dixon 2002). Their function is to facilitate consumption practices. The combined producer and consumer services sector assists consumers and producers to make decisions in relation to market, lifestyle and household management. They help align the spheres of production and consumption.

Commercially employed food-knowledge producers constitute a wider phenomenon, as identified in the sociological literature. They are responsible for undermining older forms of social authority in favour of their own expert authority. Thus, as the authority of the mother, family cook and government-employed home economist diminishes, so expert authority is increasingly being marshalled by the market (Dixon 2007). Supermarkets and fast-food chains use the producer-consumer services sector to strategically invest their capital in cultural production, in order to shape consumption discourses and practices.

The alliance between Coles and the Dietitians Association of Australia on the 7-a-day fruit and vegetable campaign is a notable example. Another partnership between supermarkets and professional authorities is the promotion by supermarket of eggs endorsed by the Royal Society for the Prevention of Cruelty to Animals (RSPCA) as produced by free-range hens. While Australian supermarkets are relative newcomers to the art of promoting themselves as ethical traders (Freidberg 2003), they are gradually adding this skill to their repertoire through promoting organic foods and animal welfare protocols: in this way, they renew their credentials as the pre-eminent family-friendly food-retailing institution.

In 2007, Woolworths held an event to support Australia's drought-stricken farmers. The company's press release began with: 'As part of a wider commitment to supporting Australia's rural communities, on January 23, 2007, Woolworths will donate its entire supermarket profits for the day to the Country Women's Association and research into sustainable farming practices' (Woolworths Limited 2007). A week after this announcement a flyer was circulating on the internet from concerned food activists asking, 'What about the other 364 days of the year?' This vignette illustrates both the opportunities and tensions that are present within the food system: here a supermarket chain was combining its economic and cultural strengths to further position itself as a guardian of Australians' well-being (for further examples, see Dixon 2007), while consumer groups were accusing the chain of farmer exploitation and of jeopardising the health of the public and the environment with its supply chain activities.

Arguably the supermarket industry as a whole benefited from this activity (a few days later Coles announced it was teaming up with the Salvation Army to work with rural Australia), providing a positive backdrop against which it quietly restructures the food system. As Burch and Lawrence (2005) note: supermarkets are using their monopsonic power to generate profits from three activities: the acquisition of food products on the best possible terms; the extraction of rent as a consequence of the ownership of critical supply chain assets, including shelf space; and generating additional revenue from supermarket home brands.

Jane Dixon

Conclusion

The essence of the cultural economy approach is the detailed and systematic analysis of the economic basis for group practices/lifestyles and of how these influence the decisions of economic actors. Using the lexicon of nutrition and consumer scientists, doing cultural economy entails making a politically critical examination of the relationships between the acceptability, availability and adoption of practices and commodities.

The table chicken case study highlights the symbiotic relationship between cultural production and capital-production activities. The growing popularity of chicken cannot be explained without exploring the cultural economy processes that have positioned it within a more general commodity context centred on 'healthy convenience'. Chicken has been a key ingredient in the marketing of convenience foods to suit the lifestyles of overcommitted family cooks: beginning with the frozen TV dinner, followed by the hot rotisserie chicken, the cook-chill meal, and more recently heat-and-serve gourmet meals. The story of the table chicken is indicative of how Australia's culinary dynamism and the balance of power in the national food system are shifting away from primary producers towards large retail traders—the supermarkets.

SUMMARY OF MAIN POINTS

- Since the 1970s, supermarkets have played the major role in positioning chicken to become Australia's preferred meat. Simultaneously, they have used chicken meals to portray themselves in the consumer consciousness as a valued social institution.
- With assistance from a range of producer and consumer services, supermarkets have claimed the balance of power in the food system because they trade not simply in goods and services but in practices, ideas and values. A range of professional services positions large retail traders at the intersection of production and consumption within a nation's culinary culture.
- Using extensive insights into the socioeconomic and psychosocial characteristics of the population, supermarkets are constantly able to 'refresh' the relevance of the products and services that they sell, and by association they renew their own centrality to the nation's food system and culinary culture.
- A cultural economy approach, with its focus on production, distribution and consumption activities, is ideally placed to examine the multifaceted nature of power, its transformation and its reproduction within the food system.
- The nascent appreciation of the value of 'doing cultural economy' will grow as the critical importance of the sphere of distribution and exchange is realised.

SOCIOLOGICAL REFLECTION

This chapter has shown how supermarkets have come to dominate the food retail sector in Australia, particularly by mediating between producers and consumers. In doing so, they are displacing independent food producers and retailers, such as the local greengrocer, butcher, 'continental deli' and fishmonger.

- What do you see as the advantages and disadvantages of the growing power of supermarket chains?
- How influential are supermarket practices on your food habits?
- Are you concerned about the demise of small, often family-run, food retailers?

DISCUSSION QUESTIONS

1. Describe the activities that comprise the spheres of food production, distribution, exchange and consumption.
2. In what ways has chicken meat become both 'good to think' and 'good to eat'?
3. When undertaking a cultural economy analysis of a commodity system, what steps would you take?
4. Do specialist food retailers operate similarly to supermarket chains? What are their points of difference?
5. Describe the contradictions in the notion of 'healthy convenience'.
6. What strategies are supermarkets using to acquire cultural and economic capital?

Further investigation

1. Take a popular commodity grouping, such as cheese, and describe the ways in which primary and secondary producers, supermarkets and specialist retail outlets, and consumers add value to the commodity.
2. Write a social history of the changes to small, family-run food retailer's since the 1950s. Are we witnessing their revival as a reaction against giant multi-chain food retailers?

FURTHER READING AND WEB RESOURCES

Books

Bourdieu, P. 1979/1984, *Distinction: A Social Critique of the Judgment of Taste*, Routledge, London

Burch, D. & Lawrence, G. (eds) 2007, *Supermarkets and Agri-food Supply Chains: Transformations in the Production and Consumption of Foods*, Edward Elgar, Cheltenham.

Jane Dixon

Dixon, J. 2002, *The Changing Chicken: Chooks, Cooks and Culinary Culture*, University of New South Wales Press, Sydney.

du Gay, P. & Pryke, M. (eds) 2002, *Cultural Economy*, Sage, London.

Humphery, K. 1998, *Shelf Life: Supermarkets and the Changing Culture of Consumption*, Cambridge University Press, Cambridge.

Websites

Agribusiness Association of Australia: www.agribusiness.asn.au. Aims to facilitate communication about the agri-food sector.

Australian Food and Grocery Council (AFGC): www.afgc.org.au/. The national food industry body representing the interests of the major food producers.

Australian Institute of Food Science and Technology (AIFST): www.aifst.asn.au/. A national body that aims to facilitate communication, learning and professional development among all people involved in the Australian food sector. Publishes the journal, *Food Australia*.

Department of Agriculture, Fisheries and Forestry (DAFF, Australia): www.daff.gov. au/. A good site to access resources on the food system.

International Journal of Sociology of Agriculture and Food: www.csafe.org.nz/ijsaf. This online refereed journal provides free access to its papers.

National Association of Retail Grocers of Australia: www.narga.com.au/. Federal body representing independently owned retail grocery businesses.

REFERENCES

ACMF—*see* Australian Chicken Meat Federation.

ACNielsen 2006a, 'What's Hot Around the Globe. Insights on Growth in Food & Beverage Products', ACNielsen Global Services, www.acnielsen.com.au.

—— 2006b, 'ACNielsen Grocery Report 2006', ACNielsen Centre, Sydney, www. acnielsen.com.au.

Amin, A. & Thrift, N. 2004, *The Blackwell Cultural Economy Reader*, Blackwell Publishing, Malden, MA, USA.

Appadurai, A. 1986, *The Social Life of Things*, Cambridge University Press, Cambridge.

Australian Chicken Meat Federation n.d., Industry Facts and Figures, www.chicken. org.au/page.php?id=4 [accessed 26/01/07].

Bailey, D. 2005, 'Beef and veal, pigs and poultry. Meat outlook 2009–2010', *Australian Commodities*, vol. 12, no. 1, pp. 65–73.

Baker, R. & Marshall, D. 1998, 'The Hilmer Paradox: Evidence from the Australian Retail Grocery Industry', *Urban Policy and Research*, vol. 16, no. 4, pp. 271–84.

Bourdieu, P. 1979/1984, *Distinction: A Social Critique of the Judgement of Taste*, Routledge, London.

Burch, D. & Goss, J. 1999, 'Global Sourcing and Retail Chains: Shifting Relationships of Production in Australian Agri-foods', *Rural Sociology*, vol. 64, no. 2, pp. 334–50.

Burch, D. & Lawrence, G. 2005, 'Supermarket Own Brands, Supply Chains and the Transformation of the Agri-food System', *International Journal of Sociology of Agriculture and Food*, vol. 13, no. 1, pp. 1–18.

—— (eds) 2007, *Supermarkets and Agri-food Supply Chains: Transformations in the Production and Consumption of Foods*, Edward Elgar, Cheltenham.

Cain, D. 1990, *History of the Australian Chicken Meat Industry 1950–1990*, Australian Chicken Meat Federation, Sydney.

Charles, N. & Kerr, M. 1986, 'Issues of Responsibility and Control in the Feeding of Families', in S. Rodmell & A. Watt (eds), *The Politics of Health Education: Raising the Issues*, Routledge and Kegan Paul, London, pp. 57–75.

Choice 2006. 'Supermarket Brands. Coles and Woolworths have launched new "private label" ranges', Online 03/06, www.choice.com.au/printFriendly.aspx?ID=105149 [accessed 26/01/2007].

CSIRO—*see* Commonwealth Scientific and Industrial Research Organisation.

Commonwealth Scientific and Industrial Research Organisation 1994, *Information Needs and Concerns in Relation to Food Choice*, CSIRO, Adelaide.

DAFF—*see* Department of Agriculture, Fisheries and Forestry.

Delforce, R., Dickson, A. & Hogan, J. 2005, 'Australia's food industry', *Australian Commodities*, vol. 12, no. 2, pp. 379–90.

Department of Agriculture, Fisheries and Forestry 2005a, *Australian Food Statistics 2005*, DAFF, Canberra.

—— 2005b, *Australian Agriculture and Food Sector Stocktake*, DAFF, Canberra.

Dawson, J. 1995, 'Food Retailing and the Food Consumer', in D.W. Marshall (ed.), *Food Choice and the Consumer*, Blackie Academic & Professional, London, pp. 77–104.

DeVault, M. 1991, *Feeding the Family: The Social Organization of Caring as Gendered Work*, University of Chicago Press, Chicago.

Dixon, J. 1999, 'A Cultural Economy Model for Studying Food Systems', *Agriculture and Human Values*, vol. 16, pp. 151–60.

—— 2002, *The Changing Chicken: Chooks, Cooks and Culinary Culture*, University of New South Wales Press, Sydney.

—— 2003, 'Authority, Power and Value in Contemporary Industrial Food Systems', *International Journal of the Sociology of Agriculture and Food*, vol. 11, no. 1, pp. 31–9.

—— 2007, 'Advisor for Healthy Life: Supermarkets as New Food Authorities', in D. Burch & G. Lawrence (eds), *Supermarkets and Agri-food Supply Chains: Transformations in the Production and Consumption of Foods*, Edward Elgar, Cheltenham.

Douglas, M. 1997, 'In Defence of Shopping', in P. Falk & C. Campbell (eds), *The Shopping Experience*, Sage, London, pp. 15–30.

du Gay, P. & Pryke, M. (eds) 2002, *Cultural Economy*, Sage, London.

Fairbrother, J. 1988, 'The Poultry Industry: Technology's Child Two Decades on', *Food Australia*, November, pp. 456–62.

Falk, P. & Campbell, C. 1997, *The Shopping Experience*, Sage, London.

Fantasia, R. 1995, 'Fast Food in France', *Theory and Society*, vol. 24, no. 2, pp. 201–43.

Featherstone, M. 1987, 'Lifestyle and Consumer Culture', *Theory, Culture & Society*, vol. 4, no. 1, pp. 55–70.

Fischler, C. 1993, 'A Nutritional Cacophony or the Crisis of Food Selection in Affluent Societies', in P. Leatherwood, M. Horisberger & W. James (eds), *For a Better Nutrition in the 21st Century*, Vevey/Raven Press, New York, pp. 57–65.

Flynn, A. & Marsden, T. 1992, 'Food Regulation in a Period of Agricultural Retreat: The British Experience', *Geoforum*, vol. 23, pp. 85–93.

Foord, J., Bowlby, S. & Tillsley, C. 1996, 'The Changing Place of Retailer-supplier Relations in British Retailing', in N. Wrigley & M. Lowe (eds), *Retailing, Consumption and Capital: Towards the New Retail Geography*, Longman, Essex, pp. 68–89.

Freidberg, S. 2003, 'Cleaning up Down South: Supermarkets, Ethical Trade and African Horticulture', *Social & Cultural Geography*, vol. 4, no. 1, pp. 27–43.

Friedland, W. 1984, 'Commodity Systems Analysis: An Approach to the Sociology of Agriculture', *Research in Rural Sociology and Development*, vol. 1, pp. 221–35.

—— 2001, 'Reprise on Commodity Systems Methodology', *International Journal of Sociology of Agriculture and Food*, vol. 9, no. 1, pp. 82–103.

Gabriel, Y. & Lang, T. 1995, *The Unmanageable Consumer*, Sage, London.

Gofton, L. 1990, 'Food Fears and Time Famines', in M. Ashwell (ed.), *Why We Eat What We Eat: The British Nutrition Foundation Bulletin*, vol. 15, no. 1, pp. 78–95.

—— & Ness, M. 1991, 'Twin Trends: Health and Convenience in Food Change or Who Killed the Lazy Housewife', *British Food Journal*, vol. 93, no. 7, pp. 17–23.

Goodman, D. & Redclift, M. 1991, *Refashioning Nature: Food, Ecology & Culture*, Routledge, London.

Goodman, D. & Watts, M. 1997, *Globalising Food: Agrarian Questions and Global Restructuring*, Routledge, London.

Halperin, R. 1994, *Cultural Economies: Past and Present*, University of Texas Press, Austin.

Harris, M. 1986, *Good to Eat: Riddles of Food and Culture*, Allen & Unwin, London.

Harvey, M. 1998, 'UK Supermarkets: New Product and Labour Market Segmentation and the Restructuring of the Supply-demand Matrix', paper presented to the International Working Party on Labour Market Segmentation Conference, Trento, Italy.

Hollander, G. 2003, 'Re-naturalizing Sugar: Narratives of Place, Production and Consumption', *Social & Cultural Geography*, vol. 4, no. 1, pp. 59–74.

Hughes, A. 1996, 'Forging New Cultures of Food Retailer-manufacturer Relations?', in N. Wrigley & M. Lowe (eds), *Retailing, Consumption and Capital: Towards the New Retail Geography*, Longman, Essex, pp. 90–115.

Humphery, K. 1998, *Shelf Life: Supermarkets and the Changing Culture of Consumption*, Cambridge University Press, Cambridge.

Jacenko, A. & Gunasekera, D. 2005, *Australia's retail food sector. Some preliminary observations*, ABARE Conference Paper 05.11, ABARE, Canberra.

Joint Select Committee on the Retailing Sector 1999, *Fair Market or Market Failure: A Review of Australia's Retailing Sector*, Parliament of Australia, Canberra.

JSCRS—*see* Joint Select Committee on the Retailing Sector.

Kingston, B. 1994, *Basket, Bag and Trolley: A History of Shopping in Australia*, Oxford University Press, Melbourne.

Kohler, A. 2003, 'Sam Walton's Long Shadow', *The Weekend Australian Financial Review*, July 26–27, p. 14.

Lash, S. 1990, *Sociology of Postmodernism*, Routledge, London.

Lash, S. & Urry, J. 1994, *Economies of Signs & Space*, Sage, London.

Lowe, M. & Wrigley, N. 1996, 'Towards the New Retail Geography', in N. Wrigley & M. Lowe (eds), *Retailing, Consumption and Capital: Towards the New Retail Geography*, Longman, Essex, pp. 3–30.

Lyons, K. 1996, 'Agro-industrialization and Social Change within the Australian Context: A Case Study of the Fast Food Industry', in D. Burch, R. Rickson & G. Lawrence (eds), *Globalization and Agri-food Restructuring: Perspectives from the Australasia Region*, Avebury, Aldershot, UK, pp. 239–50.

Mackay, H. 1992, *The Mackay Report: Food*, Hugh Mackay, Sydney.

Marshall, D. (ed.) 1995, *Food Choice and the Consumer*, Blackie Academic & Professional, London.

Mathews, J. 1989, *Tools of Change: New Technology and the Democratisation of Work*, Pluto Press, Sydney.

McMahon, S. 2005, 'Food groups unite for battle with house brands', June 18, www.theage.com.au/news/Business/Food-groups-unite-for-battle-with-house-br... [accessed 26 January 2007].

Miller, D. 1995, 'Consumption as the Vanguard of History', in D. Miller (ed.), *Acknowledging Consumption: A Review of New Studies*, Routledge, London, pp. 1–57.

Murcott, A. 1993, 'Talking of Good Food: An Empirical Study of Women's Conceptualizations', *Food and Foodways*, vol. 5, no. 3, pp. 305–18.

Murray, R. 1989, 'Fordism and post-Fordism', in S. Hall and M. Jacques (eds), *New Times: The Changing Face of Politics in the 1990s*, Lawrence and Wishart, London.

Raven, H., Lang, T. & Dumonteil, C. 1995, *Off Our Trolleys? Food Retailing and the Hypermarket Economy*, Institute for Public Policy Research, London.

RIRDC—*see* Rural Industries Research and Development Corporation.

Rural Industries Research and Development Corporation n.d., *R & D Plan for the Chicken Meat Program 2004–2009*, RIRDC, Canberra. http://www.rirdc.gov.au/pub/chick5yr.htm. Accessed 14/01/2007.

Ryan, S. & Burgess, J. 1996, 'The Supermarket Co.', in J. Burgess, P. Keogh, D. Macdonald, G. Morgan, G. Strachan & S. Ryan (eds), *Enterprise Bargaining in Three Female Dominated Workplaces in the Hunter: Processes, Participation and Outcomes* (Employment Studies Centre Working Paper Series No. 26), University of Newcastle, Australia.

SACMC—*see* South Australia Chicken Meat Council.

Santich, B. 1995, '"It's a Chore!" Women's Attitudes Towards Cooking', *Australian Journal of Nutrition and Dietetics*, vol. 52, no. 1, pp. 11–13.

Sassen, S. 1991, *The Global City*, Princeton University Press, Princeton, New Jersey.

Senker, J. 1988, *A Taste for Innovation: British Supermarkets' Influence on Food Manufacturers*, Horton Publishing, Bradford, UK.

Skurray, G. & Newell, G. 1993, 'Food Consumption in Australia 1970–1990', *Food Australia*, vol. 45, no. 9, pp. 434–8.

Smith, R. 2006, 'The Australian Grocery Industry: A Competition Perspective', *The Australian Journal of Agricultural and Resource Economics*, vol. 50, pp. 33–50.

South Australia Chicken Meat Council n.d., *Poultry meat in South Australia—strategic directions 2005–2015*, SA Chicken Meat Council and Primary Industries and Resources, SA.

Strickland, K. 1996, 'Fast Food Chains Latch onto Health', *The Australian*, 5 February, p. 3.

Symons, M. 1993, *The Shared Table*, Australian Government Publishing Service, Canberra.

Tansey, G. & Worsley, T. 1995, *The Food System: A Guide*, Earthscan Publications, London.

—— 1994, 'Consumers, Identity and Belonging: Reflections on Some Theses of Zygmunt Bauman', in R. Keat, N. Whiteley & N. Abercrombie (eds), *The Authority of the Consumer*, Routledge, London, pp. 58–73.

Watts, M. & Goodman, D. 1997, 'Agrarian Questions', in D. Goodman & M. Watts *Globalising Food*, Routledge, London, pp. 1–32.

Webb, R. 2005, 'The Supermarket Sweep', 24 July, www.theage.com.au/news/business/the-supermarket-sweep/2005/07/23/112153... [accessed 26/01/07].

Woolworths Limited 2007, 'Woolworths CEO Pledges Substantial Support for Drought Relief', Woolworths Supermarkets 1997–2007, www.woolworths.com.au/woolworths [accessed 10 January 2007].

Wrigley, N. & Lowe, M. 1996, *Retailing, Consumption and Capital: Towards the New Retail Geography*, Longman, Essex.

PART 3

Food and Nutrition Discourses, Politics, and Policies

Food is an important part of a balanced diet.

Fran Lebowitz, *Metropolitan Life* (1978)

Food is an area that brings the best and worst of politics into play; the formation of public policy and attempts to influence it by vested interest groups take place at national and international levels. The chapters in this part address the politics of food in terms of food regulations, food and nutrition policy used for health promotion, the emergence of public health nutrition as a specialist field, and the food discourses and policies relating to the feeding of infants and children. Part 3 is divided into five chapters:

- Chapter 6 examines the role of food policy in the form of dietary guidelines, exposing some of the individualistic assumptions and corporate interests that have impacted on the good intentions of government authorities and health professionals in attempting to address public health nutrition.
- Chapter 7 discusses the emergence of 'functional foods', which allegedly produce specific health benefits, and the implications these foods have for public health nutrition and food regulation policy in the face of powerful corporate interests.
- Chapter 8 explores the development and current state of the public health nutrition workforce from a sociological perspective, and examines how workforce composition influences practice.
- Chapter 9 discusses the maternal ideologies and health-related discourses surrounding the choice of method for infant feeding.
- Chapter 10 examines food discourses in the context of the family and the feeding of children.

CHAPTER 6

The Politics of Government Dietary Advice

Jennifer Lisa Falbe and Marion Nestle

OVERVIEW

- What current trends exist in development of nutrition standards, dietary guidelines and food guides?
- How do stakeholders affect the development of government dietary guidance?
- Why is dietary advice vulnerable to political influence?

Although dietary guidelines are based on science, they are also subject to pressures from food companies concerned about the commercial implications of advice to restrict certain nutrients or foods. This chapter reviews examples of food industry influence on dietary advice issued by the World Health Organization in 2004, the United States of America in 2005 and Canada in 2007. These examples suggest the need for establishing processes that keep dietary recommendations free of political influence.

Key terms

dietary guidelines
food guides
nutrient standards

Introduction

Governments issue dietary advice to their citizens in order to promote consumption of agricultural and food products as well as to improve health. In the USA, for example, the Department of Agriculture (USDA) has produced **food guides** for consumers since the early 1900s. The early guides were designed to help Americans overcome nutritional deficiencies and typically recommended increased consumption of foods from various groups. To the extent that such guides encourage eating more food to prevent nutrient deficiencies, they elicit little opposition; such advice benefits all stakeholders in the food system, from producers to consumers. However, prevention of chronic diseases—coronary heart disease, certain cancers, stroke and diabetes—sometimes requires restrictions on dietary components that raise risks for these conditions. Advice to reduce intake of energy (measured in calories or kilojoules), saturated fat, cholesterol, sugars and salt—and of their principal food sources—inevitably provokes opposition from the affected food companies (Nestle 2007).

The history of **dietary guidelines** and food guides is rife with examples of controversy over advice to 'eat less' of any nutrient or food. Food companies are businesses and, like any business in today's global marketplace, must expand sales, meet growth targets and produce immediate returns for investors. Given that all but the poorest countries in the world provide more food on average than is needed by their populations, the food industry is especially competitive. The US food supply, for example, provides 3900 calories (16 300 kilojoules) per person each day, nearly twice the average amount of energy required. Unlike the situation with shoes, clothing and electronics, consumption of food is limited even for those with the largest appetites, making competition especially intense. The need to sell more food in an overabundant marketplace explains why the annual growth rate of the American food industry is only a percentage point or two, why food companies compete so strenuously for a sales-friendly regulatory and political climate, and why they so aggressively defend the health benefits of their products and attack critics of their marketing, sales and lobbying practices (Nestle 2007).

More often than not, food industry pressures have succeeded in inducing government agencies to eliminate, weaken or thoroughly obfuscate recommendations to eat less of certain nutrients and their food sources. In part, they do so by taking advantage of current trends in nutrition science towards defining human nutritional requirements as increasingly complex and individualised. This chapter offers examples of the ways economic pressures and scientific trends affect dietary advice from three sources: the World Health Organization (WHO) in 2004, the USA in 2005 and Canada in 2007. Similar issues related to Australian dietary guidelines released in 2003 have been reviewed previously (Duff 2004). Table 6.1 summarises those guidelines.

Table 6.1   Dietary guidelines for Australian adults, 2003

Enjoy a wide variety of nutritious foods:
• Eat plenty of vegetables, legumes and fruits.
• Eat plenty of cereals (including breads, rice, pasta and noodles), preferably wholegrain.
• Include lean meat, fish, poultry and/or alternatives.
• Include milks, yoghurts, cheeses and/or alternatives. Reduced-fat varieties should be chosen, where possible.
• Drink plenty of water.
And take care to:
• Limit saturated fat and moderate total fat intake.
• Choose foods low in salt.
• Limit your alcohol intake if you choose to drink.
• Consume only moderate amounts of sugars and foods containing added sugars.
• Prevent weight gain: be physically active and eat according to your energy needs.
• Care for your food: prepare and store it safely.
• Encourage and support breastfeeding.

Source: NHMRC (2003)

The WHO Global Strategy, 2004

In the early 2000s, WHO began development of a Global Strategy to help member nations reduce the burden of death and disease related to poor diet and inactivity. The agency's intent was to provide evidence-based recommendations along with action plans and implementation policies (Waxman & Norum 2004). The process began with an Expert Consultation involving international scientists who were asked to review existing research and make recommendations. Their report, commonly referred to as 'Technical Report 916', appeared in 2003 (WHO 2003a). The process also involved stakeholder consultations with member states, UN agencies, governmental and nongovernmental organisations, the food industry and other private sector groups, as well as negotiation of co-sponsorship with the Food and Agriculture Organization (FAO). The final Global Strategy, released jointly by the two UN agencies, was ratified by member states in May 2004 (WHO 2004).

The dietary guidance components of this process proved especially contentious. In 2002, the Expert Consultation committee drafted a preliminary research review that included quantitative goals for intake of specific nutrients (see Table 6.2). To anyone familiar with the history of such recommendations, these goals should have been unremarkable; they were consistent with decades of similar targets established by numerous countries (Cannon 1992).

Table 6.2   Goals for ranges of nutrient intake recommended in the WHO/FAO consultation report

Dietary factor	Goal (% of total energy, unless otherwise stated)
Total fat	15–30%
Saturated fatty acids	<10%
Polyunsaturated fatty acids	6–10%
n-6 Polyunsaturated fatty acids	5–8%
n-3 Polyunsaturated fatty acids	1–2%
Trans fatty acids	<1%
Monounsaturated fatty acids	By difference
Total carbohydrate	55–75%
Free sugars	<10%
Protein	10–15%
Cholesterol	<300 mg per day
Sodium chloride (sodium)	<5 g per day (<2 g per day)
Fruits and vegetables	≥400 g per day
Total dietary fiber	From foods
Non-starch polysaccharides (NSP)	From foods

Source: WHO (2003a)

Nevertheless, one goal provoked unusual attention: to limit intake of 'free' sugars (those added in processing or naturally present in honey, syrups and fruit juices) to 10 per cent or less of daily caloric intake. The 10 per cent target was hardly news. The USDA's 1992 Pyramid food guide, for example, recommended a range of 7 to 13 per cent of calories from added sugars, depending on caloric needs (USDA 1992). For a diet containing 2000 calories (8400 kilojoules), the 10 per cent goal permits a daily intake of 50g of 'free' sugars, but one 20-ounce (600mL) soft drink contains more than that amount. Sugar producers and trade groups said this level of restriction was not scientifically justified as neither sugars nor their primary food sources had been shown to cause obesity (World Sugar Research Organization 2002). In the USA, lobbyists for sugar trade organisations induced the Department of Health and Human Services (HHS) to submit critiques of the draft based on materials they provided (Steiger 2002). Although sugar groups ostensibly based their arguments on science, their concerns were clearly economic. Such a recommendation, they said, would be likely to produce 'serious, detrimental and long-lasting effects on the agriculture and the economy of [sugar-producing] countries' (Khan 2003).

Just prior to release of Technical Report 916, the Sugar Association threatened not only to publicly expose flaws in the report but also to ask Congress to withdraw US funding for WHO; it demanded that WHO immediately remove the 916

Report from its website and withdraw the report. Sugar groups also induced the co-chairs of the US Senate Sweetener Caucus to ask the HHS Secretary to use his influence to have the report rescinded (Briscoe 2003). In arguing against the 10 per cent target, sugar groups invoked US standards for nutrient intake published as Dietary Reference Intakes (DRIs) by the Institute of Medicine (IOM), a scientific organisation that conducts research studies for federal agencies. In developing the DRIs, the IOM (2002) had established the safe upper limit of daily sugar intake at 25 per cent of calories, a cap established to permit diets to contain adequate levels of essential nutrients. Sugar groups, however, chose to interpret the 25 per cent cap as a recommendation. In response, the IOM president wrote to HHS to deny that his organisation endorsed 25 per cent as a goal (Fineberg 2003). Despite sugar industry pressures, the published version of Technical Report 916 included the 10 per cent goal for 'free' sugars (Table 6.2).

While development of Report 916 was underway, WHO and FAO began drafting the Global Strategy. Early in 2003, the agencies sent a 'consultation document' to member states that omitted quantitative targets for nutrient intake, and further regional consultations with the health sector were relatively uncontroversial (Norum 2005). Food industry representatives, however, continued to argue that the Global Strategy should not advise restrictions: that it should recognise that there are no good foods or bad foods, and should instead emphasise adequate nutrient intake, personal initiative, consumer education and physical activity (WHO 2003b). At the same time, industry groups were actively working to convince member states that acceptance of Technical Report 916 as the research basis for the Strategy would adversely affect the economies of sugar-producing countries. The World Sugar Research Organization, for example, distributed a report illustrating the loss to sugar producers that would occur if global consumption dropped to 10 per cent of calories. Despite flaws in this analysis, it convinced many member states to lobby against the recommendation (Waxman 2004).

Lobbying continued during preparation of the final Global Strategy document. Just prior to a meeting of the WHO Executive Board in January 2004, the US HHS continued to write to WHO restating criticisms of Technical Report 916, even after its publication (Steiger 2004a), a tactic interpreted as an attempt to stall the Global Strategy (Norum 2005). A subsequent HHS letter proposed line-by-line edits of the draft Global Strategy that repeated written statements of industry lobbyists (Steiger 2004b). These statements and correspondence were 'leaked' to the internet and made available to the press (Zarocostas 2004).

In May 2004, the 57th World Health Assembly endorsed the Global Strategy, but not without major concessions to the food industry (WHO 2004). Analysis of drafts produced between April 2003 and May 2004 provided substantial evidence of food industry influence. As ratified, the Global Strategy states that foods high in fat, sugar and salt increase the risk for non-communicable diseases, but advice about sugars is just to 'limit the intake of free sugars'. The controversial 10 per cent goal is not mentioned, and neither is any mention of Technical Report 916—not even a footnote.

US Dietary Guidelines, 2005

Since 1980, the USDA and HHS have jointly issued *Dietary Guidelines for Americans* as a policy statement on nutrition and health. The Guidelines provide dietary advice to reduce risks for chronic diseases for everyone over the age of two. Although virtually unknown to the public, the Guidelines greatly influence what the public eats, first because they govern the content of federal nutrition programs, and second because they are widely invoked by nutrition professionals, journalists and food companies. Advice to eat more of a nutrient can be used by companies to market products. But because 'eat less' advice might turn the public away from products, the Guidelines are inevitably contentious.

The Guidelines were controversial from their inception. In 1990, Congress required the two agencies to review and revise the Guidelines every five years. Each revision requires appointment of an advisory committee to review the research, hold hearings, collect testimony and write a report, and each of these steps is subject to intense lobbying by food companies and trade associations. Food companies nominate candidates for committee positions, submit research reviews on the value of their products to health, testify at hearings, and meet with agency officials to promote the health benefits of their products and the lack of evidence for adverse effects (Nestle 2007).

The politics of the 2005 Guidelines began with the process of nominating committee members. The *Federal Advisory Committee Act* of 1972 requires all such committees to be 'fairly balanced' and not 'inappropriately influenced by … any special interest' (FACA 1972), but the Center for Science in the Public Interest (CSPI), a nutrition advocacy group, charged that seven of the 13 members of the 2005 committee had financial ties to the International Life Sciences Institute, National Dairy Council or other industry groups (CSPI 2003).

Furthermore, the development of the 2005 Guidelines was politicised in unprecedented ways. Unlike previous committees, the 2005 committee was informed that it would not actually write the Guidelines. Instead, agency staff would write the report and recommendations. Moreover, the committee was instructed to take an entirely 'science-based' approach to evaluating research. Whereas previous committees were told to offer advice based on their best interpretation of existing research, the 2005 committee was to make recommendations only if justified by sound and compelling science, a subtle but important distinction. And whereas previous committees reviewed available research as the basis for recommendations, this committee was to create guidelines for diets that would meet DRI **nutrient standards**. These changes must be understood as a reflection of the industry-friendly approach of the administration of

US President George W. Bush as well as of the secrecy and level of control under which it operates and expects its agencies to operate.

The result was that the Guidelines, which are meant for policy makers and health professionals, became the second step of a three-step process. The Guidelines would have to meet the DRI standards; they would then constitute the basis of a food guide for the general public. In recent years, however, the DRIs have become extraordinarily complex. The 1989 10th edition of the Recommended Dietary Allowances (RDAs), now part of the DRIs, was a single volume of just under 300 pages. The recent DRIs, however, comprise six volumes ranging from 432 to 1331 pages each (IOM 1997-2005). As was the case with the RDAs, the DRIs are population standards set at levels likely to meet the needs of virtually all adults and, therefore, greatly exceed the needs of most individuals.

As shown in Table 6.3, the first four editions of the Guidelines included just seven recommendations (these dealt with food variety, body weight, saturated fat and cholesterol, sugar, salt, alcohol, and fruits and vegetables). The 2000 Guidelines added advice about becoming physically active, following the Pyramid food guide, and ensuring food safety (USDA & HHS 2000). The 2005 Guidelines, however, took complexity to a new level. Although the advisory committee decided that its findings supported just nine principal messages (DGAC 2004), the agencies overrode its advice and created 41 recommendations (23 for the general population and 18 for special population groups such as pregnant women and the elderly), and issued the Guidelines as a 70-page pamphlet (USDA & HHS 2005).

Table 6.3 Evolution of the US Dietary Guidelines, 1980–2005

Year	Key recommendations	Content pages
1980	7	19
1985	7	23
1990	7	26
1995	7	41
2000	10	37
2005	41	70

Source: USDA and HHS at www.health.gov/DietaryGuidelines/

Buried in this morass of information—especially in the report's Tables—are important messages: balance calories and be more active; emphasise fruits, vegetables, and whole grains; eat less of animal foods; avoid trans fats; and reduce intake of sugars and 'junk' foods (those of poor nutritional value). These, however, are difficult to distinguish from 'distracter guidelines', those that have little to do with food choices. Whereas the 2000 Guidelines included one recommendation for food

Jennifer Lisa Falbe and Marion Nestle

safety ('keep food safe to eat') and one for physical activity ('be physically active each day'), the 2005 Guidelines contain three lengthy recommendations with five sub-recommendations for food safety, and six equally lengthy recommendations with four sub-recommendations for physical activity (for example, 'To sustain weight loss in adulthood: Participate in at least 60 to 90 minutes of daily moderate-intensity physical activity while not exceeding caloric intake requirements. Some people may need to consult with a healthcare provider before participating in this level of activity'). Political influence is best detected in certain specific Guidelines, as discussed below.

Weight management

Throughout the process of developing the Guidelines, food industry groups repeatedly attempted to divert attention from food to physical activity. The American Beverage Association (2004) said that 'the guidelines should include an increased emphasis on the importance of physical activity for children, adolescents and adults', and the Grocery Manufacturers of America (2004) said, 'If Americans should be striving to improve their diets, then why would the final Report neglect to incorporate physical activity in its tables? Instead, the Report's recommendations should base dietary patterns on—at a minimum—a "low active" level of physical activity…'

Physical activity is critical for maintaining a healthy body weight, but the emphasis on such recommendations distracts attention from 'eat less' messages. Key advice about weight management in the 2005 Guidelines is to 'balance calories from foods and beverages with calories expended', and 'make small decreases in food and beverage calories and increase physical activity'. Just one sentence—not a recommendation—explains that 'the healthiest way to reduce calorie intake is to reduce one's intake of added sugars, fats, and alcohol …'

The Guidelines' advice about portion sizes also has become more complicated. In 1995, USDA and HHS recommended: 'Eat smaller portions and limit second helpings of foods high in fat and calories', and in 2000 said: 'Whatever the food, eat a sensible portion size'. The 2005 advisory committee wrote '… more calories are consumed when a large portion is served rather than a small one. Thus, steps are warranted for consumers to limit the portion size they take or serve to others …' (DGAC 2004). The agencies, however, chose to introduce the concept of portion size with a 'science-based' disclaimer: 'Though there are no empirical studies to show a causal relationship between increased portion sizes and obesity, there are studies showing that controlling portion sizes helps limit calorie intake, particularly when eating calorie dense foods …' (USDA & HHS 2005).

Sugars

The 1980 and 1985 Guideline editions concisely recommended 'avoid too much sugar', but subsequent versions became increasingly complicated, as shown in

Table 6.4. By 2005, the sugar guideline comprised 27 words, required translation (DASH is Dietary Approaches to Stop Hypertension), and was buried in a chapter on carbohydrates. The downplaying of advice to eat less sugar may have been due to the ties of some committee members to sugar industry groups, as charged by CSPI (2003), but was without question a consequence of the WHO sugar controversy discussed earlier. While officials at HHS were challenging the WHO's 10 per cent sugar recommendation, this same agency could hardly permit the Guidelines to say 'eat less sugar'.

Table 6.4   Evolution of the US dietary recommendations for sugars

Dietary guidelines	Sugar guideline or recommendation
1980	Avoid too much sugar
1985	Avoid too much sugar
1990	Use sugars only in moderation
1995	Choose a diet moderate in sugars
2000	Choose beverages and foods to moderate your intake of sugars
2005	Choose and prepare foods and beverages with little added sugars or caloric sweeteners, such as amounts suggested by the USDA Food Guide and the DASH Eating Plan.

Source: USDA and HHS at www.health.gov/DietaryGuidelines/

Meat

Guidance about meat consumption occurs in a chapter on fats. The Advisory Committee (DGAC 2004) noted the relationship between meat, intake of saturated fat and certain cancers in several statements:

- 'The major way to keep saturated fat low is to limit one's intake of animal fat …'
- 'Epidemiologic, experimental (animal), and clinical investigations suggest that diets high in … meat (both red and white) … are associated with an increased incidence of colorectal cancer'
- 'In general, fat of animal origin seems to be associated with the highest risk [of prostate cancer]'.

In commenting on the committee report, CSPI (2004) said that the guidelines ought to say 'eat less … beef, pork … and other foods that are high in saturated fat, trans fat, or cholesterol. People don't eat nutrients, they eat food'. In contrast, the National Cattlemen's Beef Association (2004) commented: 'A message to "choose lean protein sources" offers guidance consistent with the report's [other messages].' The agencies apparently agreed and their advice reads: 'When selecting and preparing meat, poultry, dry beans, and milk or milk products, make choices that are lean, low-fat, or fat-free.' That meat and dairy products are major sources of saturated fat is relegated to a table: 'Contribution of Various Foods to Saturated Fat Intake in the American Diet'.

Dairy foods

The most surprising change from earlier Guidelines was to increase the century-long recommendation of two daily dairy servings to three. The committee and agencies explained this increase as required by a near doubling of the DRI for *potassium* from 2.7 g/day in 1989 to 4.7 g/day (IOM 2004). The IOM said this increase was needed to overcome the effects of high sodium diets on blood pressure, particularly among African-Americans, but this rationale is puzzling on several grounds. The IOM based the increase on the highest amount of potassium needed to compensate for high dietary intake of sodium. However, most individuals would be expected to require much less. Furthermore, while dairy foods are good sources of potassium, they also are high in sodium and are major sources of saturated fat in US diets. Vegetables and fruits are better sources of potassium and are low in sodium. In addition, minority populations most susceptible to high blood pressure often cannot tolerate the lactose in dairy foods, and questions about the role of dairy foods in osteoporosis and other chronic diseases remain unsettled (Willett & Skerrett 2005). Nevertheless, the agencies decided that Americans would be more likely to increase potassium intake by eating more dairy foods. An investigative report by the *Wall Street Journal* attributed this decision to skilful lobbying by the National Dairy Council, as well as to the financial ties of several members of the advisory committee to dairy trade groups (Zamiska 2004).

US MyPyramid Food Guide, 2005

In the third step in the process, the USDA creates a food guide for the general public based on the Dietary Guidelines. This agency's previous Pyramid food guide was issued in 1992 after a year of controversy over its positioning of meat and dairy foods near the 'eat less' tip of the diagram (Nestle 2007). In 2005, the USDA redesigned the Pyramid and renamed it MyPyramid (USDA 2005a). Unlike the previous Pyramid, which was meant to illustrate a dietary pattern appropriate for all Americans, this one was individualised and, therefore, more complicated.

The MyPyramid design is remarkable for its lack of food. Instead, the design illustrates ribbons of colour meant to represent specific food groups. A stick figure runs up a set of stairs along the left side. To understand the meaning of this design, consumers must have access to the internet; log on to the USDA website; type in a few details about age, sex and activity level; and obtain a personalised dietary prescription at one of 12 calorie levels. Careful perusal of the website reveals that the USDA continues to promote hierarchy in food choice: 'The wider base stands for foods with little or no solid fats or added sugars. These should be selected more often. The narrower top area stands for foods containing more added sugars and solid fats' (USDA 2005b). This point, however, is easily missed.

Although influenced by politics, the process for developing the Dietary Guidelines was mostly transparent; transcripts of committee meetings and draft reports appeared promptly on the internet. In contrast, the process used by the USDA to replace its 1992 Pyramid was highly secret, and it is not obvious how agency staff made decisions. One clue comes from Porter Novelli, the public relations firm hired by the USDA to develop both the 1992 and 2005 Pyramids. The firm presented a preliminary design to the Dietary Guidelines Advisory Committee in January 2004. That design looked much like the final version with one critical exception; it illustrated hierarchy in food choice. For example, the grain band displayed whole grain bread at the bottom, pasta about half way up, and cinnamon buns at the top. The USDA chose to eliminate visible hierarchy in the final version. Because the reasons for this decision are not public, one can only presume that the agency did not wish to advise eating less of any food, useful as that advice might be to an overweight public.

Canada's Food Guide, 2007

On 5 February 2007, Health Canada released 'Eating Well with Canada's Food Guide', an update of the previous 1992 version (Health Canada 2007a). Like the US MyPyramid, this Guide offers more complicated and individualised advice and does so for many of the same reasons. Canada's Guide does not replicate MyPyramid but instead must be understood as evolving from previous Canadian Food Guides, particularly the 1992 version. Table 6.5 summarises the principal recommendations of Canadian Food Guides from 1942 to 2007.

Table 6.5   Evolution of Canada's food guide recommendations, daily servings for adults, 19 to 50+ years, 1942–2007

Year	Vegetables & Fruit	Grain Products	Milk & Alternatives	Meat & Alternatives
1942	5	5-7	1	1[†]
1944	5	5	1-2	1[†]
1949	5	5	1	1[†]
1961	5	2	1 ½	1[†]
1977	4-5	3-5	2	2
1982	4-5	3-5	2	2
1992	5-10	5-12	2-4	2-3
2007	7-10	6-8	2-3	2-3

† In addition to eggs

Source: Health Canada (2002 and 2007)

Jennifer Lisa Falbe and Marion Nestle

Like all such guides, this one is intended to improve food selection and promote nutritional health. Canada has issued food guidance since 1942, and the evolution of this advice is notable for an increase in the number of recommended servings. For the first 50 years, the guides were based on a 'foundation diet' approach designed to ensure intake of the minimum amount of food needed to meet the nutritional requirements of most people in the population (Health Canada 2002). In 1992, however, Health Canada switched the basis of the Guide to a 'total diet' approach. This called for diets that would meet energy and nutrient requirements defined by recently established Canadian standards (CIC 1990; Bush & Kirkpatrick 2003). Because these standards are based on research on single nutrients, this approach leads to apparently higher levels that encompass the nutrient needs of most individuals within a population. The 'total diet' approach resulted in advice to consume more food and, therefore, more calories. Although this advice appeared at a time when chronic diseases had replaced nutrient deficiencies as the principal public health problems related to diet, its effect was to double the recommended number of grain servings, more than double the number of vegetable and fruit servings, and increase the number of meat servings by 50 per cent.

Responses to the release of the 1992 Guide indicated substantial food industry influence on its development and content, as revealed in newspaper accounts such as 'Industry Forced Changes to Food Guide …' (Anon. 1993) and 'Food Guide Changed After Industry Outcry' (Evenson 1993). Such accounts were based on documents obtained under Canada's *Access to Information Act* that revealed earlier drafts had been altered in response to protests from beef, egg and sugar producers. The then Minister of National Health and Welfare, Benoit Bouchard (1993), defended the Guide as 'based on sound science' and reflecting the 'total diet' approach: 'There are no good foods or bad foods,' he said. 'It is the overall choices of foods made and not any one food … that determines healthful eating.' Despite this statement, the 1992 Food Guide design—a rainbow—was intended to indicate that some foods *are* better than others and should be eaten in greater quantities; its largest bands were devoted to the grain and vegetables and fruit groups.

A decade later, concerns about rising rates of obesity and chronic diseases suggested the need to revise the Guide (Shields & Tjepkema 2006). The rise in obesity had occurred in parallel with a 14 per cent increase in the calories available in the Canadian food supply (Statistics Canada 2002). Furthermore, Canada had jointly participated with the USA in development of the DRIs and had adopted these standards (Health Canada 2007b). Revising the Food Guide provided an opportunity to reverse the 'eat more' messages of the 1992 version.

To do so, Health Canada conducted a series of consultations and stakeholder sessions, and worked closely with advisory groups (Health Canada 2007b). Critics immediately complained that industry groups appeared to be overrepresented in the process. Invitational stakeholder meetings included far more industry than independent experts (Health Canada 2004a; 2004b). Critics charged that members of advisory committees had ties to food industry groups, had potential conflicts of interest, and lacked independence and expertise (Jeffery 2005; Freedhoff 2006). Although the Ontario Society of Nutrition Professionals in Public Health had nominated potential members, none of its nominees was appointed (Jeffery 2005). Meanwhile, food companies and trade associations hired lobbyists and submitted detailed briefs to ensure that the Food Guide would reflect their interests (Waldie 2007).

In late 2005, Health Canada proposed to decrease the recommended daily servings of fruits and vegetables from 5–10 to 5–8 and to increase servings of meat from 2–3 to 4 for men. This proposal was termed 'obesogenic' by commentators who calculated that following the Guide would produce diets overly high in calories (Kondro 2006). The Dairy Farmers of Canada met with Health Canada to complain that the Guide placed soy milk in the milk category (Payne 2006). How Health Canada dealt with such complaints can only be surmised. Reviewers of early drafts were required to return them, and neither draft guidelines nor transcripts of consultations or committee meetings were posted on the internet.

As published, the 2007 Guide is more complicated than the previous version. The most significant changes from 1992 are an increase in the minimum number of vegetable and fruit servings and a decrease in grain servings. Changes from the 2006 draft were a reduction in the prominence given to soy milk, and elimination of a food shopping tip to 'buy local, regional, or Canadian foods when available'. The final Guide advises consumers to be active, read food labels, limit trans fats, satisfy thirst with water, enjoy eating, and eat well. 'Eat well' includes an 'eat less' message: '[by] limiting foods and beverages high in calories, fat, sugar, or salt (sodium) such as cakes and pastries, chocolate and candies, cookies and granola bars, doughnuts and muffins, ice cream and frozen desserts, soft drinks, sports and energy drinks, and sweetened hot or cold drinks' (Health Canada 2007a). The reasons for such changes, however, are not stated.

Contradictions between the written messages and the illustrations make the Guide difficult to interpret. For example, it recommends 'Drink skim, 1%, or 2% milk each day', and 'Select lower fat milk alternatives', yet illustrates dairy products in their full fat versions. The meat illustrations do not depict red meats at all and exclusively depict meat alternatives such as fish, beans, tofu, eggs, nuts and peanut butter. The explanation of how to count Food Guide Servings is illustrated by a vegetable and beef stir-fry with rice, a glass of milk, and an apple for dessert. This meal includes a total of seven servings from the various groups plus a teaspoon of canola oil. It would take a skilled cook to stir fry 2.5 oz of lean beef and one cup of mixed broccoli, carrot and sweet red pepper in so little oil. These are small points, but potentially confusing.

Like MyPyramid, the Canadian Food Guide personalises the recommendations by creating nine diet categories based on age and gender, each with its unique allotment of servings. Also, like MyPyramid, consumers obtain this information through use of a computer. An interactive website permits users to create 'My Food Guide' (Health Canada 2007c). A woman aged 31 to 50 years, for example, is to select seven servings of vegetables and fruit, six grains, and two each of milk and meat (or alternatives) each day, which may seem like too much food. The site provides examples of foods from which to choose, but these are not distinguished by nutritional quality. One can easily select a diet that contains all of the servings from iceberg lettuce, white breads and waffles, full-fat dairy products, and high-fat red meats.

Finally, the Guide breaks precedent in suggesting that foods alone are insufficient to meet nutritional needs. It advises women capable of becoming pregnant to take a multivitamin with folic acid, pregnant women to take one with iron, and everyone over age 50 to take 400 IU of vitamin D. Advice to take supplements appears to derive from the single-nutrient focus of the DRIs and their establishment at levels that meet or exceed the 97th percentile of population requirements.

Conclusion

Nutrition scientists maintain—quite correctly—that science is complex, that individualisation makes sense for advising people about their own diets, and that dietary standards and dietary guidelines are meant as tools for professionals, not the general public. Because standards and guidelines are the basis of food guides for the general public, they need to be based not only on science but also on the need to communicate basic principles of diet and health to an increasingly confused public. As chronic diseases overtake nutrient deficiencies as public health nutrition problems, dietary guidance should encourage people to optimise eating patterns by clearly stipulating the foods best to eat on a habitual basis. Dietary guidance should also explicitly encourage people to reduce energy intake by eating less of 'junk' foods. Governments should be responsible for providing accurate and sound nutrition advice to their populations; the fact that most have difficulty doing so is an indication of the power of food companies to influence the process. Nutrition and health advocates should be diligent in encouraging governments to issue dietary advice that is clear, unambiguous and useful to the public.

SUMMARY OF MAIN POINTS

- Governments issue dietary guidance to improve the health of their populations.
- Advice to consume more of a country's agricultural and food products in order to prevent nutrient deficiencies is usually uncontroversial.
- Advice to restrict intake of certain foods to prevent obesity and chronic diseases is inevitably controversial.

- Food companies use the political process to weaken, undermine or eliminate dietary guidelines that suggest eating less of their products.
- To avoid controversy, dietary guidelines and food guides tend to reject public health messages; to express advice in terms of nutrients, not foods; and to issue more complicated and individualised advice.
- Despite political pressures, dietary guidelines and food guides invariably recommend diets based mainly on foods of plant origin: vegetables, fruit and whole grains.

SOCIOLOGICAL REFLECTION

Dietary guidelines and food guides, although apparently 'science-based', are created by individuals who serve on government committees and are subject to the same kinds of influences as any other members of society. Because the food industry is the sector of society with the strongest stake in the outcome of dietary guidance, government agencies and committee members are inevitably influenced by its concerns. Controversy over dietary advice derives from the contradiction between the health-promoting goals of public health and the profit-making goals of food companies.

- Consider the language used in the Australian Dietary Guidelines given in Table 6.1. Which of these guidelines would be most resisted by the food industry?
- How do these guidelines compare to those developed in the USA?

DISCUSSION QUESTIONS

1. Why do governments issue dietary guidelines and food guides?
2. Who are the principal stakeholders in the development of dietary guidance?
3. How important are dietary guidelines and food guides? Whose interests do they serve?
4. How do food companies and trade groups influence dietary guidance?
5. How do nutrient standards and dietary guidance illustrate trends towards the increasing complexity and individualisation of dietary advice?
6. How could public health approaches improve the development of dietary guidelines and food guides?

Further investigation

1. Why does public health nutrition policy rely so heavily on dietary guidelines? What alternative approaches could governments use to improve public health?
2. Are dietary guidelines equally useful to affluent and economically disadvantaged groups?

Jennifer Lisa Falbe and Marion Nestle

FURTHER READING AND WEB RESOURCES

Books

Lang, T. & Heasman, M. 2004, *Food Wars: The Global Battle for Mouths, Minds, and Markets*, Earthscan Publications, London.

Nestle, M. 2007, *Food Politics: How the Food Industry Influences Nutrition and Health*, Revised edition, University of California Press, Berkeley.

WHO 2003, *Diet, Nutrition, and the Prevention of Chronic Disease: Report of a Joint WHO/FAO Expert Consultation* (WHO Technical Report Series 916), WHO, Geneva, http://whqlibdoc.who.int/trs/WHO_TRS_916.pdf.

Websites

Canada's Guidelines for Healthy Eating: www.hc-sc.gc.ca/fn-an/food-guide-aliment/index_e.html

Codex Alimentarius (FAO/WHO Food Standards): www.codexalimentarius.net/web/index_en.jsp

Dietary Guidelines for Americans: www.health.gov/DietaryGuidelines/

Dietary Guidelines for Australians: www.nhmrc.gov.au/publications/synopses/dietsyn.htm

Food and Agricultural Organization (FAO)—Nutrition and Consumer Protection: http://www.fao.org/ag/agn/index_en.stm

Food Guides by Country: www.fao.org/ag/agn/nutrition/education_guidelines_country_en.stm

Food Politics: www.foodpolitics.com/

United States Food and Drug Administration (FDA)—Center for Food Safety & Applied Nutrition: www.cfsan.fda.gov/list.html

WHO Global Strategy on Diet, Physical Activity and Health: www.who.int/dietphysicalactivity/en/

REFERENCES

American Beverage Association 2004, 'Comments on the Report of the Dietary Guidelines Advisory Committee' [public comments], ABA, Washington, DC, 1 October, www.health.gov/DIETARYGUIDELINES/dga2005/comments/readComments.htm.

Anon. 1993, 'Industry Forced Changes to Food Guide, Papers Show', *The Toronto Star*, 15 January, p. A2.

Bouchard, B. 1993, 'Food-guide Advice Sound; New Philosophy Takes Broad Approach to Eating Well', *The Gazette*, 7 February, pp. B3.

Briscoe, A.C. 2003, 'Letter to Gro Harlem Brundtland, Director General, World Health Organization', The Sugar Association, Washington, DC, 14 April, www.who.int/dietphysicalactivity/media/en/gsfao_cmr_030414.pdf.

Bush, M. & Kirkpatrick, S. 2003, 'Setting Dietary Guidance: The Canadian Experience', *Journal of the American Dietetic Association*, vol. 103, no. 12, suppl. 1, pp. 22–7.

Cannon, G. 1992, *Food and Health: The Experts Agree*, Consumers' Association, London.

Center for Science in the Public Interest 2003, 'Dietary Guidelines Committee Criticized' [press release], CSPI, Washington, DC, 19 August, www.cspinet.org/new/200308191.html.

—— 2004, 'Comments on the Report of the Dietary Guidelines Advisory Committee' [public comments], CSPI, Washington, DC, 21 September, www.health.gov/DIETARYGUIDELINES/dga2005/comments/readComments.htm.

CIC—*see* Communications/Implementation Committee.

Communications/Implementation Committee 1990, *Action Towards Healthy Eating—Canada's Guidelines for Healthy Eating and Recommended Strategies for Implementation*, Department of National Health and Welfare, Ottawa, www.hc-sc.gc.ca/fn-an/nutrition/pol/action_healthy_eating_tc-action_saine_alimentation_tm_e.html.

CSPI—*see* Center for Science in the Public Interest.

DGAC—*see* Dietary Guidelines Advisory Committee.

Dietary Guidelines Advisory Committee 2004, *Report of the 2005 Dietary Guidelines Advisory Committee*, Washington, DC, September, www.health.gov/dietaryguidelines/dga2005/report.

Duff, J. 2004, 'Setting the Menu: Dietary Guidelines, Corporate Interests and Nutrition Policy', in J. Germov & L. Williams (eds), *A Sociology of Food and Nutrition: The Social Appetite*, 2nd edition, Oxford University Press, Melbourne, pp. 148–69.

Evenson, B. 1993, 'Where's the Beef? Food Guide Change after Industry Outcry', *The Ottawa Citizen*, 15 January, pp. A1.

FACA (*Federal Advisory Committee Act*) 1972. 5 U.S.C. Appendix 2 Sec. 5(b)(2).

Fineberg, H.V. 2003, 'Letter to Tommy Thompson, U.S. Secretary of Health and Human Services' [Letter], 15 April, www.who.int/dietphysicalactivity/media/en/gsfao_cmr_030415.pdf.

Freedhoff, Y. 2006, 'Big Food Has a Seat', *Weighty Matters* [Blog], 12 November, http://bmimedical.blogspot.com/2006/11/big-food-has-seat.html.

Grocery Manufacturers of America 2004, 'Comments on the Report of the Dietary Guidelines Advisory Committee', GMA, Washington, DC, 21 September, www.health.gov/DIETARYGUIDELINES/dga2005/comments/readComments.htm.

Health Canada 2002, *Canada's Food Guides from 1942 to 1992*, Health Canada, Ottawa, http://dsp-psd.pwgsc.gc.ca/Collection/H39-651-2002E.pdf.

—— 2004a, *Review of Canada's Food Guide to Healthy Eating—Stakeholder Session of January 20, 2004*, Health Canada, Ottawa, 20 January, www.hc-sc.gc.ca/fn-an/

food-guide-aliment/review-examen/meet-reunion/stake_meet_cfg-reunion_
part_inter_gac_e.html.

—— 2004b, *January 20th Stakeholder Meeting Participants' List*, Health Canada,
20 January, www.hc-sc.gc.ca/fn-an/alt_formats/hpfb-dgpsa/pdf/food-guide-
aliment/review_list_participants-examen_liste_participants_e.pdf [accessed 1
December 2006].

—— 2007a, *Eating Well with Canada's Food Guide*, Health Canada, Ottawa, www.hc-
sc.gc.ca/fn-an/food-guide-aliment/index_e.html.

—— 2007b, *The Revision Process*, Health Canada, Ottawa, www.hc-sc.gc.ca/fn-an/
food-guide-aliment/context/rev/rev_proc_e.html.

—— 2007c, *My Food Guide*, Health Canada, Ottawa, www.hc-sc.gc.ca/fn-an/food-
guide-aliment/myguide-monguide/index_e.html.

Institute of Medicine 1997–2006, *Dietary Reference Intakes*, National Academies Press,
Washington, DC, www.nap.org.

IOM—*see* Institute of Medicine.

Jeffery, B. 2005, *'Canada's Food Guide'—Promoting Health or Protecting Wealth?*
[Presentation], Centre for Science in the Public Interest Canada (CSPI Canada),
Ottawa, 16 September, at www.cspinet.org/canada/pdf/CanadaFoodGuide.ppt.

Khan, R. 2003, 'Letter to Gro Harlem Brundtland, Director General, World Health
Organization' [Letter], World Sugar Research Organisation, Reading, 25
March, www.who.int/dietphysicalactivity/media/en/gsfao_cmr_030325.pdf.

Kondro, W. 2006, 'Proposed Canada Food Guide called "obesogenic"', *Canadian
Medical Association Journal*, 28 February, vol. 174, no. 5, pp. 605–6.

National Cattlemen's Beef Association 2004, 'Comments on the Report of the Dietary
Guidelines Advisory Committee', Washington, DC, 27 September, www.
health.gov/DIETARYGUIDELINES/dga2005/comments/readComments.htm.

National Health and Medical Research Council 2003, *Dietary Guidelines for Adult
Australians*, Commonwealth of Australia, Canberra, 10 April, www.nhmrc.gov.
au/publications/_files/n33.pdf.

Nestle, M. 2007, *Food Politics: How the Food Industry Influences Nutrition and Health*,
Revised edition, University of California Press, Berkeley.

NHMRC—*see* National Health and Medical Research Council.

Norum, K.R. 2005, 'World Health Organisation's Global Strategy on Diet, Physical
Activity and Health: The Process Behind the Scenes', *Scandinavian Journal of
Nutrition*, vol. 49, no. 2, pp. 83–8.

Payne, E. 2006, 'New Rules for a Fat, Idle Nation: Once a Bible of Nutrition, can a
Single Pamphlet Possibly Satisfy Critics and a Diverse Population?', *Ottawa
Citizen*, 5 March, pp. A8.

Shields, M. & Tjepkema, M. 2006, 'Trends in Adult Obesity', *Health Reports*, Statistics
Canada, Ottawa, August, vol. 17, no. 3, www.statcan.ca/bsolc/english/
bsolc?catno=82-003-X20050039279.

Statistics Canada 2002, 'Food Consumption', *The Daily*, Statistics Canada, Ottawa, 17 October, www.statcan.ca/Daily/English/021017/d021017c.htm.

Steiger, W.R. 2002, 'To Gro Harlem Brundtland, Director General, WHO (World Health Organization)', HHS Office of International Affairs, Washington, DC, 26 April, www.who.int/dietphysicalactivity/media/en/gsfao_cmo_096.pdf.

—— 2004a, 'To J.W. Lee, Director General, WHO', HHS Office of International Affairs, Washington, DC, 2 January, www.commercialalert.org/bushadmin comment.pdf.

—— 2004b, 'To J.W. Lee, Director General, WHO', HHS Office of International Affairs, Washington, DC, 27 February, www.who.int/dietphysicalactivity/media/gseb_usa27feb.pdf.

USDA—*see* US Department of Agriculture.

US Department of Agriculture 1992, *Food Guide Pyramid*, Washington, D.C.

—— 2005a, *MyPyramid*, Washington, DC, www.mypyramid.gov.

—— 2005b, 'Anatomy of MyPyramid', Washington, DC, www.mypyramid.gov/global_nav/media_mypyramid.html.

—— & HHS (US Department of Health and Human Services) 1995, *Nutrition and Your Health: Dietary Guidelines for Americans*, 3rd edition, Washington, DC, www.health.gov/DietaryGuidelines/.

—— & HHS 2000, *Nutrition and Your Health: Dietary Guidelines for Americans*, 4th edition, Washington, DC, www.health.gov/DietaryGuidelines/.

—— & HHS 2005, *Dietary Guidelines for Americans*, 5th edition, Washington, DC, www.health.gov/DietaryGuidelines/.

Waldie, P. 2007, 'Feeding Frenzy; Companies were Quick to Praise the New Canada's Food Guide—If their Products were Included', *The Globe and Mail*, 10 February, pp. F3.

Waxman, A. 2004, 'The WHO Global Strategy on Diet, Physical Activity and Health: The Controversy on Sugar', *Development*, vol. 47, no. 2, pp. 75–82, www.palgrave-journals.com/development/journal/v47/n2/pdf/1100032a.pdf.

—— & Norum, K.R. 2004, 'Why a Global Strategy on Diet, Physical Activity and Health? The Growing Burden of Non-communicable Diseases', *Public Health Nutrition*, vol. 7, no. 3, pp. 381–3.

WHO—*see* World Health Organization.

Willett, W.C. & Skerrett, P.J. 2005, *Eat, Drink, and be Healthy: The Harvard Medical School Guide to Healthy Eating*, Free Press, New York.

World Health Organization 2003a, *Diet, Nutrition, and the Prevention of Chronic Disease: Report of a Joint WHO/FAO Expert Consultation* (WHO Technical Report Series 916), WHO, Geneva, http://whqlibdoc.who.int/trs/WHO_TRS_916.pdf.

—— 2003b, 'Meeting with Industry Associations', World Health Organization, Geneva, 17 June 17, www.who.int/dietphysicalactivity/media/en/gscon_cs_privatesector.pdf.

—— 2004, *Global Strategy on Diet, Physical Activity and Health*, WHO, Geneva, www.
who.int/entity/dietphysicalactivity/strategy/eb11344/strategy_english_web.
pdf.

World Sugar Research Organization 2002, 'Critical Commentary of the Draft Report
of WHO/FAO Joint Consultation "Diet, Nutrition and the Prevention of
Chronic Disease"', 28 May, www.who.int/dietphysicalactivity/media/en/
gsfao_cmo_108.pdf.

Zamiska, N. 2004, 'How Milk Got a Major Boost from Food Panel', *Wall Street Journal*,
30 August.

Zarocostas, J. 2004, 'WHO Waters Down Draft Strategy on Diet and Health', *The
Lancet*, vol. 363, p. 1373.

CHAPTER 7

Functional Foods and Public Health Nutrition Policy

Mark Lawrence and John Germov

OVERVIEW

- What are the public health implications of marketing foods with health claims (known as 'functional foods')?
- What controversies surround the regulation of functional foods and health claims?
- What are the implications of functional foods for individuals, food manufacturers and public health nutrition?

We are increasingly faced with a medicalised food supply, with new products marketed as health-promoting or disease-preventing foods—otherwise known as 'functional foods'. Although there remains no universal definition of functional foods, the term represents the concept that food product innovations can directly influence a person's health. This chapter reviews the controversies associated with the research and development of functional foods and their promotion using health claims, assesses the assumptions that have underpinned their emergence and explores options for the future. The functional food agenda provides a valuable case study of public policy relating to food and health. During a period of food scares and rising rates of obesity and diabetes in developed countries, there is debate over whether government food policy should preferentially seek solutions by protecting social and environmental aspects of the food and nutrition system or by promoting food innovation and marketing. The debate is taking place within a political climate characterised by the global-isation of the food trade, a reduction in public sector health spending, and market deregulation. From a sociological perspective, the functional foods agenda reflects a coalescence of the interests of food manufacturers, medical scientists and government authorities who seek to exert control over the composition and marketing of food. The increasing medicalisation of the food supply is discussed as having significant social implications, of which consumers, health professionals and government authorities should be aware.

Key terms

biomedical	functional foods/	healthism
biotechnology	nutraceuticals	medical–food–
epidemiology	health claims	industrial complex

medicalisation	new nutrition science	probiotic
molecular nutrition	novel foods	public health nutrition
neo-liberalism	nutrigenomics	reductionist
neural tube defects (NTDs)	phytosterols	risk factors

Introduction

> Let your food be your medicine, and your only medicine be your food.
>
> Hippocrates (460–360 BC)

For millennia, people have searched for miracle foods that could make them healthier, enhance performance or protect against disease. In the early 21st century, certain food manufacturers, government agencies and medical scientists argue that advances in food science and **biotechnology** enable the development of specific food products that can help promote health and prevent disease—for example, yoghurts containing **probiotic** organisms that, it is claimed, help improve immunity; and margarines with **phytosterols** that are claimed to lower cholesterol and thus help protect against heart disease. Some stakeholders predict that collectively these types of products will be worth billions of dollars for food manufacturers (Sloan 2002). The most common term used in the literature to refer to these food products is **functional foods** (also known as **nutraceuticals**), though consensus on a definition for the term remains elusive. Generally, a functional food refers to a food product that is claimed to deliver a health benefit beyond providing sustenance. In this chapter we use the term functional foods as a concept to refer to those food product innovations that claim to directly influence a consumer's health.

This focus on the potential for individual food products to promote health and prevent disease stands in stark contrast to conventional **public health nutrition** principles. Public health nutrition is concerned with the nutritional health of populations as a whole. It is holistic in the sense that food and health relationships are explained within the context of dietary patterns that reflect the concepts of balance, variety and moderation. From such a perspective, a nutrition truism is that no food in isolation can promote health or prevent disease (with the exception of breast milk in the first few months of life).

The advent of functional foods presents opportunities and challenges for public health nutrition. Are functional foods improved versions of general purpose foods? Are they simply a marketing ploy for food manufacturers? How do they differ from therapeutic agents? Will they provide solutions to contemporary health concerns such as the obesity epidemic? What is their social and environmental impact? This chapter addresses these questions, beginning with a background to functional foods, followed by an examination of public health nutrition concepts in relation to functional foods. We then consider five functional food case studies and analyse whether they represent a **medicalisation** of food, before making concluding comments about emerging challenges and possibilities for functional foods and public health nutrition policy.

The rise of functional foods

Historically, the development and marketing of food products that claimed special health properties has been fraught with controversy. Unscrupulous food adulteration and fraudulent marketing practices in the nineteenth and early twentieth centuries created the impetus for many modern food regulations to control what were little more than 'snake oil' promotions.

In contemporary times, products that claim to help promote health and prevent or treat disease are usually regulated as therapeutic goods. From a regulatory perspective, there is a continuum between foods and therapeutic goods, with an increasing number of products appearing at the interface, or 'grey' area, between foods and therapeutic goods. For example, in Australia vitamin and mineral supplements are regulated as therapeutic goods, yet when the chemicals in these supplements are added to food products such as confectionery, they are regulated as foods and classified as 'food-type dietary supplements'. Figure 7.1 illustrates the interface between foods and therapeutic goods. The interface is important from a regulatory perspective because the safety assessment and marketing of products varies depending upon which 'side' of the interface the product is located. It is anticipated that functional foods will be regulated as foods, albeit closer to the interface than conventional general purpose foods.

Figure 7.1   The regulatory interface between foods and therapeutic goods

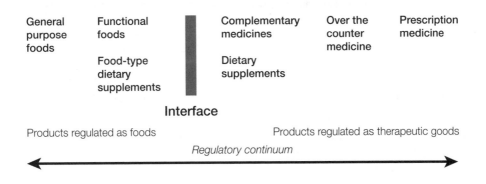

Designer foods are not new—selective breeding and food fortification have existed for some time. However, the increasing sophistication of **molecular nutrition**

and biotechnology is now enabling scientists to investigate, in considerable detail, the functional characteristics of food ingredients and their effects on the human body. Some scientists predict that increased genetic knowledge about humans, diseases and food ingredients, combined with advances in food technology, will make it possible to construct functional foods that prevent and even treat specific diseases (Thomas & Earl 1994). However, other scientists are sceptical of such claims, warning against overly simplistic assumptions that suggest the expansion of our genetic information knowledge-base will so readily translate into health gains (Cole & Comuzzie 2007).

The existence and promulgation of functional foods are dependent upon there being food regulations permitting the use of **health claims** (see Box 7.1) on food product labels and in advertising. Food manufacturers state candidly that if they are not allowed to use health claims to promote the potential health benefits of their products to consumers, research and development of functional foods is unlikely to proceed. In the United States of America, researchers have described health claims as the 'engine that powers' functional food development (Hasler et al. 1995).

BOX 7.1

What is a food-related health claim?

According to the international food standards agency, the Codex Alimentarius Commission (Codex), a health claim 'means any representation that states, suggests, or implies that a relationship exists between a food or a constituent of that food and health' (CAC 2004). Traditionally, countries prohibited the use of health claims on food products based on the fundamental public health nutrition principle that total diet, not individual foods, influences health and illness. Instead, most countries permitted the more general nutrient content claims (for example, 'this product is high in calcium'; 'cholesterol free'; 'low fat'), often on the condition that a nutrition information panel was also included on food packaging that specified levels of energy (kilojoules), protein, saturated and total fats, sugars, total carbohydrate and sodium (salt).

Many countries and international agencies such as Codex are now reviewing their food regulation policies in relation to health claims (Hawkes 2004). In recent years, the USA, Canada, Sweden and Japan have developed regulatory frameworks that permit certain health claims to be made, albeit within strict guidelines. In Australia, discussion on health claims began in the late 1980s, gained momentum after a number of policy documents in the 1990s (see Table 7.1 for a chronology of key events), and culminated in a new food standard: Standard 1.2.7—Nutrition, Health and Related Claims planned for introduction in mid 2008 (see Box 7.2).

Table 7.1 Functional foods and health claims in Australia: Timeline of key developments

1986	The Australian *Food Standards Code* adopted by state and territory governments—includes Standard A1(19), prohibiting health claims.
1988	National Health and Medical Research Council (NHMRC) Nutrition Committee discusses the possibility of reviewing the health claims prohibition.
1991	National Food Authority (NFA) established.
1994	Discussion Paper on Functional Foods (NFA 1994).
1996	Concept Paper on Health and Related Claims (NFA 1996).
1997	NFA renamed the Australia New Zealand Food Authority (ANZFA), reflecting increased cooperation on food regulation between the two countries.
1998	Pilot of new health claim framework—folate/NTD health claim allowed on certain foods.
1999	Evaluation of health claims pilot completed; folate/neural tube defects (NTDs) health claim permission subsequently extended several times to bring it into line with the gazettal of proposed food Standard 1.2.7 in mid-2008.
2001	ANZFA renamed Food Standards Australia New Zealand (FSANZ).
2001	Inquiry Report—Proposal P153: Review of Health and Related Claims (ANZFA 2001) recommends the adoption of new health claims standard allowing health claims to be approved in Australia on a case-by-case basis.
2002	*Australia New Zealand Food Standards Code* comes into full effect on 20 December 2002, ending a transition phase that began in 2000.
2002	Standard 1.1A.2, the Transitional Standard—Health Claims, added to the Australia New Zealand Food Standards Code; initially in place for a two-year transitional period and subsequently extended. The standard incorporates clause 19 of Standard A1 of the old Code, which includes the general prohibition on health claims, with the addition of the pilot folate/ NTD health claim.
2003	The Australian and New Zealand Food Regulation Ministerial Council endorsed a policy guideline for nutrition, health and related claims that includes provisions that, for the first time, permit the use of health claims in Australia and New Zealand. The Ministerial Council then directs FSANZ to develop a Standard to regulate nutrition, health and related claims.
2004	FSANZ prepares, and releases for public consultation, an Initial Assessment Report for Proposal P293—Nutrition, Health and Related Claims that specifies a number of options for managing the introduction of health claims within a food standard.
2005	A draft assessment report for proposal P293 detailing FSANZ's preferred regulatory option as well as a draft Standard 1.2.7—Nutrition, Health and Related Claims to be added to the Food Standards Code is released for further public consultation.
2007	Preliminary Final Assessment Report for Proposal P293 is released for public comment.
2008	Standard 1.2.7—Nutrition, Health and Related Claims to be added to be Food Standards Code.

Sources: FSANZ (2005a; 2007a, b)

Mark Lawrence and John Germov

An analysis of the role of functional foods within public health nutrition policy is invariably vexed because it engages competing views towards the relationship between food and health and competing interests towards food's role as a profitable commodity. The diversity of views towards functional foods as a health commodity range from perceiving them as little more than 'quackery' (Jacobson & Silverglade 1999) to arguing that access to such products is a social right (O'Connell 2001). Some advocates for functional foods have gone so far as to suggest that regulatory restrictions on their promotion may be contributing to health inequalities across society (Williams 1998). However, opponents express concern that the marketing

BOX 7.2

The proposed Australia and New Zealand health claims framework

A food regulation, entitled Standard 1.2.7—Nutrition, Health and Related Claims, will be added to the Australia New Zealand Food Standards Code in 2008. It includes three levels of claims:

1. 'Nutrient content claims': describe the presence or absence of a nutrient in a food product (for example, 'This food is high in iron').
2. 'General level health claims': describe the function of a food component in terms of its effect on the body (for example, 'This food is high in calcium, which is good for strong bones'; 'This food gives you energy'; 'This food may improve gut function and reduce the risk of an upset stomach').
3. 'High level health claims': describe the function of a food component in relation to a serious disease (for example, 'This food is high in X, which as part of a diet low in saturated fat and high in soluble fibre may reduce your risk of heart disease') or a biomarker of a serious disease (for example, 'This food is low in sodium. A diet low in sodium may assist to reduce blood pressure'). The claims can refer to risk reduction, illness reduction or health improvement.

All claims must be scientifically substantiated and all food products must contain a sufficient amount of the specified component to achieve the claimed benefit. Claims are not permitted on alcohol and infant food products. Nutrient content and general level health claims will not require premarket approval by Food Standards Australia New Zealand (FSANZ), but must be supported by evidence in the scientific literature and must meet specified qualifying criteria. High level health claims must be preapproved by FSANZ, after which they will be added to the food Standard. FSANZ has already substantiated the following five diet–disease relationships that are likely to form the basis of initial high level health claims:

BOX 7.2

- consumption of foods with low amounts of sodium (with or without potassium) may help to prevent hypertension
- increased consumption of fruit and vegetables may help to prevent coronary heart disease
- foods with low levels of saturated fat and/or trans fat may prevent increases in serum cholesterol or reduce the risk of heart disease
- foods with certain amounts of calcium (with or without vitamin D) may prevent osteoporosis
- foods with folic acid may prevent **neural tube defects**.

It is worth noting that the inclusion of fruit and vegetables in the above list was only made in response to the submissions of public health bodies, who pointed out that earlier drafts had an inordinate focus on processed foods (which are clearly of interest to the food industry).

Source: FSANZ (2007a)

of such products is based on scaremongering in that it panders to consumer anxiety about food and health relationships and creates confusion by blurring the distinction between food and drugs. Conversely, proponents of functional foods believe that they offer consumers increased choice for selecting a healthy diet and that health claims are a legitimate nutrition education tool, which will help to inform consumers of the health benefits of certain food products.

From a food industry perspective, functional foods represent the creation of a food category for product differentiation, 'value-adding', sales growth and ultimately increased profit (Childs 1998). It is estimated that the global functional food market is worth US$30–50 billion and is growing at a rate of 8 to 14 per cent per year (Euromonitor 2004). The arguments that are presented in support of functional foods generally include: that there is scientific evidence that food may provide health benefits beyond nutritive value; greater social emphasis on personal responsibility for health, escalating health care expenditure (particularly in the context of an ageing population); the potential for food industry development and export dollars (see Invest Australia 2007); and increasing consumer interest in the relationships between diet and disease.

When setting legally binding standards (rules), most national food standards agencies are required to abide by a primary objective that is to protect public health and safety. Some agencies argue that their role also includes intervening proactively for the benefit of public health and safety. For example, according to FSANZ, 'While any individual or organisation can apply to amend the Food Standards Code, the vast majority of changes are initiated by the food industry, or by FSANZ itself in the interests of public health and safety' (FSANZ 2007c). Hence, it might be expected that during the development of a standard for health claims (and by extension, functional foods) any potential public health and safety concerns would be taken into account.

The challenge for food standards agencies is that the objective 'to protect public health and safety' has not been defined and hence is open to interpretation. This lack of definition means that the decision-making process for setting food standards is vulnerable to political influence. This vulnerability has been especially pronounced since the 1990s when the food regulatory systems of most countries with advanced economies have operated within a **neo-liberal** climate of reduced public sector expenditure and deregulation. It is not uncommon for certain food manufacturers to lobby for a liberalisation of food regulations, such as the prohibition on health claims, which they perceive as restricting their ability to market their food products.

How do we make sense of these competing views and claims about functional foods? How might functional foods be regulated to help promote public health nutrition while protecting public health and safety? In the next section of this chapter we outline what is public health nutrition and the contrasting paradigms that shape its policy and practice. The purpose of this outline is to provide a framework against which expectations for functional foods might be placed in perspective.

Contrasting paradigms of public health nutrition

Public health nutrition has been defined in the constitution of the World Public Health Nutrition Association as:

> The promotion and maintenance of nutrition related health and well-being of populations through the organised efforts and informed choices of society (Barcelona Declaration 2006).

Public health nutrition (and the work of public health nutritionists) is described and discussed in detail in Chapter 8.

The contemporary understanding of public health nutrition policy and practice is being developed by research activities pursued within the context of two contrasting paradigms:

- **new nutrition science**
- molecular nutrition.

In 2005, a workshop was held at the University of Giessen, Germany, to agree on principles, definitions and dimensions of the 'new nutrition science'. Emerging from the workshop was *The Giessen Declaration*, which proposes a holistic foundation for a new approach towards nutrition science as a whole, defined as:

> the study of food systems, foods and drinks, and their nutrients and other constituents; and of their interactions within and between all relevant biological, social and environmental systems. The purpose of nutrition science is to contribute to a world in which present

and future generations fulfil their human potential, live in the best of health, and develop, sustain and enjoy an increasingly diverse human, living and physical environment (The Giessen Declaration 2005, p. 786).

The new nutrition science is holistic in the sense that it is informed by an analysis of the food and health relationship based on integrating social and environmental dimensions, with the 'classical' biological dimension. The Declaration was published as part of a whole issue dedicated to the new nutrition science in the journal *Public Health Nutrition* (Cannon & Leitzmann 2005) and continues to be the subject of significant debate in that and other journals. By integrating a sociological and environmental perspective into nutritional science, *The Giessen Declaration* marks a major shift away from nutrition science's **biomedical** and **reductionist** traditions. However, it is worth pointing out that such a perspective has been advocated by other commentators, including the editors of this book(!) (see Germov & Williams 1999; 2004), since the mid 1990s (see Germov & Williams 1996; Germov 1997).

The new nutrition science is a formal recognition of public health nutrition interventions that have attempted to address the social, economic and cultural circumstances in which people live (see Lawrence & Worsley 2007). This is illustrated by the fact that populations with lower socioeconomic status suffer a disproportionate burden of ill health and disease (Wilkinson & Marmot 2006; Townsend et al. 1992). Therefore, interventions to promote the health of populations need to address the underlying social, economic and cultural determinants of health. The priority interventions are those that aim to ensure access to affordable, nutritious and safe food.

By contrast, molecular nutrition refers to the science that extends our knowledge of nutrition-related molecular, cellular and genomic mechanisms. The completion of the Human Genome Project has raised expectations among some scientists that genetic variants responsible for the expression of complex phenotypes (the manifestation of multiple genes interacting with environmental stimuli), including those associated with diet-related diseases such as obesity, diabetes and heart disease, will be identified. Proponents of the burgeoning discipline of **nutrigenomics**, which examines the relationship between nutrients and genetics, speculate that it will not be too long before knowledge about the human genome can be applied to assess an individual's dietary requirements (IFIC 2006). Some researchers go so far as to predict that such knowledge will be applied to the development of specially formulated food products tailored to an individual's needs to help treat disease (Debusk et al. 2005).

Molecular nutrition is an inherently reductionist approach to the investigation of food and health relationships. From this perspective, food is viewed as a composite of chemical constituents and its importance lies in the impact it has on the physiological functioning of individual bodies (Cannon & Leitzmann 2005), and is thus abstracted from its social, cultural and political context. Yet, public health

Mark Lawrence and John Germov

nutrition conceptualises the population as an integrated whole, with interventions addressing social and environmental dimensions. Therefore, the capacity of molecular nutrition to make substantial impacts on public health nutrition is not immediately apparent. Stakeholders who subscribe to molecular nutrition as a basis for improving population health regard public health nutrition, in a narrow sense, as the sum of the health of individuals. Subsequently, public health nutrition interventions based on molecular nutrition aim to address individuals' physiological **risk factors** and genetic disposition associated with disease, by focusing on changing dietary intake. In this context, food is regarded as a commodity that may be modified to assist the dietary reform process and as such it is claimed functional foods will contribute to the development of a healthier food supply, and by consequence, healthier individuals.

Extrapolating scientific evidence from one paradigm to another can be problematic and may falsely raise expectations. For example, caution is needed in applying the findings of molecular nutrition research based on trials on individuals to generate public health nutrition policy intended for the total population. This is because scientific findings that are established under controlled experimental or clinical settings do not necessarily directly translate to the 'real world', where people consume varied diets and adopt a wide range of lifestyles. It is with this precaution in mind that the likely impact of functional foods should be considered.

Case studies of functional food

The functional foods agenda is raising both expectations and concerns among different stakeholders about risks and benefits for public health nutrition. In this section we critically analyse the concept of functional foods against public health nutrition policy principles. The analysis is conducted by examining five case studies: folic acid, psyllium, phytosterols, the fortification of fruit juice with calcium, and the endorsement of certain McDonald's meals by the National Heart Foundation (NHF) in Australia.

Folic acid fortified foods and neural tube defects (NTDs)

Folate is one of the water-soluble B group vitamins. Folic acid is the synthetic form of the vitamin that is used in nutrient supplements and food fortification. During the 1980s and 1990s, the findings from 13 of 14 **epidemiological** trials provided compelling evidence that an increase in a mother's folic acid intake during the 'periconceptional period' (one month before through to three months after conception) may help reduce the risk of her giving birth to a baby with an NTD (for example, Medical Research Council 1991; Czeizel & Dudas 1992). The actual biological mechanism that underlies this protective action is not yet understood. It would appear that increased exposure to a 'dose' of synthetic folic acid is likely to be compensating for a congenital defect affecting a biochemical pathway involved in folate metabolism in certain susceptible women. Effectively, the folic acid is acting more as a therapeutic agent than as a conventional nutrient. Hence, food products fortified with folic acid might be considered to be prime examples of foods with specific functional properties.

There are challenges for policy makers in translating the epidemiological findings about the relationship between folic acid and NTDs into public health nutrition policy. First, the genetic condition that predisposes some women to giving birth to a baby with an NTD is not fully understood and cannot be detected. Second, a significant proportion of pregnancies are unplanned. Third, the neural tube closes by approximately the end of the fourth week after conception, a period during which many women may be unaware that they are pregnant and do not realise they needed to increase their exposure to folic acid. Consequently, those interventions that may best target individuals—nutrition education and the promotion of folic acid-supplement consumption—may not achieve maximum coverage. By contrast, folic acid fortification of staple food products is likely to reach most individuals at risk. However, such fortification exposes everyone in the population to raised levels of folic acid in the food supply.

The policy response of several governments to the epidemiological evidence has been to encourage folic acid fortification of staple foods (voluntary or mandatory) to reduce the risk of NTDs. This policy has created a unique opportunity for proponents of functional foods and health claims. For example, in Australia in November 1998, these developments resulted in an exemption being made to the existing prohibition on health claims to permit a pilot study of a folate-NTD health claim (ANZFA 1998). The use of a health claim to complement the voluntary folic acid fortification intervention was intended, first, to assist the targeted individuals by informing them of the benefit of consuming fortified products and, second, to provide manufacturers with an incentive to implement government policy (where fortification is a voluntary recommendation) and invest in research and development (USDHHS 1996; Lawrence 1997). A further proposed benefit was that it may help to mitigate the concern that fortification is a non-specific intervention; a health claim on a folic acid fortified food product could inform those individuals who wish to avoid such products. Eight years after the introduction of the folate-NTD health claim in Australia, the intervention was being poorly implemented with just two food products using the health claim (Lawrence 2006). Yet, the folate-NTD health claim intervention was hailed a success and used as evidence to support the removal of the prohibition on health claims in Australia and New Zealand (FSANZ 2007a).

Neural tube defects are a relatively rare condition in most countries including Australia, where it is estimated there are approximately 350 cases each year (FSANZ

2006). Nevertheless, NTDs are especially tragic for affected individuals and their families. These circumstances raise ethical issues for policy making in relation to attempting to protect at-risk individuals at the same time as avoiding exposing the population as a whole to raised levels of folic acid, and possible other health risks. Potential health risks associated with increased exposure to folic acid for the population as a whole include promoting the progression of colorectal cancer (Van Guelpen et al. 2006; Cole et al. 2007), masking the symptoms of vitamin B12 deficiency (Savage & Lindenbaum 1995) and increasing the likelihood of multiple births (Lumley et al. 2003). Given the scientific and ethical uncertainties associated with raised exposure to folic acid it was alarming that in June 2007 the Australia New Zealand Food Regulation Ministerial Council approved the mandatory fortification of all wheat flour for bread-making with folic acid (with an exemption for organic wheat products). What is essentially a population-wide intervention is being used to address a medical condition in a relatively small number of at-risk individuals (Lawrence 2003).

Psyllium and risk of coronary heart disease

Psyllium is a rich source of soluble fibre and has been included as an ingredient in some breakfast cereals. Feeding trials have indicated that a psyllium-based breakfast cereal reduced cholesterol levels by approximately 9 per cent when consumed as part of a low-fat diet (Anderson et al. 1988; Greenberg et al. 1994). A food manufacturer urged the US Food and Drug Administration (FDA) to allow the following health claim regarding the relationship between psyllium and coronary heart disease (CHD) (USDHHS 1993a): 'Low-fat diets that include foods high in soluble fiber from psyllium may help lower blood cholesterol levels, which are among the risk factors for heart disease'.

The following questions are raised by this scientific data, and by any health claims resulting from it:

1. How relevant are the findings to the majority of the population? The feeding trials involved middle-aged men who were hypercholesterolaemic (that is, had a high cholesterol level). Is it appropriate to extrapolate these findings to men who are not hypercholesterolaemic, or to women? Is it desirable to expose children to products that might lower their cholesterol levels?
2. Are there special considerations that need to be taken into account? The studies reported that between three and five serves of the breakfast cereal per day were required to achieve the 9 per cent reduction in cholesterol levels.

Despite these unresolved issues, in early 1998 the FDA approved a health claim stating that the consumption of grain products that contain psyllium may help to reduce the risk of heart disease.

Phytosterols and cholesterol reduction

Phytosterols (plant stanol or sterol esters) are not naturally occurring components in edible vegetable oils. Phytosterols were initially approved for use in Australia in a limited range of edible oil spreads (margarines). Evidence from clinical trials indicates that high doses of plant sterols or stanols may lower serum cholesterol concentrations by 8–15% (Law 2000). Phytosterols reduce serum cholesterol by inhibiting the absorption of dietary cholesterol. The dietary phytosterol contribution from edible oil spreads required to lower cholesterol levels is significantly higher than would otherwise typically be consumed. Edible oil spreads with added phytosterols are primary candidates for health claims (and classification as functional foods).

Among the strongest advocates in Australia for the use of phytosterol related food products to protect against heart disease is the Commonwealth Scientific and Industrial Research Organisation (CSIRO). The CSIRO's Food Futures Flagship program receives support for conducting research and the promotion of such food innovations through its collaborative work with food manufacturers as well as being allocated government funding. According to the CSIRO, 'Sterol-fortified margarine trials conducted by the Centre confirmed that LDL or "bad" cholesterol can be reduced by up to 10 per cent within three weeks. To optimise this effect however, an individual would have to eat at least 20g or four teaspoons of sterol-fortified margarine a day' (CSIRO 2007). This risk-based approach to reducing heart disease stands in contrast to the work of Syme (2007) who points out that, even when all known risk factors for heart disease, including smoking, high blood pressure and blood cholesterol, are taken into account the majority of heart disease cases remain unexplained.

There are safety concerns about exposure to high levels of dietary phytosterols (see Baker et al. 1999). In addition, public health practitioners have raised concerns about the broader public health implications of the marketing and widespread use of such expensive and highly processed food products. They also highlight the contradictions implicit in promoting a high-fat product as a commodity that will help reduce risk of heart disease when high fat intakes are associated with obesity, itself a risk factor for heart disease.

In June 2001, the Australia New Zealand Food Regulation Ministerial Council approved vegetable oil-derived plant sterol esters as a **novel food** ingredient in edible oil spreads and required that such products carry an advisory statement. The advisory statements should recommend that 'these products are not appropriate for infants, children and pregnant and lactating women and that people using cholesterol reducing medication should seek medical advice before using the spreads' (FSANZ 2001a). Permission was recently extended for the use of the phytosterol esters in a broader range of foods products, such as fibre-increased bread, low-fat milk and low-fat yoghurt.

Mark Lawrence and John Germov

Food products with added phytosterols sit in the grey area between food and drugs (see Figure 7.1). On the one hand, they have the appearance of a food product; on the other hand, they have been developed to serve a physiological role beyond the provision of nutrients. The achievement of this physiological role requires a dosage and advisory statement of usage. Food products with added phytosterols represent an example of the potential benefits and risks associated with functional foods. Although there is no evidence that such products offer any health benefit to the population at large, or to individuals who do not have raised cholesterol levels, they may (as a component of a healthy diet) provide some medical benefit to individuals with raised cholesterol levels. From a public health and safety perspective, the regulation of food products with added phytosterols needs to ensure that the potential risks do not outweigh the potential medical benefits for certain individuals.

Calcium fortified fruit juice to help prevent osteoporosis—chalk and cheese?

In December 2001, FSANZ received an application (A424) from Nutrinova Australasia and Arnott's Biscuits Ltd requesting a variation be made to the Food Standards Code to permit the voluntary addition of calcium to a variety of foods such as fruit and/or vegetable juices to 25% Recommended Dietary Intake/reference quantity (FSANZ 2005b); a level that allows a 'good source' nutrient content claim.

The application highlights issues at the heart of the tension between food innovation and public health nutrition interests in the functional foods debate. The applicant argued that changes to the Food Standards Code would support food innovation to produce functional food-type products that could provide a public health nutrition service. The argument was that such food innovation would offer more opportunity for consumers to achieve nutrition reference standards for calcium intake. However, not all stakeholders believed that it was appropriate public health nutrition policy to permit these products. The opposition centred on concerns that:

- there was a lack of evidence of the need for increased dietary calcium consumption among the population
- fruit juices contain high levels of sugar and are associated with increasing dental caries and obesity among children
- dairy products may be substituted with fruit/vegetable juices, resulting in dietary imbalances of essential nutrients found in dairy products, especially protein, calcium, riboflavin and vitamin D in children.

The application proved to be controversial and its consideration extended over the next five years. Over 30 different stakeholders made submissions to FSANZ during the public consultation periods. Most public health and consumer organisations and professionals opposed the application. Most submissions from food manufacturers

Table 7.2   Stakeholder arguments for and against calcium fortification of fruit juices

Main arguments against fortification	Main arguments for fortification
Food supply already contains sufficient products that are naturally rich sources of calcium. There is a lack of evidence of calcium deficiency among the population.	Provide alternative sources of calcium for consumers.
Lack of evidence of efficacy and represents a 'band-aid' solution to a multifactorial public health nutrition concern.	Will aid in the prevention of osteoporosis.
Excessive consumption of fruit juice is associated with the onset of other chronic health problems (dental caries and obesity).	Will address population groups who are low consumers of dairy products.
Is inconsistent with existing dietary guidelines and may cause consumer confusion and dietary distortions.	Current labelling requirements and consumer knowledge is sufficient to ensure dairy substitution does not occur.
Proposed food vehicles are non-traditional and therefore the bioavailability of calcium in these products is unknown.	Nutrient claims will provide sufficient information.

supported the application. The respective arguments for and against voluntary calcium fortification of fruit and/or vegetable juices are listed in Table 7.2.

On 11 October 2005, an amended food standard that permitted wider permissions for calcium fortification of fruit and/or vegetable juices was gazetted and became law. In approving these changes to the Food Standards Code, FSANZ stated the following reasons that illustrate how the tension between food innovation and protecting public health nutrition was assessed:

- there was a lack of evidence of harm of calcium fortified fruit juices (food manufacturers were not required to demonstrate evidence of a need for calcium fortification and harm was measured in terms of relatively immediate toxicological risks, rather than considering potential longer-term nutrition risks among the population and children in particular)
- the food standards code permits other food products, such as breakfast cereals, to be fortified with calcium
- it will bring Australia in line with other countries and has the potential to open up new markets for industry (FSANZ 2005b).

What this case study highlights in relation to the relationship between functional foods and public health nutrition policy is that:

- The decision was based on a technical analysis of toxicological risks associated with their use (and nothing found).

- A policy approach of 'no harm' complemented with risk management prevails over the need for evidence of efficacy.
- The risk management approach appears hollow given the lack of nutrition surveillance and investment in nutrition education.
- Broader health concerns were not considered, particularly given recent evidence linking fruit juice consumption with obesity (Sanigorski et al. 2007).

Functional meals? The National Heart Foundation endorsement of McDonald's meals

Since the 1990s there has been an increasing number of endorsement activities promoting food products and meals to consumers. One of the most well-known endorsement programs in Australia has been the National Heart Foundation's (NHF) 'Tick Program'. The Tick Program enables food manufacturers and food service establishments to submit products to the NHF for approval against specified nutrition standards such as level of salt in a reference quantity. Once the food producer has paid the required licence fee, those submitted products or meals that meet the standards are permitted to display the Tick symbol as an NHF endorsement that the products or meals are consistent with its health criteria.

Implicitly, the NHF's Tick endorsement program relates to the functional foods agenda. Broadly speaking, the nutrition standards used in the Tick Program are based on dietary guideline concepts (see Chapter 6). Also, the objective for the program is to shift consumers' choices within food categories in the direction of the dietary guidelines (for example, from a fatty meat to a less fatty meat). However, in contrast to conventional public health nutrition approaches, the program focuses on endorsing individual foods or meals, rather than total diets. In addition, concerns have been expressed about the program's reliance upon a licensing fee that creates the potential for distortions in the public health message. For example, two products with an identical composition might be perceived differently by consumers if one has paid for and then displayed the Tick symbol and the other has chosen not to pay the licence fee for the symbol. Such endorsement programs privilege larger food companies that can better afford the expense of the licence fee.

One of the more controversial aspects of the Tick Program is its linkage with McDonald's restaurants. In early 2007 McDonald's Australia announced it had paid the NHF a licence fee of $330 000 in return for endorsing nine 'Tick-approved' meals at its restaurants. Each of these endorsed meals contains less than 2 per cent saturated fat, virtually no trans fat, at least one serve (75g) of vegetables and provides less than a third of a person's daily energy needs (NHF 2007). According to the NHF, McDonald's spent 12 months modifying its recipes and meal combinations to comply with the NHF standards and 'With more than one million customers through the doors of McDonald's every day, these changes result in real improvements to public health' (NHF 2007).

Dr Mukesh Haikerwal, the then president of the Australian Medical Association (AMA), wondered if the NHF had been naïve in this partnership arrangement and effectively enabled its name to be exploited to buy good public relations for McDonald's while at the same time tarnishing its own image (*The Age* 2007a). However, David Lloyd, the chief operating officer at the Baker Heart Research Institute in Melbourne, saw no such conflict when he said, 'There's not much point going into the lion's den and then announcing you won't deal with lions. Chances are they'll eat you and your principles for dinner.' Instead, he said the problem with the licensing arrangement was that 'the leverage the foundation undoubtedly had over McDonald's in these discussions appears to have been spent for so little gain (for funding for education and research programs)' (*The Age* 2007b). Previously, McDonald's had introduced salad meals as healthier alternatives for its customers. While the sales of the salads were impressive, the sales of high fat, salt and sugar products apparently has not changed significantly, suggesting that such programs create a halo effect for McDonald's whereby many consumers do not distinguish the endorsement of specific products from an endorsement for the restaurant chain overall. Indeed, one study found that around one-third of people misinterpreted the Tick logo, and 14 per cent of men and 5 per cent of women thought foods with the tick logo could be consumed without limitation (Mhurchu & Gorton 2007).

Towards the medicalisation of food

The functional foods agenda presents a novel challenge to public health nutrition. There are few precedents upon which to base an assessment of whether it is likely to have public health and safety consequences. The main concern we raise in this chapter relates to the general theme of 'medicalising' the food supply—producing and marketing food that approximates drugs—and the possible detrimental implications this has for population health.

Peter Conrad (1992) defines 'medicalisation' as the process of adopting medical terminology and treatment for non-medical, social problems. The medicalisation of food involves treating food like a drug with therapeutic properties in order to prevent disease. Such a view represents a pathologised and reductionist approach to public health nutrition. A preoccupation with the consumption of individual foods for their hypothetical health benefits ignores the fact that disease causation is multifactorial and the outcome of wider social influences. Therefore, universal claims of the health benefits resulting from consumption of functional foods are oversimplified and give a misleading message by overemphasising dietary risk factors at the expense of others (for example, smoking and hypertension are also risk factors for heart disease). As Tillotson bluntly admits, 'the overriding purpose of the claim is commercial—to sell a *food product*. Any collateral public health or consumer education that occurs is necessarily secondary' (Tillotson 2003, p. 60, original italics).

Mark Lawrence and John Germov

If government authorities were really serious about the role of food in health and disease (rather than in promoting food as a lucrative industry), they would also consider 'disease claims' on food products. If the policy rationale for health claims is about achieving public health goals, then why not introduce warning statements about the potential disease outcomes of consuming certain food products, such as those high in fat, salt and sugar? If the manufacturers of certain food products are permitted to make dietary-guideline-type claims, it would appear logical to mandate that manufacturers also include 'disease claims' on their labels where there is evidence that a product may be inconsistent with dietary-guideline recommendations. An example of a possible disease claim could be: 'This food is high in salt; high salt foods eaten frequently are a risk factor for hypertension'.

The other implicit message of the functional food-health claims agenda is what Richard Crawford (1980) refers to as **healthism**; a belief that health attainment and maintenance should be primary human values. The key philosophical principle underpinning healthism is self-responsibility. This belief is based on an idealised 'health consumer' who, in this case, consciously responds to health education messages by modifying his/her individual food choices. Such a conceptual model does not account for the manipulation of 'choices' or for obstacles to exercising choice, such as the social inequalities suffered by marginalised groups (especially given functional foods are likely to be marketed as premium, and thus high-priced goods, restricting access for low socioeconomic groups). It is not difficult to envisage a not too distant future of victim-blaming individuals for not choosing to consume appropriate functional foods.

The functional foods–health claims agenda reflects a coalescence of the interests of food manufacturers, pharmaceutical companies, some medical scientists and government agencies who seek to exert control over the composition and marketing of food. The impetus for governmental support appears to be the potential economic gain, particularly the export dollars that the pundits predict the development of functional foods will bring, as well as the alleged long-term savings in health care costs. Together these stakeholders constitute a new **'medical–food–industrial complex'**.

Scientific substantiation will be essential to the success of functional foods and health claims, with a considerable amount of trust placed with food manufacturers to act ethically and abide by the regulations (see Box 7.3 for a cautionary tale). Invariably, substantiation is conducted within a biomedical setting, in which findings relate to risk factors in individuals; while the broader public health impact is generally not studied or considered. As Alan Petersen and Deborah Lupton (1996) point out, medical and epidemiological findings are often oversimplified by the media, corporations and health authorities, such that tentative conclusions come to be presented to the public as unquestionable 'facts'. Yet the relationship between food and health is complex, and thus does not lend itself to simple cause-and-effect explanations.

As the Ribena scandal highlights, one of the fundamental issues in the debate over functional foods is the difference in ethical standards of the marketing and

The Ribena scandal: Can we trust the claims of food manufacturers?

BOX 7.3

Ribena is a blackcurrant-based fruit juice made by the multinational pharmaceutical company GlaxoSmithKline (GSK). For decades Ribena was marketed to parents as a healthy and nutritious drink for children based on the claim that blackcurrants in Ribena had four times the vitamin C of oranges. In 2004, a science project undertaken by two 14-year-old school girls from New Zealand put the claim to the test and found that the level of vitamin C was barely detectable. After approaches to the company by the students were unsuccessful, a TV program reported the story, which spread worldwide in 2007. The company was fined around $200 000 dollars for misleading and deceptive advertising, issued a public apology, and revised its marketing claims (see ACCC 2007; Commerce Commission 2007). In its public apology, GSK claimed it had been unaware that the testing method used as the basis of the vitamin C claim had been unreliable (GlaxoSmithKline 2007).

The marketing of the product played on parents' health anxieties, based on unproven assertions that high vitamin C consumption promoted well-being. Furthermore, many fruit drinks are also high in sugar and low in fibre and nutrients. Daily requirements of vitamin C can be obtained by consuming two serves of fruit and five serves of vegetables per day. Given the many years over which the unproven claims were promoted, the Ribena scandal provides a cautionary lesson about poor compliance with food labelling regulation. Also, it highlights the lack of monitoring that is undertaken in the marketplace. It was not until the two school girls conducted the relatively straightforward experiment that the false claims were exposed, and even then it was several more years before enforcement was exercised. Without effective monitoring and independent testing, a proliferation of health claims in ensuing years may have to rest on the old maxim—'buyer beware'.

science communities (Miller 1991). An Australian survey of health claims made on food company websites found a number of clear breaches of the Food Standards Code, suggesting which existing monitoring efforts are ineffective, and indicating the potential for exaggerated or unapproved claims (Dragiecevich et al. 2006). Public health researchers have reported that some sections of the community are becoming sceptical about diet and health messages, and that in some cases a backlash against dietary recommendations has been observed (Patterson et al. 2001). Nevertheless, marketing analysts provide many examples of food products, such as grape juice and breakfast cereal, which have shown a significant increase in sales when a health claim has been displayed on their food label (Leighton 2002).

Functional foods with health claims are not a panacea given that their use in the USA since the early 1990s has shown little positive impact on diet-related disease.

Mark Lawrence and John Germov

The food label is just one tool that can complement public health nutrition initiatives. While some consumers assiduously read food labels, studies have shown many others are clearly overwhelmed and confused when confronted with the bewildering array of messages, often couched in technical language (Cowburn & Stockley 2005; Mhurchu & Gorton 2007). The danger is that the marketing of functional foods will oversimplify the diet–disease link in the public mind, providing a false sense of security in terms of protection against disease.

There are many aspects of the relationship between food and health that remain poorly understood. It is premature to start predicting the public health impact of novel changes to the food supply. The reduction of public health nutrition to the analysis of how single foods or nutrients may influence population health is problematic, since the introduction of one intervention can have broader and more profound effects, particularly by distorting nutrient metabolism. For example, the interaction between nutrients may affect their bio-availability (the amount of nutrients that are absorbed), as occurs when excessive calcium intake interferes with iron absorption (Hallberg et al. 1992).

Functional foods can play a valid role in clinical practice when recommended to patients as a component of a prescribed therapeutic diet. Rather than blindly supporting or resisting functional foods, we propose that a third way in this debate is possible, based on establishing a secure framework within which manufacturers could pursue research and development, while protecting public health and safety. This can be achieved by food regulators placing the functional foods–health claims agenda into a coherent public health nutrition policy perspective. Specifically, the concept of functional foods, and specific products such as margarines with added phytosterols, should be conceptualised as sitting in the 'grey area' between food and drugs (as shown in Figure 7.1). We suggest that foods with such potential therapeutic benefits should be regulated as therapeutic products (just like medicines), rather than as foods per se. Conceptualising such products as existing at the interface of foods and drugs provides a relevant perspective for anticipating their public health efficacy and preparing regulatory measures to protect public health and safety, provide consumer information and prevent misleading conduct.

Conclusion: Challenges and possibilities

Public health nutrition policy is frequently required to contend with the competing agendas of food innovation and the protection of public health and safety; this is no more evident than in the debate over functional foods and health claims. Functional foods represent food innovations that, it is claimed, will help prevent disease and promote health. As such, the functional foods agenda presents one of the most complex and political public health nutrition policy debates confronting governments today. It engages the competing values, interests and beliefs of different stakeholders about the relationship between food and health. Intense lobbying of government by the food industry to permit health claims, the promise of huge profits, the scepticism of consumer groups and public health activists, and the consequent need for research and government regulation, have resulted in heated debate. At a technical level, the debate concerns the safety of such products for the population as a whole, as well as their efficacy in terms of the appropriateness of applying medical research data, most often derived from trials on small, specific groups, to justify changes to public health nutrition policy intended for society as a whole.

This chapter has challenged the assumption that the functional foods agenda is exclusively about benefits to population health, and instead exposed its commercial and philosophical underpinnings. As we have argued, there is a lack of empirical evidence to support the argument that functional foods with health claims will significantly or equitably reduce health care costs or improve population health. The paradigm of molecular nutrition that informs the functional foods agenda is inadequate to deal with, or substantially affect, health outcomes at a population level. Rather, there may be benefits for certain individuals, particularly those with the resources to afford to incorporate functional foods into their diet.

Evidence from the introduction of functional foods in local and overseas markets indicates challenges for public health nutrition policy, whereby investment in the production and promotion of highly processed and expensive functional food products disadvantages core foods such as fruits and vegetables (due to the lack of resources to do the research and development, as well as the logistics of packaging to display a claim). A secondary concern is increasing consumer confusion due to distorted health messages taken out of context (that is, that individual foods can act like medicines and prevent or cure health problems).

The policy challenge for food regulators is to establish a strong regulatory framework within which food manufacturers can develop functional foods with health claims, while ensuring that public health and safety is protected. This could be achieved by substantiating the public health benefit and ensuring claims are not misleading to consumers. Regulatory reform might then offer at-risk individuals more choice in constructing a therapeutic diet consistent with dietary advice to help prevent or treat disease.

The functional foods policy agenda heralds a significant transition in the composition, marketing and regulation of many food products. This transition must be adequately resourced to manage the implementation and enforcement of food regulations, along with complementary nutrition education, monitoring and evaluation activities. From a sociological perspective, the functional foods–health claims agenda represents the coalescence of medical, food and government interests over the composition and marketing of food, resulting in a medicalisation of the food supply.

Mark Lawrence and John Germov

SUMMARY OF MAIN POINTS

- It is claimed that functional foods are food products that will provide health benefits beyond the provision of nutrients.
- The functional foods–health claims agenda is being driven by medical research in the area of molecular nutrition and food science biotechnologies.
- Food manufacturers predict that functional foods will be a lucrative new market of goods and be a source of significant profit in the future.
- Critics of functional foods suggest they represent an unnecessary and misguided medicalisation of the food supply.
- The political environment in which food regulation policy is being developed is characterised by a desire to take economic advantage of opportunities emerging from the globalisation of food trade, in parallel with a neo-liberal philosophy of self-responsibility for health.
- The potential benefits of functional foods need to be kept in perspective; while some functional foods may provide some health benefits for some people in some circumstances, overall they present social, environmental and public safety challenges.
- In the future, challenges associated with functional foods will include: appropriate scientific substantiation, effective monitoring and evaluation of their impact, and appropriate nutrition education of consumers.

SOCIOLOGICAL REFLECTION

- What are some examples of functional foods available in your country? Do you, or would you, consume functional foods? Why or why not?
- Functional foods represent an interesting example of the structure–agency debate. On the one hand, they allegedly offer people choice to exercise their agency and literally 'consume health', while at the same time altering the structure of the food supply for the whole population to potentially improve public health without individuals changing their lifestyle or food habits. Do you believe that functional foods, on balance, will be a benefit or a risk for public health nutrition?

DISCUSSION QUESTIONS

1. What implications, both positive and negative, for public health nutrition do functional foods present?
2. Who are the key stakeholders in the functional foods debate and what are their respective views?

3. Food regulation is a political process. What does the functional foods and health claims debate reveal about the operation of the food regulatory system? What does it say about the role of different stakeholders and their influence on the decision-making process?

4. How can government protect public health and safety while managing the introduction of functional foods?

5. What do you think should be the respective roles of the public and private sectors in nutrition education, monitoring and evaluation of functional foods?

6. What do you expect would be the impact (positive and/or negative) of the introduction of functional foods and health claims? Consider your answer in terms of the impact on:
    a. consumers
    b. food manufacturers
    c. public health
    d. public health practitioners
    e. the food supply
    f. the food regulatory system.

Further investigation

1. Functional foods are illusory 'magic bullets' and health claims are little more than marketing tools that lead to the medicalisation of the food supply and create consumer confusion. Discuss.

2. Do you believe that there is a role for functional foods and, if so, what are the characteristics of a regulatory framework that facilitates this role while still protecting public health and safety? (Consider scientific substantiation, nutrition education, monitoring and enforcement.)

3. Is it inevitable that the social and cultural agenda of food and health and the economic agenda of food and trade will be in conflict? How might public policy makers resolve this dilemma?

4. Are public health nutrition challenges such as the obesity and diabetes epidemic best addressed by focusing on social and environmental determinants or promoting food innovation and marketing?

FURTHER READING AND WEB RESOURCES

Books

Belasco, W. 2006, *Meals to Come: A History of the Future of Food*, University of California Press, Berkeley.

Lang, T. & Heasman, M. 2004, *Food Wars: The Global Battle for Mouths, Minds, and Markets*, Earthscan Publications, London.

Mark Lawrence and John Germov

Lawrence, M.A. & Worsley, A. (eds) 2007, *Public Health Nutrition: From Principles to Practice*, Allen & Unwin, Sydney.

Nestle, M. 2007, *Food Politics: How the Food Industry Influences Nutrition and Health*, Revised edition, University of California Press, Berkeley.

Websites

Codex Alimentarius Commission: www.codexalimentarius.net

Dietitians Association of Australia: www.daa.asn.au

Food and Agricultural Organization (FAO) – Nutrition and Consumer Protection: www.fao.org/ag/agn/index_en.stm

Food Standards Australia New Zealand: www.foodstandards.gov.au

Institute of Food Science & Technology: www.ifst.org

International Union of Nutritional Sciences: www.iuns.org/

National Centre of Excellence in Functional Foods: www.nceff.com.au/

Public Health Association of Australia: www.phaa.net.au

United Kingdom Food Standards Agency: www.food.gov.uk

United States Food and Drug Administration (FDA)—Center for Food Safety & Applied Nutrition: www.cfsan.fda.gov/list.html

WHO Global Strategy on Diet, Physical Activity and Health website: www.who.int/dietphysicalactivity/en/

REFERENCES

ACCC—*see* Australian Competition and Consumer Commission.

Anderson, J., Zettwoch, N., Feldman, T., Tietyen-Clark, J., Oeltgen, P. & Bishop, C. 1988, 'Cholesterol-lowering Effects of Psyllium Hydrophilic Mucilloid for Hypercholesterolemic Men', *Archives of Internal Medicine*, no. 148, pp. 292–6.

ANZFA—*see* Australia New Zealand Food Authority.

Australia New Zealand Food Authority 1998, *ANZFA News: The Monthly Newsletter of the Australian and New Zealand Food Authority*, no. 4, August.

—— 2001, *Inquiry Report—Proposal P153: Review of Health and Related Claims*, Australia and New Zealand Food Authority, Canberra.

Australian Competition and Consumer Commission 2007, 'Ribena Vitamin C claims "may have misled consumers"', *Australian Competition and Consumer Commission—News releases*, www.accc.gov.au/content/index.phtml/itemId/783192/fromItemId/2332, [accessed 19 August 2007].

Baker, V.A., Hepburn, P.A., Kennedy, S.J. et al. 1999, 'Safety Evaluation of Phytosterol Esters: Part 1. Assessment of Oestrogenicity Using a Combination of In Vivo and In Vitro Assays', *Food Chemical Toxicology*, vol. 37, pp. 13–22.

Barcelona Declaration on the formation of the World Public Health Nutrition Association 2006, 'Inaugural Planning Meeting', 30 September, Barcelona.

CAC—*see* Codex Alimentarius Commission.

Cannon, G. & Leitzmann, C. 2005, 'The New Nutrition Science Project', *Public Health Nutrition*, vol. 8, no. 6A, pp. 673–94.

Childs, N. 1998, 'Public Policy Approaches to Establishing Health Claims for Food Labels: An International Comparison', *British Food Journal*, vol. 100, no. 4, pp. 191–200.

Codex Alimentarius Commission 1996, *Report of the Twenty-fourth Session of the Codex Committee on Food Labelling, Ottawa, Canada, 14–17 May 1996* (ALINORM 97/22), Food and Agriculture Organization of the United Nations, World Health Organization, Geneva.

—— 2004, Guidelines for Use of Nutrition and Health Claims, *CAC/GL 23-1997, Rev. 1-2004*, Food and Agriculture Organization of the United Nations, World Health Organization, Geneva.

Cole, B.F., Baron, J.A., Sandler, R.S., Haile, R.W., Ahnen, D.J., Bresalier, R.S. et al. 2007, 'Folic Acid for the Prevention of Colorectal Adenomas: A Randomized Clinical Trial', *Journal of the American Medical Association*, vol. 97, pp. 2351–9.

Cole, S. & Comuzzie, A.G. 2007, 'The End of the Beginning', *American Journal of Clinical Nutrition*, vol. 86, pp. 274–5.

Commerce Commission 2007, 'Ribena Vitamin C Claims False and Misleading', Commerce Commission—Media Releases, www.comcom.govt.nz//Media Centre/MediaReleases/200607/ribenavitamincclaimsfalseandmislea.aspx [accessed 19 August 2007].

Conrad, P. 1992, 'Medicalization and Social Control', *Annual Review of Sociology*, vol. 18, pp. 209–32.

Cowburn, G. & Stockley, L. 2005, 'Consumer Understanding and use of Nutrition Labelling: A Systematic Review', *Public Health Nutrition*, vol. 8, no. 1, pp. 21–8.

Crawford, R. 1980, 'Healthism and the Medicalisation of Everyday Life', *International Journal of Health Services*, vol. 10, no. 3, pp. 365–88.

CSIRO—*see* Commonwealth Scientific and Industrial Research Organisation.

Commonwealth Scientific and Industrial Research Organisation 2007, 'Functional Foods: Separating Food Fact from Fiction', www.foodscience.csiro.au/ functional-foods.htm [accessed 9 August 2007].

Czeizel, A. & Dudas, I. 1992, 'Prevention of the First Occurrence of Neural-tube Defects by Periconceptional Vitamin Supplementation', *New England Journal of Medicine*, vol. 327, pp. 1832–5.

Debusk, R.M., Fogarty, C.P., Ordovas, J.M. & Kornman, K.S. 2005, Nutritional Genomics in Practice: Where Do We Begin?', *Journal of the American Dietetic Association*, vol. 105, no. 4, pp. 589–98.

Dragiecevich, H., Williams, P. & Ridges, L. 2006, 'Survey of Health Claims for Australian Foods Made on Internet Sites', *Nutrition & Dietetics*, vol. 63, pp. 139–47.

Euromonitor 2004, *Global Market Review of Functional Foods: Forecasts to 2010*, AROQ Ltd.

Food Standards Australia New Zealand 2001a, 'Media Releases & Publications', www.foodstandards.gov.au/mediareleasespublications/mediareleases/ mediareleases2001/foodstandardsministe118.cfm.

—— 2001b, 'Standard 2.6.4: Formulated Caffeinated Beverages', *Australia New Zealand Food Standards Code*, Food Standards Australia New Zealand, Canberra.

—— 2005a, *Draft Assessment Report, Proposal P293: Nutrition, Health and Related Claims*, FSANZ, Canberra.

—— 2005b, *Second Review Report, Application A424: Fortification of Foods with Calcium*, FSANZ, Canberra

—— 2006, *Final Assessment Report Proposal P295: Consideration of Mandatory Fortification with Folic Acid. Report 7-06*, FSANZ, Canberra.

—— 2007a, *Preliminary Final Assessment Report, Proposal P293: Nutrition, Health and Related Claims*, FSANZ, Canberra.

—— 2007b, *Nutrition, Health and Related Claims: A Guide to the Development of Food Standard for Australian and New Zealand*, FSANZ, Canberra.

—— 2007c, *FSANZ Considers a New GM Food and Other Changes to Food Laws*, FSANZ, Canberra, www.foodstandards.gov.au/newsroom/mediareleases/mediareleas es2007/8august2007fsanzcons3635.cfm [accessed 10 August 2007].

FSANZ—*see* Food Standards Australia New Zealand.

Germov, J. 1997, '"Whetting the Appetite": A Taste of the Sociology of Food and Nutrition', *Annual Review of Health Social Sciences*, vol. 7, pp. 35–46.

—— 1999, 'Introducing the Social Appetite: Why do we Need a Sociology of Food and Nutrition?', in J. Germov & L. Williams (eds), *A Sociology of Food and Nutrition: The Social Appetite*, Oxford University Press, Melbourne, pp. 1–9.

—— 2004, 'Introducing the Social Appetite: Towards a Sociology of Food and Nutrition', in J. Germov & L. Williams (eds), *A Sociology of Food and Nutrition: The Social Appetite*, 2nd edition, Oxford University Press, Melbourne, pp. 3–26.

—— & Williams, L. 1996, 'The Epidemic of Dieting Women: The Need for a Sociological Approach to Food and Nutrition', *Appetite*, vol. 27, pp. 97–108.

GlaxoSmithKline 2007, 'Ribena: Keeping you Informed', *Ribena*, www.ribena.com. au/ [accessed 19 August 2007].

Greenberg, E., Baron, J., Tosteson, T. et al. 1994, 'A Clinical Trial of Antioxidant Vitamins to Prevent Colo-rectal Adenoma', *New England Journal of Medicine*, vol. 331, pp. 141–7.

Hallberg, L., Rossander-Hulten, L., Brune, M. & Gleerup, A. 1992, 'Inhibition of Haem-Iron Absorption in Man by Calcium', *British Journal of Nutrition*, vol. 69, pp. 533–40.

Hasler, C., Huston, R. & Caudill, E. 1995, 'The Impact of the Nutrition Labeling and Education Act on Functional Foods', in R. Shapiro (ed.), *Nutrition Labeling Handbook*, Marcel Dekker, New York.

Hawkes, C. 2004, *Nutrition Labels and Health Claims: The Global Regulatory Environment*, World Health Organization, Geneva. Available online: http://whqlibdoc.who. int/publications/2004/9241591714.pdf.

IFIC—see International Food Information Council.

International Food Information Council 2006, *Functional Foods: Backgrounder*, www. ific.org/nutrition/functional/index.cfm [accessed 14 August 2007].

Invest Australia 2007, *Nutraceuticals/Functional foods* [web page], www.investaustralia. gov.au/index.cfm?id=557A6FB2-508B-A0EB-683DCBB697269F6B [accessed 14 August 2007].

Jacobson, M. & Silverglade, B. 1999, 'Functional Foods: Health Boon or Quackery?', *British Medical Journal*, vol. 319, pp. 205–6.

Law, M. 2000, 'Plant Sterol and Stanol Margarines and Health', *British Medical Journal*, vol. 320, pp. 861–4.

Lawrence, M. 1997, 'Highlight Interview', *Food Australia*, vol. 49, no. 3, p. 106.

—— 2003, 'Folate Fortification: A Case Study of Public Health Policy-making in a Food Regulation Setting', in V. Lin, B. Gibson & J. Daly (eds), *Evidence-based Health Policy*, Oxford University Press, Melbourne.

—— 2006, 'Evaluation of the Implementation of the Folate–Neural Tube Defect Health Claim Pilot and its Impact on the Availability of Folate-fortified Food in Australia', *Australian and New Zealand Journal of Public Health*, vol. 30, no. 4, pp. 363–8.

—— & Rayner, M. 1998, 'Functional Foods and Health Claims: A Public Health Policy Perspective', *Journal of Public Health Nutrition*, vol. 1, no. 2, pp. 75–82.

—— & Worsley, A. (eds) 2007, *Public Health Nutrition: From Principles to Practice*, Allen & Unwin, Sydney.

Leighton, P. 2002, 'Selling Wellness leads to Greener Pastures', *Functional Foods & Nutraceuticals*, November, pp. 24–6.

Lumley, J., Watson, L., Watson, M. & Bower, C. 2003, 'Periconceptional Supplementation with Folate and/or Multivitamins for Preventing Neural Tube Defects (Cochrane Review)', in *The Cochrane Library*, issue 1.

Medical Research Council 1991, Vitamin Research Group, 'Prevention of Neural Tube Defects: Results of the Medical Research Vitamin Study', *Lancet*, no. 338, pp. 131–7.

Miller, S. 1991, 'Health Claims: An Ethical Conflict?', *Food Technology*, vol. 45, May, pp. 130–56.

Mhurchu, C.N. & Gorton, D. 2007, 'Nutrition Labels and Claims in New Zealand and Australia: A Review of Use and Understanding', *Australian and New Zealand Journal of Public Health*, vol. 31, no. 2, pp. 105–12.

National Food Authority 1994, *Discussion Paper on Functional Foods*, Australian Government Publishing Service, Canberra.

—— 1996, *Review of the Food Standards Code: Concept Paper on Health and Related Claims*, Australian Government Publishing Service, Canberra.

National Heart Foundation 2007, *The Tick Update*, National Heart Foundation, February, www.heartfoundation.org.au/document/NHF/tick_hpn_mcd_specialedition_feb07.pdf [accessed 14 August 2007].

NFA—*see* National Food Authority.

NHF—*see* National Heart Foundation.

O'Connell, M. 2001, 'Nutraceuticals and Social Ethics: An Introductory Inquiry into the Relationship Between Functional Foods and Economic Justice', *Journal of Nutraceuticals, Functional and Medical Foods*, vol. 3, pp. 27–42.

Patterson, R., Satia, J., Kristal, A., Neuhouser, M. & Drewnowski, A. 2001, 'Is There a Consumer Backlash Against the Diet and Health Message?', *Journal of the American Dietetic Association*, vol. 101, no. 1, pp. 37–41.

Petersen, A. & Lupton, D. 1996, *The New Public Health: Health and Self in the Age of Risk*, Allen & Unwin, Sydney.

Sanigorski, A.M., Bell, C. & Swinburn, B. 2007, 'Association of Key Foods and Beverages with Obesity in Australian Schoolchildren', *Public Health Nutrition*, vol. 10, no. 2, pp. 152–7.

Savage, D.G. & Lindenbaum J. 1995, 'Folate-cobalamin Interactions', in L.B. Bailey (ed.), *Folates in Health and Disease*, Marcel Dekker, New York, pp. 237–85.

Sloan, A.E. 2002, 'The Top 10 Functional Food Trends: The Next Generation', *Food Technology*, vol. 56, no. 4, pp. 32–57.

Syme, L.S. 2007, 'The Prevention of Disease and Promotion of Health: The Need for a New Approach', *European Journal of Public Health*, vol. 17, no. 4, pp. 329–30.

The Age 2007a, 2 July.

The Age 2007b, 2 September.

The Giessen Declaration 2005, *Public Health Nutrition*, vol. 8, no. 6A, pp. 783–86. Also available at: www.iuns.org/features/05-09%20NNS%20Declaration.pdf.

Thomas, P. & Earl, R. (eds) 1994, *Opportunities in the Nutrition and Food Sciences: Research Challenges and the Next Generation of Investigators*, National Academy Press, Washington, DC.

Tillotson, J.E. 2003, 'Does Nutrition Sell? Do Health Claims Work? Part 2', *Nutrition Today*, vol. 38, no. 1, pp. 6–10.

Townsend, P., Davidson, N. & Whitehead, M. (eds) 1992, *Inequalities in Health: The Black Report and the Health Divide*, Penguin Books, London.

US Department of Health and Human Services 1993a, 'Food and Drug Administration, Final Rules to Amend the Food Labeling Regulations', *Federal Register*, vol. 58, no. 3, pp. 2533–620.

US Department of Health and Human Services and Food and Drug Administration 1996, 'Food Labeling; Health Claims and Label Statements; Folate and Neural Tube Defects, and Food Standards: Amendments of Standards of Identity for Enriched Grain Products to Require Addition of Folic Acid, Final Rules', *Federal Register*, vol. 61, no. 44, pp. 8749–807.

USDHHS—*see* US Department of Health and Human Services.

Van Guelpen B., Hultdin J., Johansson I., et al. 2006, 'Low Folate Levels May Protect Against Colorectal Cancer', *Gut*, April 26 [Advanced online publication].

Wilkinson, R.G. & Marmot, M. (eds) 2006, *Social Determinants of Health*, 2nd edition, Oxford University Press, Oxford.

Williams, P. 1998, 'Health Claims and Functional Foods: Time for Regulatory Change', *Australian Journal of Nutrition and Dietetics*, vol. 55, no. 2, pp. 87–90.

CHAPTER 8

The Public Health Nutrition Workforce: A Sociological Review

Roger Hughes

OVERVIEW

- What is public health nutrition? What is the public health nutrition workforce?
- How can a sociological analysis of the public health nutrition workforce help us to identify factors that affect its capacity and performance?
- Why is the sociological perspective important in examining the development of the public health nutrition workforce?

The public health nutrition workforce represents a social organisation of human resources with the specific purpose of providing services that address the determinants of nutrition-related health issues and in the process prevent disease and enhance health and well-being. This chapter focuses on the public health nutrition workforce to illustrate the importance of sociological scholarship in building the capacity of society to combat population health problems. It will explore the historical, cultural and structural determinants of workforce performance and provide a critical analysis of the factors that currently limit the capacity of this workforce to effectively address public health nutrition issues. As a result, it will cover a range of issues relevant to students and practitioners who have an interest in developing careers in this important field of nutrition practice.

Key terms

competencies

continuing competency
   development

dietitian

health promotion

medical model

population health

primary prevention

public health nutrition

socio-ecological model

Introduction

Readers of this book with plans to become a nutrition professional such as a **dietitian** or a nutritionist might wonder about the relevance of sociological studies to their own competency development. Those who are already experienced nutrition professionals will, on reflection, acknowledge the importance of the sociological perspective as one of the approaches to developing knowledge that can be applied to solving nutrition-related problems. For many, this realisation has come more from experience and learning in the workplace than from formal education methods and mediums such as courses and textbooks. This may be because the existing workforce received inadequate sociological education in their training, or it may simply reflect a reality that learning about sociological phenomena requires the learner to be embedded in the phenomena and to learn from experience.

The sociological imagination template, introduced in Chapter 1, provides a framework for interpreting the public health nutrition workforce, its historical development, the cultural factors that influence its effectiveness and actions, and the structural factors that limit or enhance the workforce's capacity to effectively address food and nutrition problems in society. This sociological perspective enables a critical analysis and interpretation of the workforce development needs that has implications not only for students but also for the contemporary workforce.

Before a sociological analysis of the public health nutrition workforce can be adequately performed, a definition of '**public health nutrition**' needs to be developed.

Defining 'public health nutrition'

Common use of 'public health nutrition' as a term to describe a field of practice or the workforce employed in this field is a relatively recent development. However, the application of prevention principles to prevent diet-related disease has a centuries-long history. Eighteenth-century English naval officer Captain James Cook's attempt to prevent the vitamin C-deficiency disease scurvy by promoting the consumption of vitamin C-rich foodstuffs among his sailors is a famous example of a public health nutrition intervention involving food supply changes, supported by policy and enforced with the threat of punitive action. Enforcing the consumption of lime juice and sauerkraut through the threat of 50 lashes for malingerers is a strategy rarely available to contemporary health promoters. While population-based approaches have been a mainstay of nutrition work for decades in many countries, the popular use of the title 'public health nutritionist' for nutrition practitioners has only recently been adopted in countries such as Australia and the United Kingdom.

Roger Hughes

Preventative and population-based approaches to dealing with nutrition issues to enhance public health have recently become more accepted in those Western countries that have experienced increases in the social and financial burdens associated with diseases of affluence (sometimes called 'affluenza'), such as obesity, heart disease, some cancers and diabetes. This acceptance is linked to a realisation that countries cannot afford to sustain the cost of treatment of these diseases, and that investment in effective prevention makes good sense economically as well as socially. There is evidence that countries worldwide are putting more money and effort into the development of the public health nutrition workforce (Landman 2001), in order to deal with the spiralling social costs of these largely preventable health problems. Unfortunately, this investment in prevention and capacity building is not always applied equally and is often applied in an ad hoc nature.

During the last decade there have been various attempts in the international literature to define 'public health nutrition' as a field of nutrition practice distinct from the well-established professional practice of clinical nutrition and dietetics (Hughes & Somerset 1997; Rogers & Schlossman 1997; Landman et al. 1998; Yngve et al. 1999; Johnson et al. 2001). This literature has developed from considerable effort and debate among professionals and organisations in response to health-service policy shifts consistent with the public health, **health promotion** and primary health care movements. It has also been in response to efforts to raise people's awareness of public health nutrition as a distinct profession or mode of practice delineated from clinical practice paradigms (Hughes & Somerset 1997; Landman et al. 1998).

In the late 1990s the Nutrition Society in the United Kingdom identified the need for a definition of 'public health nutrition' to make explicit the broad vision, intention, character, and commitment to popular service values associated with the field (Landman et al. 1998). Statements that define a field of practice or a type of work are important in workforce development because they help describe the work needed, and in turn provide direction about the type of worker and competency mix required for that work. Definitions serve as a statement of intent, philosophy and method, important for communication of what the field entails. They have implications for marketing, development of professional identity, and systematic workforce development.

Table 8.1 lists the definitions found in the international literature since 1997 and includes the definition adopted for the national public health nutrition strategy in Australia (SIGNAL 2001a; 2001b). This definition differs from the others in that it makes a point of specifying what public health nutrition is not (in the words, 'rather than the specific needs of individuals') in order to delineate public health nutrition from clinical dietetic modes of service. It also includes the most recent iteration of public health nutrition as defined by the recently formed World Public Health Nutrition Association (WPHNA), an international body formed to support public health nutrition action and practitioners on a global scale.

Table 8.1   Definitions of 'public health nutrition'

Publication and country	Definition
Hughes & Somerset 1997 (Australia)	'Public Health Nutrition is the art and science of promoting population health status via sustainable improvements in the food and nutrition system. Based upon public health principles, it is a set of comprehensive and collaborative activities, ecological in perspective and intersectoral in scope, including environmental, educational, economic, technical and legislative measures.'
Rogers & Schlossman 1997 (USA)	'The term "public nutrition" has been defined as a new field encompassing the range of factors known to influence nutrition in populations, including diet and health, social, cultural, and behavioural factors; and the economic and political context. Like public health, public nutrition would focus on problem solving in a real-world setting, making its definition an applied field of study whose success is measured in terms of effectiveness in improving nutrition situations.'
Landman et al. 1998 (UK)	'Public health nutrition focuses on the promotion of good health through nutrition and the primary prevention of diet-related illness in the population. The emphasis is on the maintenance of wellness in the whole population.'
Yngve et al. 1999 (EU)	'Public health nutrition focuses on the promotion of good health through nutrition and physical activity and the prevention of related illness in the population.'
Johnson et al. 2001 (USA)	'Public health nutrition practice includes an array of services and activities to assure conditions in which people can achieve and maintain nutritional health, including surveillance and monitoring nutrition-related health status and risk factors, community or population based assessment, program planning and evaluation, leadership in community/population interventions that collaborate across disciplines, programs and agencies, and leadership in addressing the access and quality issues around direct nutrition services to populations.'
SIGNAL 2001a (Australia)	'Public health nutrition focuses on issues affecting the whole population rather than the specific dietary needs of individuals. The impact of food production, distribution and consumption on the nutritional status and health of particular population groups is taken into account, together with the knowledge, skills, attitudes and behaviours in the broader community.'
APHNAC 2005 (Australia)	'Public health nutrition is the organized effort of society in the areas of food and nutrition to promote and protect the health of populations.' (Hughes 2005)
WPHNA 2007 (International)	'Public health nutrition is the promotion and maintenance of nutrition related health and well-being of populations through the organised efforts and informed choices of society.'

Roger Hughes

Close assessment of the descriptors used in these definitions reveals a number of consistent elements, suggesting that there is international consensus about public health nutrition as a field of practice. This observation has been tested as part of an international Delphi study (see Box 8.1) among an international panel of public health nutrition experts in 2002/3 to assess the level of agreement about how 'public health nutrition' is defined (Hughes 2003a). This study, conducted among 24 public health nutrition experts from Portugal, Spain, Sweden, Finland, Iceland, England, Switzerland, Belgium, South Africa, the United States of America and Australia, identified key descriptors of public health nutrition, as an alternative to a prescribed definition. The agreed descriptors of this field of practice included the following:

- being population-based
- applying public health principles
- focusing on **primary prevention**, health promotion and wellness
- using a food and nutrition systems approach that utilises environmental, political, behavioural and inter-sectoral strategies.

Having identified the nature of public health nutrition work, we will now examine and delineate the composition of the public health nutrition workforce.

The Delphi Technique

BOX 8.1

The Delphi Technique is a research strategy that was developed by the RAND Corporation as a forecasting tool in the 1960s to measure or develop agreement about issues. It uses multiple survey rounds among an anonymous group of experts. Controlled feedback between survey rounds is provided by the researcher in the form of statistical summaries of the previous round's results, and this is followed by further ratings by experts. This process continues until there is stability in responses and consensus is achieved.

Source: Rowe & Wright (1999)

Workforce composition

The public health nutrition workforce is a social organisation of human resources with the role of enhancing public health by addressing the determinants of nutrition-related health problems. This emphasis on identifying, understanding and addressing the determinants of public health problems is consistent with the **socio-ecological model** of public health, a model that underpins much of the public health movement internationally (Gebbie et al. 2002).

Numerous factors, such as workforce composition, level of collaboration, **competencies**, practice methods, information access, resource allocation and organisational issues, are likely to affect the capacity of the workforce to effectively address population nutrition problems (Hughes 2004a). An analysis of this workforce capacity using a socio-ecological analytical approach has recently been published (Hughes 2006). It is important to consider the composition of this workforce, so that specific workforce development initiatives can be targeted to groups within the workforce with the greatest opportunity to affect the desired outcomes or possessing the greatest need.

An inclusive and simplistic approach would be to argue that the public health nutrition workforce includes all those who make a contribution to organised efforts to prevent diet-related disease and promote health. This could include nutritionists, dietitians, teachers, nurses, medical practitioners, town planners, food-industry staff and advertisers, to name a few. This approach is not very helpful if the objective is to identify and target factors that influence the capacity and development needs of the workforce. It also does not fit the realities of workforce organisation, in which workers are usually categorised on the basis of work tasks and roles, employing agency, professional background, credentials or competencies.

Previous attempts to conceptualise the composition of the public health, health promotion and public health nutrition workforces in Australia (PHAA 1990; NHMRC 1996; Campbell et al. 1997) have resulted in the recognition of multiple workforce tiers that consistently differentiate between specialist and generalist categories. There is a developing consensus, at least in Australia, that the public health workforce can be categorised into a number of workforce categories or tiers, with different professional backgrounds, development needs, roles and functions, but all part of, and contributing to, the collective capacity of the workforce (PHAA 1990; Campbell et al. 1997).

One approach is to consider the workforce in terms of its employers. It is naive to assume that organised efforts to influence population or societal dietary behaviour only originate in the health sector or that such efforts have health promotion as their driving agenda. Marion Nestle's exposé of the food industry in America highlights the significant influence of this sector on **population health** and nutrition (Nestle 2002). Nestle demonstrates that the food industry spends huge amounts of money each year on lobbying and on marketing foods that can only be classified as 'junk food'. The industry employs an army of workers (including nutrition professionals) to ensure that their market is protected and expanded. Should nutritionists working in the food industry be considered part of the public health nutrition workforce, despite the fact that they are employed by an industry whose primary objective is shareholder profits rather than the public good?

The first argument worth considering is that nutritionists employed in the food industry can promote public health from within this sector by, for example, reducing the fat or salt content of food products (and thus changing to the food supply) or by conducting nutrition education/marketing programs that increase consumer awareness about healthy diets and products (Tapsell & de Groot 1999). The counter

Roger Hughes

argument is that nutritionists in the food industry are confronted with a conflict of interests (corporate profit versus public health) in their role (Niall & O'Dea 1997) and that this conflict means that, in reality, the ability of nutrition professionals 'embedded' in the food industry to promote public health is limited.

An alternative approach to viewing the workforce in relation to the employer is to consider what group in the workforce is the lead group in terms of employment, competency mix and capacity to initiate population-level action. There have been only a few specific studies published that describe national public health workers specialising in nutrition or occupying designated public health nutrition positions— in the USA (Kaufman et al. 1986; Haughton et al. 1998), Canada (Gatchell & Woolcott 1992), Britain (Adamson & Cowburn 1996) and Australia (Hughes 2004b). These studies consistently identify practitioners with dietetic professional backgrounds as the dominant professional group occupying designated public health nutrition work roles. The reasons for this will be considered in the sociological analysis of the workforce that follows.

A historical perspective

Little has been published on the historical development of the public health nutrition workforce. In any case, the relative stage of workforce development tends to vary between countries. The USA, for example, has a relatively large and well-developed public health nutrition workforce that has developed over the past 50 years, whereas in countries such as Australia and the United Kingdom the development of public health nutrition as a professional grouping or a specific workforce is in its infancy. In the European Union, there is considerable variability and inequity in terms of population access to public health nutrition services because of the complexity of different health systems, resource allocation to workforce and national policies. The recently funded JobNut Project (funded by the EU Commission's Leonardo Da Vinci Program), aims to explore public health nutrition labour market issues in an attempt to enhance workforce capacity in Europe.

Public health nutrition as a discipline in many countries is more appropriately described as an offshoot of public health and/or the dietetic profession. There are, however, indications that there is a desire for recognition of public health nutritionists as a professional group distinct from other public health and dietetic professionals. In the United Kingdom, the Nutrition Society has established a registration program for public health nutritionists that confers registration as a credential of competency in this field (Landman 2001). There is also a concerted move at a global level to establish a World Public Health Nutrition Association, an initiative that has developed from the First Global Congress in Public Health Nutrition held in Barcelona in 2006. If we limit our discussion of the public health nutrition workforce to the designated workforce (that is, those workers with designated positions with a full-time work mandate for preventative and population-based practice), the historical development of the public health nutrition workforce is closely linked to that of the dietetic profession.

A cultural perspective

It is often difficult to separate historical from cultural perspectives because they are interrelated. In the case of the public health nutrition workforce, it can be argued that, in Australia at least, public health nutritionists as distinct nutrition practitioners have evolved out of the dietetic profession in response to changes in the professional, policy and funding environments. This relates to the dominance of dietetic training as a background for work in public health nutrition, identified in workforce enumeration studies internationally (Gatchell & Woolcott 1992; Haughton et al. 1998; Hughes 2004b). This suggests that dietetic professional culture would have a strong influence on the culture of the public health nutrition workforce. In many cases it probably has. Values such as a commitment to the public good, social justice, ethical practice, evidence-based practice and advocacy for the public are strong features of the public health nutrition workforce culture and are consistent with those of dietetics and health professions generally.

Some differences, however, can be observed in the public health nutrition workforce as a result of this evolution of practice from clinical practice based on a **medical model** to public health practice based on a socio-ecological model. Many of the contemporary public health nutrition workers in Australia report having 'evolved' through work as clinical dietitians to public health nutrition work because of frustration with the (perceived) ineffectiveness of a treatment paradigm for preventable diseases. Evolution in this sense does not imply that public health nutrition is a more advanced version of practice, but a product of natural selection of career paths based on interests and circumstances. This evolution influences work culture, as is illustrated by the following quote from a high-level Australian public health nutritionist: 'I got pretty sick of going to ICU every morning and realising that much of the problems presenting there were preventable ... ' (quoted in Hughes 2003b).

Public health nutritionists appear to have moved on from the philosophies they learned during their professional socialisation as a dietitian. There is evidence that individual professionals are rejecting the medical model and embracing what they consider to be a more holistic, socially empowering and appropriate approach to public health improvement: 'I could see solutions to problems like obesity come through public health efforts in communities ... the clinical model is a limited model for dealing with complex social phenomena like obesity' (Hughes 2003b). Qualitative investigation of the career paths of advanced public health nutrition practitioners in Australia (Hughes 2003b) has also shown that this evolution has largely been opportunistic and unplanned. This reflects the lack of coordinated workforce development at a national level in Australia.

Roger Hughes

Public health nutrition is a field of practice that is currently in the process of defining and delineating its professional boundaries. There is, for example, whispered debate in Australia about the appropriateness of employment stipulations requiring applicants for public health nutrition positions to be qualified in dietetics: why not instead hire people with a demonstrated competency in public health nutrition and recruit people from diverse backgrounds rather than from a specific professional group? Part of the problem is that there has been no consensus about which public health nutrition competencies are required for effective practice, and a lack of clarity about what constitutes effective practice. In an effort to address this limitation, a group of Australian public health nutrition academics (the Australian Public Health Nutrition Academic Collaboration, or APHNAC) published, in 2005, a competency framework for public health nutrition workforce development (www.aphnac.com) (Hughes 2005). It is still unclear whether the dietetic profession in Australia has come to terms with a developing workforce (and mode of practice) that requires more than the traditional competencies developed in dietetic training and practice.

Clearly, the culture of the public health nutrition workforce is still evolving, borrowing heavily from dietetics and public health, but responding to events as they arise.

A structural perspective

Structural factors relevant to the analysis of the public health nutrition workforce include the policy and strategic environment within government, the size of the workforce, employment requirements, workforce organisation and systems for workforce development.

Policy and strategic framework

Government policy is a structural determinant of the workforce's activity, structure and development. Government policy and the strategic plans that are developed to put policy into practice have important influences on the activity of the nutrition workforce. These plans (such as Australia's *National Public Health Nutrition Strategy: Eat Well Australia* released in 2001) aim to provide 'a coherent national approach to the underlying causes of the preventable burden of diet-related disease and early death, providing a set of interlinked initiatives for the prevention and management of these diseases' (SIGNAL 2001b, p. 2). This strategic framework influences the workforce because it guides the actions of employers, such as state-government health departments (many of which have developed a state version of the national strategy), and influences resource allocation. Many similar action plans have been developed at a national level since the early 2000s, particularly in Europe (refer to:

http://data.euro.who.int/nutrition/ for analysis of European nutrition strategies and action plans).

Size and characteristics of the workforce

Workforce scholarship in the USA (Gebbie & Merrill 2001; Kennedy & Moore 2001) has recently focused on enumerating and profiling the public health workforce in order to plan for workforce development. There have been only a few specific studies published that describe national public health workers specialising in nutrition in the USA (Kaufman et al. 1986; Haughton et al. 1998), Canada (Gatchell & Woolcott 1992) and Britain (Adamson & Cowburn 1996). Until recently the information about the public health nutrition workforce in Australia was limited to grey literature (that is, unpublished reports) (Steele 1995; Anthony & Cooper 1998) and information gleaned from workforce studies in the nutrition and dietetics and public health fields. Workforce studies in nutrition and dietetics in Australia (Scott & Binns 1988, 1989; Williams 1993; Hughes 1998; AIHW 2000; Meyer et al. 2002) make little reference to public health nutrition practice.

In order to garner more information about the public health nutrition workforce in Australia, a mixed-method study of the public health nutrition workforce was recently conducted (Hughes 2004a). Data from this study—and various studies done in other countries—relevant to the analysis of the composition and nature of the public health nutrition workforce are summarised in Box 8.2.

Summary of data relating to compositional analysis of the public health nutrition workforce in Australia, the USA and Canada

BOX 8.2

- The public health nutrition workforce is seen by most within the public health nutrition community as multidisciplinary, with many 'players'.
- There are multiple workforce tiers, each tier having different roles, competency needs and mandates for public health nutrition action.
- A key constituent of the public health nutrition workforce is the nutrition 'specialist'.
- Practitioners who have a dietetics background and who work in community health settings are the dominant workforce constituent in Australia and in most countries for which there are available data.
- Most employers recruiting health professionals to public health nutrition positions in Australia stipulate dietetic qualifications.

▶

Roger Hughes

BOX 8.2 CONTINUED

- Other key workforce constituents include individual care dietitians, health promotion officers, academics, managers, nurses and home economists.
- The existing Australian community and public health nutrition workforce is predominantly female and most workers have entry-level dietetic qualifications as their highest qualification.
- Inconsistent and variable position nomenclature is used for the 'designated' public health nutrition workforce tier. Use of the title 'public health nutritionist' is increasing.
- Almost half of the workers are in temporary or part-time positions and most are employed in the government health sector.
- Public health nutrition work is only a part of the role of most of those in the community and public health nutrition workforce in Australia, with most having clinical responsibilities also. This is a potential limitation on the capacity for public health nutrition efforts.
- The public health nutrition workforce is dynamic and evolving. Some 35 per cent of the Australian workforce reported that they expected to change jobs in the next two years and only 18 per cent expected to be in their current job for another five years or more.
- The workforce responsible for addressing public health nutrition in Australia is small relative to the size of the problems, and self-reported capacity is low.

Sources: Kaufman et al. (1986); Gatchell & Woolcott (1992); Steele (1995); Adamson & Cowburn (1996); Campbell et al. (1997); Hughes (2003b, 2003c, 2003d)

Table 8.2 provides data from an Australian study attempting to enumerate and delineate between different public health nutrition workforce groups, and illustrates the relatively small number of positions dedicated to public health nutrition work. This suggests that the current workforce in Australia is less than 40 per cent of projected need based on established staff-to-population ratios used in the USA (Dodds & Kaufman 1991).

Employment requirements

Employers' expectations of and requirements for public health nutrition positions are important structural factors influencing the composition and nature of the workforce. Position descriptions are an instrument of human resource management used by employers to define the roles and responsibilities, credentials and competency requirements of a position. They define a position and express the organisational expectations of the position, and are the standard against which employers recruit, and assess the performance of, the public health nutrition workforce (Hughes

Table 8.2 Calculations of adjusted national full-time-equivalent positions dedicated to public health nutrition (PHN) practice: Australian Public Health Nutrition Workforce Study, November 2001–February 2002

Position	A Number	B Mean hours worked	C FTE positions (AxB/38)	D Assumed proportion of work dedicated to PHN practice	E FTE positions dedicated to PHN practice (CxD)	F Total FTE positions, adjusted for survey response rate (E/0.87)
PHN in regional/zonal	15	33.0	13.0	1.0	13.0	14.9
PHN in NGO	10	36.1	9.5	1.0	9.5	10.9
PHN in state health department	18	36.2	17.1	1.0	17.1	19.7
Community dietitian/nutritionist in community health	81	30.3	64.6	0.5	32.3	37.1
Community dietitian/nutritionist in hospital	14	31.7	11.7	0.5	5.9	6.8
Project officer in health promotion	20	33.9	17.8	1.0	17.8	20.5
Regional dietitian/nutritionist	16	34.3	14.4	0.5	7.2	8.3
Hospital-based dietitian with community role	13	32.8	11.2	0.5	5.6	6.4
Nutritionist in academic institution	11	31.6	9.1	0.5	4.6	5.3
Nutritionist on project grant	11	27.3	7.9	1.0	7.9	9.1
Nutritionists working with food industry	2	31.0	1.6	1.0	1.6	1.8
Other*	19	33.0	16.5	0.5	8.3	9.5
Total	****239**		**194.4**		**130.8**	**150**

FTE = full-time equivalent; PHN = public health nutrition; NGO = non–government organisation

* Includes eleven staff from Food Standards Australia New Zealand

** One missing response (total response sample = 240)

Source: Hughes (2004b)

Roger Hughes

2004c). They also provide an organisational mandate for a particular type of practice. The importance of this codified mandate has been demonstrated in a study of the Victorian public health nutrition workforce: community-based dietitians reported being limited in their capacity to perform public health nutrition roles because position descriptions and organisational expectations did not provide support for services that were not clinical in nature (Hughes & Woods 2003). Box 8.3 summarises the results of a recent review of public health nutrition position descriptions in Australia that identified consistent job roles (functions) and key selection criteria (credentials and competencies). The fact that dietetic qualifications are required for most of the positions in this study suggests that:

- this credential is valued by employers as a benchmark of competency and workforce preparation
- these position descriptions (or this credential requirement) are based on dietetic position descriptions
- the professionals or employers who develop these instruments of staff recruitment are dietitians.

The development of a position description implies that the person developing it has adequate knowledge of the work required and the competency requirements needed to effectively do this work. This assumption is questionable. Regardless of the limitations of analysis based on position descriptions, this structural factor limits the access of nutritionists not trained as dietitians to public health nutrition work, because of the widespread dietetic credential requirement. This may explain the dominance of dietetic professionals in the designated public health nutrition workforce, which will be discussed further in the critical-perspective section.

BOX 8.3

Employers' expectations about public health nutrition workforce functions, credentials and competencies

Most common functions:

- team building
- program planning
- program evaluation
- providing nutrition advice/support
- program implementation
- human resource management
- needs assessment
- strategy design

▶

- training other professionals
- continuing professional development
- conducting local research
- community development
- dietary education of individuals
- grantsmanship (submission writing)
- quality management.

BOX 8.3

Most common credentials (listed in at least 33 per cent of position descriptions):

- dietetic qualifications
- eligibility for Dietitians Association of Australia (DAA) membership
- current driver's licence.

Most common competency requirements (listed in at least 33 per cent of position descriptions):

- experience in and knowledge of public health nutrition intervention management (planning, implementation and evaluation)
- consultation and negotiation skills
- interpersonal communication skills
- ability to work in a multidisciplinary manner
- knowledge of public health nutrition issues and strategies
- being an independent and self-directed worker
- cultural competency.

Source: Hughes 2004c (based on analysis of 46 position descriptions reviewed between February and August 2002)

Workforce organisation

The organisation of the public health nutrition workforce—in terms of location, setting of practice, accountability and funding source—may have important effects on its composition, practice culture and overall effectiveness. Profiling studies of the Australian public health nutrition workforce indicate that the publicly funded health sector is the main employer, with most of the workforce employed and located in community health services and reporting to health managers without nutrition qualifications (Hughes 2004b). The workers in this setting experience considerable pressure from managers and the community to provide clinical services that address the short-term needs of individuals, reflecting the traditional culture of community health services in many parts of Australia. This limits their ability to plan and develop interventions that address long-term population needs (Hughes & Woods 2003).

Roger Hughes

Recent workforce developments in some Australian states have placed new public health nutritionists in public health units that have a mandate for public health surveillance, planning, intervention and evaluation at a zonal or state level (Lee 2002). This organisational positioning of practitioners in a practice culture consistent with public health is likely to be more conducive to an effective public health nutrition effort.

Systems for workforce development

There are a number of systems that are used to recruit and develop workforces, one of which has already been discussed (position descriptions). Other examples include codifications or statements of the core functions and competencies required for effective practice.

Core function statements have recently been developed for the broad area of public health work in a number of countries (NPHP 2001; CLBAPHP & HRSA 2002) to help define the core or essential functions of the public health workforce. The following list of core public health nutrition functions (Box 8.4) has been developed in Australia (Hughes 2004a) based on a mix of research methods, including literature review, position description auditing, national workforce surveying, practitioner consultation and consensus development. These functions represent the consistent function categories identified following triangular analysis of data from these different methods.

BOX 8.4

Proposed core public health nutrition workforce functions

Research and analysis

- Monitor, assess and communicate population nutritional health needs and issues.
- Develop and communicate intelligence about determinants of nutrition problems, policy impacts, intervention effectiveness and prioritisation through research and evaluation.

Building capacity

- Develop the various tiers of the public health nutrition workforce and its collaborators through education, disseminating intelligence and ensuring organisational support.
- Build community capacity and social capital to formulate and implement solutions to nutrition problems.
- Build organisational capacity and systems to facilitate and coordinate effective public health nutrition action.

▶

Intervention management

- Plan, develop, implement and evaluate interventions that address the determinants of priority public health nutrition problems.
- Enhance and sustain population knowledge and awareness of healthy eating so that dietary choices are informed choices.
- Lobby for food- and nutrition-related government policy and action that protects and promotes health.
- Promote, develop and support healthy growth and development throughout all life stages.
- Promote equal access to safe and healthy food so that healthy choices are easy choices.

BOX 8.4

Workforce practices are a factor affecting human resource contributions to the structural capacity of the public health system (Handler et al. 2001). Box 8.5 presents a hypothetical scenario to illustrate how these core functions are applied in practice and how the public health nutrition mode of practice differs from the traditional clinical dietetic approach. As the scenario demonstrates, the practice approach used to address nutrition problems will influence the effectiveness of the work. A large workforce that practices in a way that is inconsistent with disease prevention (for example, one-on-one dietary counselling to prevent obesity) may have low overall effectiveness in disease prevention because of poor reach and/or efficacy.

Competencies: The architecture for workforce development

The public health nutrition scenario in Box 8.5 illustrates the extensive interaction with stakeholders in communities that is required to successfully implement solutions to nutrition problems. Public health nutritionists have to be in touch with their community, build trust in relationships and be culturally competent, and be committed to community development—all qualities that depend on their having advanced social skills—in order to be able to understand and effectively interact with community members.

Public health workforce development scholarship over the last few years has emphasised the importance of developing a competent public health workforce as a precursor to increasing societal capacity to protect and promote public health (CDC & ATSDR 2001; Kennedy & Moore 2001; Lichtveld et al. 2001; Gebbie et al. 2002; Riddout et al. 2002). As a result, there has been an emphasis on developing competency standards to provide the architecture for workforce development in the fields of public health (Healthwork UK 2001; CLBAPHP & HRSA 2002), preventive medicine (Lane

Roger Hughes

BOX 8.5

A comparison of the traditional and public health nutrition approaches to dietetics

The traditional dietetic approach

Tony is a dietitian employed by the Gosford Community Health Centre. Data produced by the Area Health Epidemiology Unit has identified a recent increase in the prevalence of overweight and obesity in the area population and this finding is supported by an increasing rate of referral of overweight and obese clients to the health centre by general practitioners (GPs). Tony's initial response is to work with the other staff in the Community Health Centre to establish a multidisciplinary weight-reduction clinic, linking with the local Division of General Practice. This results in a streamlined service that provides services for an average of 60 individuals a week and that occupies three days a week of his time. He notices that each individual needs an average of six visits spread over two to three months to successfully stabilise their weight and sustain changes to related behaviours (the desired outcome), so there are 10 outcomes per week. Realising that this method requires significant resources for the limited population reach, he reorganises the service into a group-education format, increasing the client service rate to 120 per week for the same time investment and for twice as many outcomes per week (20). At this rate he will achieve about 1000 outcomes per year.

The public health nutrition approach

Tess is a public health nutritionist working for the Central Coast Area Health Service of New South Wales and has decided to develop a public health nutrition response to the spiralling rates of overweight and obesity in her community. The following account describes how each of the core functions listed in Box 8.4 applies to this scenario.

Tess decides to act after analysing recently collected data from her epidemiology unit that shows that the rates of overweight and obesity are increasing at an alarming rate, particularly among school-aged children. Her first step is to consult key stakeholders in her community and form a representative taskforce to assist in planning a community-wide intervention to address the problem. At the same time as this taskforce is being established and commencing discussions, Tess lobbies her local public health unit to provide research support and some seed funding for the community taskforce to develop and implement its initial strategies.

With the public health epidemiologist, Tess summarises the available public health data about overweight and obesity in a report that is used to inform the taskforce's deliberations and to communicate this information to the local health workforce. The taskforce then undertakes a determinant analysis (consultation, research and discussion

▶

BOX 8.5

to identify determinants of overweight and obesity in its community) assisted by Tess and staff from the public health unit. This analysis finds that sedentary lifestyles and increasing reliance on takeaway food are the major direct determinants of increasing adiposity. Indirect determinants include a lack of community facilities for exercise, such as safe pathways, organised sport and affordable gym access. The increasing reliance on takeaway food is considered to be the result of time poverty among working parents, limited food preparation skills, the saturation of the local community environment with fast-food advertising, and the high number of fast-food outlets.

The taskforce develops a community strategy with the help of Tess, who informs them about earlier interventions and their effectiveness and other possible options. This strategy forms the basis of a submission for funding from the state government to develop a community-wide obesity-prevention strategy. Among other things, the strategy mix includes:

- working with local government to develop policies and invest in safe pathways and regulate fast-food outlet locations through town planning
- a train-the-teacher program in district schools and health centres, so that teachers and health workers can implement a healthy meal preparation skills development program for students, parents and other community members
- developing a community sports organisation to coordinate community-wide physical activity for people of all ages (assisted by the Department of Sport and Recreation).

On receipt of the government funding, Tess works with the taskforce and community stakeholders to implement the program, making a concerted effort to keep the stakeholders engaged in and informed about the project. The project team also develops community organisation systems and seeks funding to sustain the project after the government funding ends. On completion of the intervention funding, Tess works with stakeholders to evaluate the intervention and reports widely on its outcomes and lessons.

Comparison of approaches

The difference between these two approaches relates not only to the reach of the interventions, but also to the types of changes achieved, the determinants addressed, and the competencies required to successfully implement them.

et al. 1999; Gebbie et al. 2002), health promotion (Howat et al. 2000; Precision Consultancy 2000) and health education (NCHEC 2002). This has also been of interest to public health nutrition scholars (Rogers & Schlossman 1997; Landman et al. 1998; Pew Health Professions Commission 1998; Dodds & Polhamus 1999; Nutrition Society 2000).

Roger Hughes

Table 8.3   Competency domains identified by an international public health nutrition expert panel

Competency domain	Example units
Analytical	Nutrition monitoring and surveillance, applied research, needs assessment, evaluation
Sociocultural and political processes	Advocacy, policy development and analysis, building capacity, cultural awareness
Public health services	Intervention planning, strategy design, workforce development, intervention research, health promotion
Communication	Interpersonal and scientific communication skills, media and writing skills, grantsmanship
Management and leadership	Strategic planning, team building and staff management, negotiation, collaboration
Nutrition sciences	Nutrition assessment, food guidance and goals, lifespan nutrition and requirements
Professionalism	Ethics, quality assurance, evidence-based practice, reflective practice, commitment to lifelong learning

Source: Hughes (2003c)

Competencies reflect the knowledge, skills and attitudes required to be able to effectively perform the required work. Table 8.3 lists the broad competency domains considered by an international group of public health nutrition experts as essential for effective public health nutrition practice (Hughes 2004d). There is a strongly held view among advanced public health nutrition practitioners in Australia that competencies in the nutritional sciences are essential and distinguish the public health nutritionist from the rest of the public health workforce (Hughes 2003b).

Although there is a developing literature about competency standards and the needs of the public health nutrition workforce, few studies have focused on how workforce competencies are best developed. This leads us to the critical phase of the sociological analysis.

A critical perspective

The level of competence possessed by the public health nutrition workforce at any given time is a product of the interaction between, and effects of, workforce education and training processes and workforce management processes (Kennedy & Moore 2001). Competency development can therefore be temporally compartmentalised into pre-employment education and training (such as university programs) and postgraduate **continuing competency development** (CCD). Postgraduate CCD takes many forms, including further university-based course work, research higher degrees and workplace-based CCD.

The adequacy of workforce preparation

Given the dominance in the contemporary public health nutrition workforce of workers from a dietetic training background—with most having entry-level dietetics training as their highest qualification (Hughes 2004b)—it is important to consider the adequacy of this preparation for competency in public health nutrition practice. Two recent studies of the CCD needs of this workforce provide evidence that dietetic training is inadequate preparation for effective public health nutrition work (Hughes 2004d; 2003b). This suggests that there may need to be a review of existing competency standards and of how training programs meet those standards relevant to public health nutrition practice.

In response to a question asking public health nutrition workers with dietetic qualifications to list the advantages of dietetic training, the most commonly cited benefits were the strong grounding in nutrition knowledge and the wide range of skills attained, including health promotion skills, basic research skills and problem-solving skills. The most commonly mentioned disadvantages of dietetic training were its clinical bias and narrow focus, the inadequate training in public health approaches, and the inadequate public health nutrition work experience (Hughes 2003b). In the same study, when respondents were asked to rate the adequacy of dietetic training as preparation for public health nutrition practice, 57 per cent rated it as inadequate to very inadequate.

The (perceived) inadequacy of dietetic training as preparation for public health nutrition work may be due to the fact that dietetic education is designed to produce entry-level graduates, not specialists. It is now recognised that public health nutrition competency is considered to be an advanced qualification, or a specialised practice area, which, by definition, builds on experience and more generic professional proficiencies (Hughes 2003c). It is also recognised that public health nutrition competency development is best facilitated by experiential and problem-orientated learning in a work setting (Pelletier 1997; Hughes 2003b), making it more suited to practice-based learning and consistent with the principles of self-directed learning and adult learning (Kaufman 1990). The existing workforce has privileged access to work situations that encourage CCD via these learning styles (Hughes 2004d). Evidence from recent Australian studies suggests that competency development among the public health nutrition workforce has been largely unplanned, uncoordinated and probably inefficient (Hughes 2004b, 2004d).

The necessity of integrated learning systems

There is therefore a need for integrated learning systems that facilitate CCD among the existing workforce and future workers. A recent study (Hughes 2003d) has shown that the most common motivations to further develop competencies in public health nutrition in the Australian workforce were intrinsic motivations (such as a desire to

Roger Hughes

learn more and a desire to be more effective), consistent with the features of adult and self-directed learning (Kaufman 2003). The reported barriers to continuing professional development were similar to those found in American studies of the dietetic workforce (American Dietetic Association 2000; Manning & Vickery 2000). Time poverty in the workplace and financial constraints may reflect a lack of employer support for CCD and suggest that workforce development strategies should focus on creating a workplace environment that supports and encourages ongoing education and competency development. This means that organisational and cultural change within the workplace may be needed, rather than more CCD courses and training programs.

A practitioner's confidence in their own ability and skills may be an important variable affecting practices (Hughes 2004b). This notion is based on the concept of self-efficacy, which asserts that an individual's judgment of their own ability to deal with certain situations is central to their actions (Kaufman 2003). Self-reported confidence levels may also be used as an indicator of competency development needs and has been used in CCD needs assessment studies in the public health workforce (Corby 1997). The confidence deficits reported most frequently by Australian public health nutritionists in a recent national survey (Hughes 2004d) were in analytical and policy-process competency areas.

Formal training to develop public health nutrition competencies needs to be flexible and student-centred if it is to successfully engage the workforce (Hughes 2003d). Most of this workforce is currently employed in the public health nutrition field and further study must be integrated into their existing work. This will require greater interaction between universities and employers. It also provides an opportunity to apply teaching and learning strategies that reflect contemporary views about health-profession competency development, such as problem-based learning (Vernon & Blake 1993), situated learning (Grant 2002), and self-directed learning and reflective practice (Kaufman 2003). The recent funding of an advanced public health nutrition training program by the Commonwealth's Public Health Education and Research Program (PHERP) may provide the opportunity to develop integrated learning systems that address these issues.

Constraints on workforce development imposed by current recruitment stipulations

The common inclusion of dietetic credentials as a key selection criterion, discussed earlier, is potentially a problem for workforce development in public health nutrition. It assumes that dietetic qualifications provide appropriate preparation for public health nutrition work and does not recognise that it is possible to develop competencies in public health nutrition via other routes. The evidence discussed previously seriously challenges this assumption.

Workforce development efficiency: Up-skilling dietitians

Workforce development rarely involves starting with a clean slate that allows the development of a workforce tailor-made for the work needed. The work that the public health nutrition workforce in Australia must perform does not always match the competency or practice mix available among the existing workforce. Hughes (2004b) argues that the existing infrastructure and outcomes associated with dietetic training and the dietetic profession should be built on to improve the capacity of the public health nutrition workforce. This would entail targeting dietitians and dietetic graduates for advanced competency development via integrated learning systems—such as linking work with further studies, linking novices with mentors, and developing systems that increase worker access to public health information.

Dietitians as a professional group have been recognised as priority (but not exclusive) targets for ongoing public health nutrition workforce development in Australia. Underpinning this view is a consistent qualifier that workforce development targeting dietitians should not be exclusive or limited to this professional group (Hughes 2004a, 2003b). An inclusive view is consistent with the multidisciplinary model of public health nutrition workforce development and practice (Rogers & Schlossman 1997).

Conclusion

This chapter has illustrated how sociological analysis can be used to identify and describe the determinants that affect the capacity of the public health nutrition workforce. Consideration of the historical, cultural, structural and critical factors that affect the actions and effectiveness of the public health nutrition workforce is an important step in effective workforce development. This will ultimately bolster society's capacity to address public health nutrition issues.

SUMMARY OF MAIN POINTS

- The public health nutrition workforce is that group within the health workforce that focuses on addressing the determinants of population-level nutrition and health problems, on preventing diet-related disease, and on promoting health and well-being.
- Dietitians are the dominant professional group in the designated public health nutrition workforce. They have also been identified as a priority target for public health nutrition workforce development, in recognition of this existing workplace positioning, their training background and competency development needs.

Roger Hughes

- The public health nutrition workforce is influenced by a range of factors that influence its capacity to effectively address public health nutrition issues. The major capacity determinants identified in this sociological analysis were structural, including small workforce size, existing practices that do not align with agreed core functions, inadequacies in workforce preparation, and a lack of consensus on workforce competencies.

SOCIOLOGICAL REFLECTION

- Reflect on how you conceptualise the nutrition workforce in terms of its composition and structure. Include how you see your role within this workforce.
- Reflect on your own competency mix (existing or developing). Do you have the competencies to be effective in public health nutrition?
- For those who have been, or are being, educated as a dietitian, reflect on the adequacy of your education for public health nutrition practice.

DISCUSSION QUESTIONS

1. What workforce groups (other than dietitians) are important constituents of the public health nutrition workforce?
2. What competency strengths and deficits are these practitioners likely to have in terms of effective public health nutrition practice?
3. What strategies, other than further competency development for dietitians, do you think are required to enhance the capacity of the public health nutrition workforce?
4. Review the definitions of 'public health nutrition' given in the chapter. Which of these definitions would you use? Justify your answer.
5. What are the main differences between the practice of public health nutrition and that of clinical dietetics?
6. Why is consideration of the capacity of the workforce important in the context of addressing public health nutrition issues such as obesity?

Further investigation

1. To what extent can a dietitian working in a community health setting reorient their services away from the traditional clinical role to working as a public health nutritionist?
2. What structural and cultural barriers might hamper the reorientation from clinical to public health nutrition work?

FURTHER READING AND WEB RESOURCES

Books and reports

Commonwealth Department of Housing, Health and Community Services 1992, *Food and Nutrition Policy*, Australian Government Publishing Services, Canberra.

Commonwealth of Australia 2001, *Food Regulation in Australia: A Chronology*, Department of the Parliamentary Library, Canberra.

Hughes R. 2005, *A Competency Framework for Public Health Nutrition Workforce Development*, Australian Public Health Nutrition Academic Collaboration, November, www.aphnac.com.

Lester, I. 1994, *Australia's Food and Nutrition*, Australian Institute of Health and Welfare, Canberra, available online at www.aihw.gov.au.

National Health and Medical Research Council (NHMRC) 1997, *Acting on Australia's Weight: A Strategic Plan for the Prevention of Overweight and Obesity*, NHMRC, Canberra, available online at www.nhmrc.gov.au/publications/synopses/n21syn.htm.

—— 2003, *Dietary Guidelines for Adult Australians*, NHMRC, Canberra (including appendices on the Nutrition of Aboriginal and Torres Strait Islander Peoples; Social Status, Nutrition and the Cost of Healthy Eating; and Dietary Guidelines and the Sustainability of Food Systems), available online at www.nhmrc.gov.au/publications/synopses/dietsyn.htm.

Nestle, M. 2007, *Food Politics*, Revised edition, University of California Press, California.

Strategic Inter-Governmental Nutrition Alliance (SIGNAL) 2001, *Eat Well Australia: A Strategic Framework for Public Health Nutrition 2000–2010*, National Public Health Partnership, Canberra, available online at www.nphp.gov.au/publications/index.htm#signal.

—— 2001, *National Aboriginal and Torres Strait Islander Nutrition Strategy and Action Plan, 2000–2010*, National Public Health Partnership, Canberra, available online at www.nphp.gov.au/publications/index.htm#signal.

Wahlqvist, M. & Kouris-Blazos, A. 2002, 'Food and Nutrition Policies in the Asia-Pacific Region: Nutrition in Transition', in M. Wahlqvist (ed.), *Food and Nutrition: Australia, Asia and the Pacific*, 2nd edition, Allen & Unwin, Sydney, pp. 575–98.

Journals

Australia and New Zealand Journal of Public Health: www.blackwellpublishing.com/journal.asp?ref=1326-0200&site=1

Critical Public Health: www.criticalpublichealth.net

Public Health: http://intl.elsevierhealth.com/journals/pubh/default.cfm

Public Health Nutrition: http://journals.cambridge.org/action/displayJournal?jid=PHN

Websites

Australian Institute of Health and Welfare (AIHW): www.aihw.gov.au

Australian Public Health Nutrition Academic Collaboration (APHNAC): www.aphnac.com

Codex Alimentarius Commission: www.codexalimentarius.net/

Food and Agriculture Organization (FAO): www.fao.org

Food Standards Australia New Zealand (FSANZ): www.foodstandards.gov.au

National Health and Medical Research Council (NHMRC, Australia): www.nhmrc.gov.au

Public Health Association of Australia (PHAA): www.phaa.net.au

WHO Global Strategy on Diet, Physical Activity and Health: www.who.int/dietphysicalactivity/en/

REFERENCES

Adamson A. & Cowburn G. 1996, 'Community Nutrition and Dietetics: A Survey of Nutrition Group Members in 1995', *Journal of Human Nutrition and Dietetics*, vol. 9, pp. 339–48.

AIHW—*see* Australian Institute of Health and Welfare.

American College of Preventive Medicine 2002, *Core Competencies and Performance Indicators for Preventive Medicine Residents*, American College of Preventive Medicine, Washington, DC.

American Dietetic Association 2000, 'Report on the American Dietetic Association's Member Needs Assessment/Satisfaction Survey', *Journal of the American Dietitians Association*, vol. 100, pp. 112–16.

Anthony H. & Cooper C. 1998, *Summary Report on Public Health and Community Nutrition Activities Carried Out by Victorian Members of the Dietitians Association of Australia*, Dietitians Association of Australia (Vic. Branch), Melbourne.

Australian Institute of Health and Welfare 2000, *Profile of Dietitian Labour Force Australia 1996*, Australian Institute of Health and Welfare, Canberra.

Campbell K., Steele J., Woods J. & Hughes R. 1997, *Developing a Public Health Nutrition Workforce in Australia: Workforce Issues*, National Specialty Program in Public Health and Community Nutrition, Melbourne.

CDC & ATSDR—*see* Centers for Disease Control and Prevention & Agency for Toxic Substances and Disease Registry.

Centers for Disease Control and Prevention & Agency for Toxic Substances and Disease Registry 2001, *Strategic Plan for Public Health Workforce Development*, US Department of Health and Human Services, Washington, DC.

CLBAPHP & HRSA—*see* Council on Linkages Between Academic and Public Health Practice & Health Resources and Services Administration.

Corby, L. 1997, 'Assessment of Community Development and Leadership Skills Required by Caribbean Nutritionists and Dietitians: Research and International Collaboration in Action', *Journal of Nutrition Education*, vol. 29, no. 5, pp. 250–7.

Council on Linkages Between Academic and Public Health Practice & Health Resources and Services Administration 2002, *Core Competencies for Public Health Professionals: 2002*, CLBAPHP & HRSA, Rockville, Maryland.

Dodds J. & Kaufman M. 1991, *Personnel in Public Health Nutrition for the 1990s: A Comprehensive Guide*, Public Health Foundation, Washington, DC.

Dodds J. & Polhamus B. 1999, 'Self-perceived Competence in Advanced Public Health Nutritionists in the United States', *Journal of the American Dietetic Association*, vol. 99, no. 7, pp. 808–12.

Gatchell S. & Woolcott D. 1992, 'A Demographic Profile of Canadian Public Health Nutritionists', *Journal of the Canadian Dietetic Association*, vol. 53, pp. 30–4.

Gebbie K. & Merrill J. 2001, 'Enumeration of the Public Health Workforce: Developing a System', *Journal of Public Health Management Practice*, vol. 7, no. 4, pp. 8–16.

Gebbie K., Rosenstock L. & Hernendez L. 2002, '*Who Will Keep the Public Health? Educating Public Health Professionals for the 21st Century*', Institute of Medicine National Academic Press, Washington, DC.

Grant, J. 2002, 'Learning Needs Assessment: Assessing the Need', *British Medical Journal*, vol. 321, pp. 156–9.

Handler A., Issel M. & Turnock B. 2001, 'A Conceptual Framework to Measure Performance of the Public Health System', *American Journal of Public Health*, vol. 91, no. 8, p. 1235–9.

Haughton B., Story M. & Keir B. 1998, 'Profile of Public Health Nutrition Personnel: Challenges for Population/System-focused Roles and State-level Monitoring', *Journal of the American Dietetic Association*, vol. 98, no. 6, pp. 664–70.

Healthwork UK 2001, *National Standards for Specialist Practice in Public Health: An Overview* (Approved Version), Healthwork UK, London, p. 7.

Howat P., Maycock B., Jackson L., Lower T., Cross D., Collins J. & van Asselt K. 2000, 'Development of Competency-based University Health Promotion Courses', *Promotion & Education*, vol. VII, no. 1, pp. 33–8.

Hughes R. 1998, 'An Omnibus Survey of the Australian Rural Health Dietetic Workforce', *Australian Journal of Nutrition and Dietetics*, vol. 55, no. 4, pp. 163–9.

—— 2003a, 'Definitions for Public Health Nutrition: A Developing Consensus', *Public Health Nutrition*, vol. 6, no. 6, pp. 615–20.

——2003b, 'Public Health Nutrition Workforce Composition, Core Functions, Competencies and Capacity: Perspectives of Advanced Level Practitioners in Australia, *Public Health Nutrition*, vol. 6, pp. 607–13.

—— 2003c, 'Competency Development in Public Health Nutrition: Reflections of Advanced Level Practitioners in Australia', *Nutrition & Dietetics*, vol. 6, pp. 607–13.

—— 2003d, 'Competency Development Needs of the Australian Public Health Nutrition Workforce,' *Public Health Nutrition*, vol. 6, pp. 839–47.

—— 2004a, *Public Health Nutrition Workforce Development: A Blue-print for Australia*, School of Health Science, Griffith University, Gold Coast.

—— 2004b, 'Enumerating and Profiling the Australian Public Health Nutrition Workforce', *Nutrition & Dietetics*, vol. 61, pp. 162–71.

—— 2004c, 'Employers' Expectations of Core Functions and Competencies for Public Health Nutrition Practice in Australia', *Nutrition & Dietetics*, vol. 61, pp. 105–11.

—— 2004d, 'Competencies for Effective Public Health Nutrition Practice: A Developing Consensus', *Public Health Nutrition*, vol. 6, pp. 839–47.

—— 2005, 'A Competency Framework for Public Health Nutrition Workforce Development', Australian Public Health Nutrition Academic Collaboration, November, www.aphnac.com.

—— 2006, 'A Socio-ecological Analysis of the Determinants of National Public Health Nutrition Workforce Capacity: Australia as a Case Study', *Family & Community Health*, vol. 29, pp. 55–67.

—— & Somerset S. 1997, 'Definitions and Conceptual Frameworks for Public Health and Community Nutrition: A Discussion Paper', *Australian Journal of Nutrition and Dietetics*, vol. 54, no. 1, pp. 40–5.

—— & Woods J. 2003, *A Needs Assessment for Public Health Nutrition Workforce Development in Victoria: Report 2 of the Victorian Public Health Nutrition Workforce Development Initiative*, Monash University, Melbourne.

Johnson D., Eaton D., Wahl P. & Gleason C. 2001, 'Public Health Nutrition Practice in the United States', *Journal of the American Dietetic Association*, vol. 101, no. 5, pp. 529–34.

Kaufman D. 2003, 'Applying Educational Theory in Practice', *British Medical Journal*, vol. 326, pp. 213–16.

Kaufman M. (ed.) 1990, *Nutrition in Public Health: A Handbook for Developing Programs and Services*, Aspen Publishers, Gaithersburg, New York State.

——, Heimendinger J., Foerster S. & Carroll M. 1986, 'Survey of Nutritionists in State and Local Public Health Agencies', *Journal of the American Dietetic Association*, vol. 86, pp. 1566–70.

Kennedy V. & Moore F. 2001, 'A Systems Approach to Public Health Workforce Development', *Journal of Public Health Management Practice*, vol. 7, no. 4, pp. 17–22.

Landman J. 2001, 'Training in Public Health Nutrition: Symposium at the 17th International Congress of Nutrition, Vienna', *Public Health Nutrition*, vol. 4, no. 6, pp. 1301–2.

——, Buttriss J. & Margetts B. 1998, 'Curriculum Design for Professional Development in Public Health Nutrition in Britain', *Public Health Nutrition*, vol. 1, no. 1, pp. 69–74.

Lane D., Ross V., Chan D. & O'Neill C. 1999, 'Core Competencies for Preventative Medicine Residents: Version 2', *American Journal of Preventive Medicine*, vol. 16, no. 4, pp. 367–72.

Lee A. 2002, 'Enhanced Investment in Nutrition in Queensland Health', *Foodchain*, vol. 9.

Lichtveld M., Cioffi J., Baker E., Bailey S., Gebbie K., Henderson J., Jones D. & Kurz R. 2001, 'Partnership for Front-Line Success: A Call for a National Action Agenda on Workforce Development', *Journal of Public Health Management Practice*, vol. 7, no. 4, pp. 1–7.

Manning C. & Vickery C. 2000, 'Disengagement and Work Constraints are Deterrents to Participation in Continuing Professional Education Amongst Registered Dietitians', *Journal of the American Dietetic Association*, vol. 100, pp. 1540–2.

Meyer R., Gilroy R. & Williams P. 2002, 'Dietitians in NSW: Workforce Trends 1984–2000', *Australian Health Review*, vol. 25, no. 3, pp. 122–30.

National Commission for Health Education Credentialing 2002, *Responsibilities and Competencies for Health Educators*, NCHEC, Allentown, Philadelphia.

National Health and Medical Research Council 1996, *Promoting the Health of Australians: A Review of Infrastructure Support for National Health Advancement: Final Report*, Australian Government Publishing Service, Canberra.

National Public Health Partnership 2001, *Public Health Practice in Australia Today: Core Functions*, National Public Health Partnership, Melbourne.

NCHEC—*see* National Commission for Health Education Credentialing.

Nestle M. 2002, *Food Politics: How the Food Industry Influences Nutrition and Health*, University of California Press, Los Angeles.

NHMRC—*see* National Health and Medical Research Council.

Niall M. & O'Dea K. 1997, 'Viewpoint Article: Definitions and Conceptual Framework for Public Health and Community Nutrition' [letter to editor], *Australian Journal of Nutrition and Dietetics*, vol. 54, no. 4, pp. 208.

NPHP—*see* National Public Health Partnership.

Nutrition Society 2000, *How to Specify Levels of Learning Outcome in Public Health Nutrition*, Nutrition Society, London.

Pelletier D. 1997, 'Advanced Training in Food and Nutrition: Disciplinary, Interdisciplinary, and Problem Orientated Approaches', *Food and Nutrition Bulletin*, vol. 18, no. 2, pp. 134–45.

Pew Health Professions Commission 1998, *Recreating Health Professional Practice for a New Century: Fourth Report of the Pew Health Professions Commission*, Pew Health Professions Commission, San Francisco.

PHAA—*see* Public Health Association of Australia.

Precision Consultancy 2000, *Draft Health Promotion Competency Standards*, Precision Consultancy, Melbourne.

Public Health Association of Australia 1990, *Workforce Issues for Public Health: The Report of the Public Health Workforce Study*, Public Health Association of Australia, Canberra.

Riddout L., Gadiel D., Cook K. & Wise M. 2002, *Planning Framework for the Public Health Workforce: Discussion Paper*, National Public Health Partnership, Melbourne.

Rogers B. & Schlossman N. 1997, '"Public Nutrition": The Need for Cross-disciplinary Breadth in the Education of Applied Nutrition Professional', *Food and Nutrition Bulletin*, vol. 18, no. 2, pp. 120–33.

Rowe G. & Wright G. 1999, 'The Delphi Technique as a Forecasting Tool: Issues and Analysis', *International Journal of Forecasting*, vol. 15, pp. 353–75.

Scott J. & Binns C. 1988, 'A Profile of Dietetics in Australia: Part 1—Demography and Educational Characteristics', *Journal of Food and Nutrition*, vol. 45, no. 3, pp. 77–9.

—— 1989, 'A Profile of Dietetics in Australia: Part 2—Employment Characteristics', *Australian Journal of Nutrition and Dietetics*, vol. 46, no. 1, pp. 14–17.

SIGNAL—*see* Strategic Inter-Governmental Nutrition Alliance.

Steele J. 1995, *Towards a Public Health Nutrition Human Resource Infrastructure in Queensland*, Master of Public Health Program, University of Queensland, Brisbane, p. 158.

Strategic Inter-Governmental Nutrition Alliance 2001a, *Eat Well Australia: Strategic Framework for Public Health Nutrition 2000–2010*, National Public Health Partnership & Department of Health and Aged Care, Canberra.

—— 2001b, *Eat Well Australia: An Agenda for Action for Public Health Nutrition 2000–2010*, National Public Health Partnership & Department of Health and Aged Care, Canberra.

Tapsell L. & de Groot, R. 1999, 'Dietitian-nutritionists in the Australian Food Industry: An Educational Needs Assessment', *Australian Journal of Nutrition and Dietetics*, vol. 56, no. 2, pp. 86–90.

Vernon D. & Blake R. 1993, 'Does Problem-based Learning Work? A Meta-analysis of Evaluation Research', *Academic Medicine*, vol. 68, pp. 550–3.

Williams P. 1993, 'Trends in the New South Wales Dietetic Workforce 1984–1991', *Australian Journal of Nutrition and Dietetics*, vol. 50, no. 3, pp. 116–19.

Yngve A., Sjostrom M., Warn D., Margetts B., Rodrigo C. & Nissinen A. 1999, 'Effective Promotion of Healthy Nutrition and Physical Activity in Europe Requires Skilled and Competent People: European Masters' Programme in Public Health Nutrition', *Public Health Nutrition*, vol. 2(3a), pp. 449–52.

CHAPTER 9

Risk, Maternal Ideologies and Infant Feeding

Elizabeth Murphy

OVERVIEW

- How and why is infant feeding seen as a social problem in industrialised countries?
- How can we understand policy responses to the 'problem' of infant feeding?
- How do mothers respond to the demands that such policies and associated professional practices place on them?

The decline in the frequency and duration of breastfeeding in industrialised countries during the early twentieth century was a concern to policy makers. While breastfeeding rates in most industrialised countries have increased since 1970, many mothers continue to feed their babies in ways experts see as suboptimal. Currently around 30 per cent of mothers in the United Kingdom and less than 40 per cent of American mothers breastfeed babies for the recommended period. Rather more Australian mothers breastfeed, but a significant proportion do not. This situation concerns policy makers and health professionals because of evidence of the nutritional and health benefits of breastfeeding.

Breastfeeding promotion is emblematic of many areas where individuals are presented with expert assessments of risk and encouraged to modify their behaviour accordingly. Risk assessment and avoidance have been elevated to the status of moral obligations and, in the case of infant feeding, this obligation is intensified by the intersection of the discourse of risk with those surrounding expertise and motherhood. I consider the ways in which, both historically and currently, the 'problem' of infant feeding has been individualised and transformed into a question of maternal morality. I consider how experts are invested with power to define standards of 'good mothering' and how mothers seek to re-establish positive identities when they fail to live up to these standards. I suggest that mothers' accounts of feeding decisions can be read as displays of morality and responsibility in the face of expectations about what it means to be a good wife or girlfriend and a good woman, as well as a good mother.

Key terms

deviance   medicalisation   risk discourse

Introduction

'One must feel an absolute failure or feel that you are letting your baby down in some way if you don't breast-feed.'

'You've got to say "yes" or you're some kind of monster.'

One of the most immediate decisions facing a new mother in contemporary industrialised societies concerns whether to breastfeed or formula feed. As illustrated by the above excerpts from interviews with first-time mothers, this decision raises profound issues of morality and maternal responsibility. Medical opinion and health and nutrition policy are unequivocal: breast is best. Internationally, the WHO (2001) and UNICEF (2006) are committed to promoting breastfeeding. This pro-breastfeeding stance is reflected in government policies. In both the UK and the USA exclusive breastfeeding for six months is recommended (DoH 2003; AAP 2005) and this is reflected in national health objectives (DoH 1999, 2004; US Department of Health and Human Services 2000). Similarly, guidelines from the Australian National Health and Medical Research Council (2003) emphasise that 'exclusive breastfeeding until around six months should be the aim for every infant'.

Breastfeeding promotion is directed towards reducing risks to babies' short-, medium- and long-term health. These include:

- respiratory, urinary tract and gastro-intestinal infections (Howie et al. 1990; Lopez-Alarcon et al. 1997; Heinig 2001; Marild et al. 2004)
- allergies such as eczema, asthma and food intolerance (Saarinen & Kajosaari 1995; Gdalevich et al. 2001; Chulada et al. 2003)
- insulin-dependent diabetes (Virtanen et al. 1991; Jones et al. 1998)
- Chron's disease and cancers (Lawrence 1995; Davis et al. 1988; Bener et al. 2001)
- sudden infant death syndrome (Ford et al. 1993; McVea et al. 2000; see also Golding 1993 and British Paediatric Association 1994)
- impaired mother–infant bonding and lowered self-esteem (Lawrence 1995).

Breastfeeding is also credited with improving cognitive development and thus intelligence in adulthood (Mortensen et al. 2002).

Contemporary patterns of infant feeding

Despite strong scientific support, current breastfeeding initiation rates are relatively low in most industrialised countries. UK and US rates increased markedly after 1970, reaching 60 per cent in the USA by 1984 (Hartley & O'Connor 1996) and 67 per cent in the UK by 1980 (Martin & Monk 1982). Hopes of further improvements have not entirely been fulfilled. In 1990, 64 per cent of mothers in England and Wales initiated breastfeeding. Apparent increases to 68 per cent in 1995 and 71 per cent in 2000 (Foster et al. 1997; Hamlyn et al. 2002) disappear when standardised for age and occupational class. The US situation has been more volatile (Ryan et al. 2002). After declining to 51 per cent in 1990 (Hartley & O'Connor 1996), the most recent data show an upswing to 73 per cent in 2005 (CDCP 2006). In Australia, breastfeeding rates on hospital discharge have risen, from 40 to 45 per cent in the 1970s to 83 per cent in 2001, one of the highest breastfeeding initiation rates in the world (ABS 2001).

Concerns also centre on mothers who breastfeed for less than the recommended length of time. In 2000, only 29 per cent of British mothers breastfed to four months (Hamlyn et al. 2002). The percentage of women who were exclusively breastfeeding their babies is unknown but is probably considerably less. In the USA, in 2005, 39 per cent of babies were breastfed and 14 per cent exclusively breastfed at six months (the recommended duration in the USA) (CDCP 2006). Once again, figures for Australia are somewhat higher, with 48 per cent of mothers breastfeeding their babies to the recommended six months, although all of these were offering other foods as well (ABS 2001).

Breastfeeding and the privatisation of risk

Infant feeding raises profound issues of morality and responsibility. As such, breastfeeding is emblematic of the way in which **risk discourses** dominate a wide range of political programs and professional practices (Giddens 1991). In many areas, from mobile phones to pension provision, individuals are confronted with expert assessments of risk and are called upon to modify behaviour accordingly. Expert risk calculations are particularly prevalent in the health field, where individuals are warned about lifestyle risks—including those related to diet, exercise, smoking, alcohol and sexual behaviour—and are urged to reform their lifestyles. This contributes to the 'privatisation of risk management', characteristic of contemporary liberal societies (Rose 1996, p. 58).

Health is increasingly understood as something to be chosen (Greco 1993). The citizen no longer simply enjoys good health or suffers poor health. An individual can, through self-control, foster personal well-being. Citizens are expected to 'adopt a calculative, prudent personal relation to fate now conceived in terms of calculable dangers and avertable risks' (Rose 1996, p. 58).

Obligations to exercise prudence in the light of expert risk assessments are strongly moral (Nettleton 1997; Petersen 1997). Good health is a visible sign of 'initiative, adaptability, balance and strength of will ... a free and rational agent' (Greco 1993, p. 370). Health-compromising practices raise questions about mastery and self-control (Ogden 1995). Engaging in risky behaviours places one in potential 'moral danger' (Lupton 1993, p. 425), for neglecting to 'take care of self' (Greco 1993, p. 357). Failing to live up to the liberal ideal of the rational, responsible individual invites moral judgment (S. Carter 1995).

The excerpts above suggest this moral obligation to exercise prudence is intensified in the case of infant feeding. I propose that this is for two reasons. First, the potential consequences arising from 'risky' infant-feeding 'choices' (Murphy et al. 1998b) are borne not by the mother but by someone to whom she owes a duty of care. As I have argued elsewhere (Murphy 2000), special censure is reserved for those who knowingly put others at risk. Mary Douglas (1990) has gone so far as to suggest that being put at risk is the equivalent of being sinned against.

Second, such moral obligations are intensified by the cross-cutting of contemporary discourses of risk by an ideology of motherhood that holds mothers responsible for their children (Phoenix & Woollett 1991) and insists they need expert advice to carry out their responsibilities (Apple 1987). Mothers' main function is assumed to be maximising the short- and long-term physical and psychological welfare of their children (Hays 1996; Ribbens McCarthy et al. 2000). Locating infant feeding at this intersection between the powerful and mutually reinforcing discourses of risk, responsibility and motherhood places mothers who formula feed in particular moral jeopardy. Later, I examine how such mothers deal with this threat to their identities.

Breastfeeding 'failure': A historical perspective

Concern about mothers who 'fail' to breastfeed is not new. While policy makers sometimes reminisce about a golden age before formula feeding, anxiety about women's failure to breastfeed is longstanding (Arnup 1990; Lewis 1990; Fildes 1992; P. Carter 1995). In the eighteenth century, this focused on wet-nursing (Maher 1992; P. Carter 1995). Rousseau (cited in Kukla 2006) attributed the degeneration of 'the whole moral order' to this practice. In 1747, William Cadogan, a physician, ascribed wet-nursing to women's reluctance to 'give up a little of the Beauty of her Breast to feed her off-spring' (quoted in P. Carter 1995, p. 7). Although Cadogan attributed wet-nursing to female vanity, modern commentators point to husbands' insistence on sexual privileges and the belief that sexual intercourse would 'spoil the milk' (Maher 1992).

Katherine Arnup (1990), Jane Lewis (1990) and Valerie Fildes (1992) all show that failure to breastfeed caused public and professional anxiety in the early twentieth century in the United Kingdom and Canada. Fildes (1992) reports doctors' concerns about the decline of breastfeeding in the UK. Arnup (1990) relates the preoccupation with mothers who did not breastfeed to wider public anxieties about national adequacy. In the UK the discovery, during Boer War recruitment, that many working-class men were unfit for military service provoked concern. In Canada, similar issues arose during the World War I. In both countries, attention focused on high rates of infant mortality, which were attributed to women's failure to breastfeed their babies.

The Canadians established a complex public health bureaucracy (Arnup 1990), emphasising prevention. Experts insisted most infant deaths were avoidable. However, the concept of prevention was limited. While acknowledging that a range of factors, including poverty, overcrowding and malnutrition, were associated with infant mortality, reformers focused on changing maternal behaviour—in particular, on promoting breastfeeding. As Arnup acknowledges, the reformers were right to view breast-feeding as the safest form of infant feeding. However, their exclusive focus on maternal behaviour diverted attention from social and material causes of infant mortality, making mothers exclusively responsible. Individualising the problem of infant feeding is, as we shall see, also characteristic of contemporary approaches to breastfeeding.

Jane Lewis (1990) describes similar concerns in England during the same period. Working-class women were seen as particularly problematic, and their education and reform as the key to improving the nation's health. Once again, by focusing upon the supposed 'ignorance and carelessness of mothers' (G. Newman 1906, quoted in P. Carter 1995, p. 41), such policies diverted attention from wider causes of infant mortality. As Lewis observes, 'The fault lay not in offering mothers information on child rearing, which they welcomed, but in subordinating the material conditions of their lives—the poverty and unsanitary living conditions—which were also at the root of the problem and which early twentieth century medical reports adequately diagnosed, to an individualist solution' (Lewis 1990, p. 6). Such individualisation is politically expedient. Emphasising the one aspect over which mothers may, superficially at least, be said to exercise control, renders other sources of morbidity and mortality invisible. Infant feeding becomes a problem of individual morality and responsibility.

Contemporary policy responses to the 'problem' of infant feeding

Infant feeding continues to be an intransigent problem for policy makers and health care practitioners. Despite expert consensus about the benefits of breastfeeding, most mothers feed their babies in ways that are judged suboptimal. Extensive efforts to educate mothers about the benefits of breastfeeding and the risks of formula feeding have not changed this situation. There is evidence that mothers have heard and understood these expert views and yet do not necessarily follow them (Murphy 1999; 2000; 2003; Kukla 2006), with implications for the health of the citizenry and future welfare expenditure (DoH 1994).

For contemporary liberal governments, reluctant to intervene directly in the private sphere and committed to upholding the autonomy of individuals and families, possibilities for improving childhood nutrition are limited. During the last century, a few direct welfare interventions were attempted. For example, in the UK, universal free school milk was introduced (and subsequently abandoned). More recently, the National Fruit Scheme provides every child aged between four and six with a free piece of fruit each day at school. However, government policy continues to invest mothers with the responsibility for feeding their babies in ways that foster short- and long-term health. Thus, despite recent rhetorical shifts, government policy in the UK (DoH 2004) and Australia continues to perpetuate the individualising approach to health promotion criticised by Arnup and Lewis (Wall 2001; Kukla 2006).

This devolution of responsibility to mothers persists despite substantial evidence that initiation and duration of breastfeeding are associated with social positioning. Older, better educated, white women, from higher occupational classes, living with partners on higher incomes are more likely to start breastfeeding and to continue breastfeeding for longer (White et al. 1992; Lowe 1993; Pessl 1996; Piper & Parks 1996; Foster et al. 1997; Hamlyn et al. 2002; Ryan et al. 2002). Women who can least afford to buy infant formula, and whose babies are in greatest need of the protective and health-promoting qualities of breast milk, are least likely to breastfeed.

Professional and governmental responses to socioeconomic variations in infant feeding have largely been restricted to educating and 'targeting' mothers (Kukla 2006). Professionals are encouraged to direct education towards groups with low breastfeeding rates. Interventions sometimes include 'support' for disadvantaged women but this is generally limited to verbal encouragement rather than modifying the conditions under which women feed their babies. Once again, the problem of infant feeding is individualised. While research informing such interventions refers to 'determinants' of infant feeding practices (for example, Salt et al. 1994), these tend to be seen as immutable. Little attention is paid to disadvantages that constrain mothers' decisions, and even less has been done to overcome these, other than encouraging individual mothers to compensate for them. There is little recognition that the ability to make the 'right choice' is a privilege that is unevenly distributed (Knaak 2005).

Establishing breastfeeding makes heavy demands on mothers' time and energy (Murphy et al. 1998b). The American Academy of Pediatrics (2005) recommends up to 12 feeds a day, allowing no more than four hours between each, even if the baby is sleeping peacefully. Optimal infant nutrition is only one of the (sometimes competing) tasks that mothers must perform (Murphy et al. 1998a). The ability to meet such demands is inextricably linked to human and material resources. A new mother supported by her partner, family, and friends can breastfeed while others run the home. Later, when time between feeds is at a premium, access to a car allows women to combine breastfeeding with essential trips to the supermarket or the health centre.

The romanticisation of breastfeeding (Kukla 2006) may obscure not only such material constraints on maternal 'choice', but may also trivialise both physical discomforts and the impact of cultural imperatives derived from the sexualisation of breasts, that mean that some women risk accusations of inappropriate sexual display if they breastfeed in front of others. Linda Blum (1999) has reported that, for some women at least, the cost of transgressing such imperatives goes beyond disapproval to physical violence.

Mothers' responses to expert advice on infant feeding

The **medicalisation** of infant feeding is one aspect of expert involvement in child-rearing and family life. Dorothy Chunn (1990) describes the impact of this new 'cadre of experts': 'Good mothering, parenthood, marital sex were not simply a matter of following biological instinct: they were activities requiring the most specialised knowledge and training' (p. 92). Thus, as Lynn Jamieson and Claire Toynbee (1990) argue, children's needs are now defined by professionals rather than by parents, and experts can undermine parents' definitions of reality. Parents, and in particular mothers, bear the responsibility of meeting expert-defined needs, in expert-approved ways, rather than identifying and interpreting their children's needs for themselves. More traditional sources of information, such as family and friends, have been displaced (Arnup 1990). Stephanie Knaak's historical analysis of selected editions of Dr Spock's influential child care manual, from 1946 to 1998, shows how discourses around infant feeding have shifted over the period (Knaak 2005). In the 1998 edition few situations are recognised as justifying formula feeding and breastfeeding is increasingly associated with notions of good, child-centred motherhood. The dominance of science and technology has led to an assumption that lay people, particularly parents, need expert guidance. In infant feeding, as elsewhere, children's needs and the optimal means of meeting those needs are now defined by experts.

While recognising that infant feeding has become an 'expert domain', we should not exaggerate the power of experts to control infant feeding (Murphy 2003). Women are not passive recipients of expert directives. In practice, their exposure to surveillance and control is limited. While women's feeding practices are subject to social, cultural and material constraints, it is mothers who are in day-to-day control of feeding (Maher 1992). Experts may recommend exclusive breastfeeding, but mothers can ignore such advice. This is reflected in the relatively small numbers of women who actually meet current recommendations for exclusive breastfeeding. Mothers can and do resist attempts to direct infant feeding.

The force of expert advice lies not in compelling women to conform, but in setting a moral context within which women negotiate their identities as mothers. Just because women do not always follow expert recommendations does not mean such recommendations have no impact. Their power lies not in making women do what they would otherwise not have done, but in their authority to define standards by which mothers' feeding is judged, by others and by the women themselves.

Elizabeth Murphy

The categorical nature of expert advice on breastfeeding makes failing to follow it particularly transparent. Either babies are exclusively breastfed for the recommended period or they are not. Failure to breastfeed lays one open to the charge of being a 'poor mother' (P. Carter 1995). However, simply breastfeeding one's child is not in itself constitutive of good mothering. 'Good mothers' not only breastfeed their babies, but they must do so 'successfully', so that the baby thrives. As Oakley comments: 'A baby that is feeding and growing "well" is … a tangible token of her love and work. Conversely, a baby who gains weight more slowly than it "should", and who perhaps cries a lot and seems unsatisfied is … a sign of maternal failure' (1979, p. 165). Infant feeding is not simply a practical activity; it is a moral undertaking. The way a mother feeds her baby becomes a symbol of her general ability to care for her child (Lupton 1996).

Dealing with moral jeopardy

The force of expert definitions of breastfeeding and formula feeding as 'good' and 'bad' respectively, and the implications of such definitions for the self-evaluations of mothers, were illustrated in a recent longitudinal study of mothers' decisions about feeding their babies (Murphy et al. 1998a; 1998b; Murphy 1999; 2000; 2003; 2004; 2007). Thirty-six first-time mothers living within 10 miles of Nottingham, England, were interviewed at six intervals between late pregnancy and their babies' second birthdays. Quota sampling was used to ensure heterogeneity in terms of both the age and occupational class of the women. (Full details can be found in Murphy 1999, 2000.) The data discussed below are from the first two interviews, one shortly before the births and the other two months afterwards.

Antenatally, most women (29) intended to breastfeed; six to formula feed; and one to combine breastfeeding and formula feeding. Those planning to breastfeed emphasised the health benefits to the baby, reflecting current expert opinion. One said, 'I just think it's healthy for the baby; it gets all the, the goodness from the breast … because at the beginning the first lot of milk, it's got all the extra vitamins and nourishment which the baby needs and also, er whatever it is, antibodies, whatever to protect it from diseases and bugs.' These women were able to present themselves unproblematically as 'good mothers' who prioritised their babies' needs. Their intentions converged with expert advice and their explanations can be read as straightforward claims to responsible motherhood.

By contrast, despite the interviewers' self-consciously neutral stance, the talk of five of the six women intending to formula feed appeared to be formulated in response to the putative charge that formula feeding is irresponsible or inappropriate, evidence that the woman will be a 'bad mother'. These women treated their decision to formula-feed their babies as morally accountable, as an 'untoward act' (Scott & Lyman 1963). The sixth woman's talk differed from all the others in the study. She acknowledged that breastfeeding was 'supposed to be more good for the baby', but did not treat either her decision to formula-feed or any other decision about her baby as needing justification.

The remaining five women who intended to formula-feed acknowledged their deviation from expert recommendations and sought to counter any consequent suggestion that they were not 'good mothers'. Their ripostes took different forms. First, they challenged expert claims that 'breast is best', often using the quasi-scientific language of 'nutrients' and 'vitamins'. One woman said, 'There's the same nutrients in both … they say breast milk is better because it's yours and it's nature … there's definitely the same nutrients in both.' Formula feeding was presented as more reliable, because 'at least you know how much it's getting'. Breastfeeding mothers ran the risk of underfeeding their babies:

> Like sometimes a woman's had a poor diet through pregnancy or if she has a poor diet when she's had a baby because probably she is rushing around after the baby, then her milk could be poor if she was breastfeeding the baby. So the baby might be starving you know. It might not be getting the right, or gaining weight properly. So I think it's better bottle.

Here, the 'good mother' is redefined as one who ensures her baby receives sufficient milk, rather than one who uses a particular type of milk. The women bolstered the legitimacy of formula feeding by pointing to 'perfectly healthy' babies who have been formula fed.

The women's second challenge to the implied charge of irresponsibility was to question experts' authority in defining the best interests of their particular child. They appealed to their own authority as mothers ('I don't care what everybody else says, it's what I feel is better for my child') and to the expertise of their family and friends ('I think my family knows best').

These women also justified their decision in terms of responsibilities to others. Breastfeeding would exclude their partners or other family members. One explained, 'But you see, if I was breastfeeding he'd feel left out because he wouldn't be able to feed his baby.' This reminds us that the moral responsibilities of mothers extend beyond their babies. Not only did these women have to be 'good mothers', but they were also expected (and expected themselves) to be 'good partners'. Harriette Marshall's analysis of child-care manuals shows how women are required to insulate their partners from any negative consequences of the baby's arrival. It is for women to reconcile the baby's and the father's interests, however much these conflict (Marshall 1991).

While women who intended to breastfeed their babies did not have to justify this decision per se, a number emphasised their continued commitment to their partners, confronting the potential charge that breastfeeding would lead to neglect or exclusion of partners. Thus, the defence invoked by formula-feeders became, for some breastfeeders, a challenge to be addressed. A number described plans to express breast milk to avoid the father feeling 'left out'. One said, 'I intend, as

Elizabeth Murphy

early as possible, to start expressing and giving it bottles of breast milk so that Ray [her partner] can have that [the opportunity to feed the baby]'. Another said, 'I was worried he'd feel a bit left out, but I've bought a breast pump anyway and I've got some bottles and a sterilising unit'.

As well as dealing with the moral injunctions to be 'good mothers' and 'good partners', mothers must also be 'good women'. The 'sexualisation' of women's breasts (Kukla 2006) means that breastfeeding women risk being seen as immodest or indiscreet. Those intending to formula-feed also justified their decision in terms of modesty. One explained, 'I'm self-conscious about my body … I'm not going to have to get my boobs out in the middle of Nottingham'. Another had been 'quite put off' by seeing a woman breastfeeding in public and insisted breastfeeding women should 'hide away'.

Conversely, several women intending to breastfeed distanced themselves from any suggestion of brazenness or immodesty. They stressed measures they would take to avoid giving offence:

> When I'm out in public, I don't like the idea of that … I couldn't just openly do it in public … I'd feel conscious if I was out and the baby wanted to feed, and I'd want some kind of privacy, because it's like flashing your flesh to everyone.

As we have seen, the women who had decided against breastfeeding their babies were vulnerable to the charge of being 'bad mothers'. Their reasons for formula feeding can be read as a rebuttal of a potential charge of **deviance**. However, mothers who prolong breastfeeding, particularly for more than one year, may also incur disapproval (Hills-Bonczyk et al. 1994; Kendall-Tackett & Sugarman 1995). A number of women distanced themselves from being the 'sort of woman' who prolonged breastfeeding. They referred to such behaviour as 'not very dignified' and 'very, very distasteful'. One woman said, 'Our midwife told us that somebody breastfeeds when they are three. That to me is absolutely revolting, for mother and child, because it's not natural'.

Of the 30 women intending to breastfeed, only six went on to meet current UK recommendations for exclusive breastfeeding for a minimum of four months. The other 24 women breastfed from four hours to 14 weeks, with half stopping before two weeks after the birth and 21 before two months. These women described, in detail, their disappointment and distress at not feeding their babies for as long as they intended. They detailed their sense of failure and judgment by both professional and lay people (Murphy 2000).

Women who reverted to formula feeding faced particular difficulties in establishing themselves as responsible and morally adequate mothers. They had, in the antenatal interviews, endorsed expert opinion that breast milk was nutritionally superior and reduced the risks to the health of babies. Often they had framed breastfeeding in moral terms. One had said, 'I think sometimes you've got to be not selfish and consider the baby's health'. Breastfeeding had been presented as a subordination of mothers' interests to those of babies (Murphy et al. 1998b). As such, antenatally, they framed their feeding intentions squarely within the ideology of motherhood discussed above. Their subsequent decision to formula feed raised doubts about their maternal credentials and required renegotiating moral meanings (Douglas 1990). The postnatal interviews became occasions when mothers reconstructed images of themselves as normal, moral, responsible and good mothers in the face of doubts provoked by formula feeding.

In reconstructing identities as good mothers, these women accounted for formula feeding in various ways (Murphy 2000; 2003). Whereas, antenatally, they drew on expert assessments to assert the superiority of breastfeeding, they now appealed to knowledge based on experience rather than statistics to defend using formula. They cited both the experience of friends and relatives and their own experience to argue that formula feeding was best for their child. Babies who were unhappy or failing to thrive were presented as settling and thriving once formula milk was introduced. Many detailed difficulties that made introducing formula milk inevitable. These included the extreme nature of both the baby's hunger and the physical distress to the woman herself from breastfeeding. They pointed to others' contribution to failed breastfeeding. They told 'atrocity stories' (Webb & Stimson 1976) in which they and their babies were victims of insensitive, careless, ignorant or negligent behaviour of others, both professional carers and lay contacts.

As we have seen, the moral obligations confronting a new mother are both complex and weighty. To be a 'good mother', a woman must breastfeed her baby for an extended period. To be a 'good mother' who is also a 'good partner', she must breastfeed without allowing her husband or boyfriend to feel neglected or displaced. To be a 'good mother' and a 'good wife' who is also a 'good woman' is even more demanding. She must avoid offending others by breastfeeding in public or beyond the age when it is socially acceptable. The space within which she can simultaneously be a 'good mother', a 'good partner', and a 'good woman' is extremely limited. Many women in the Nottingham study were actively engaged in moral repair work, both before and after their babies' births. Faced by potential threats to their identities as good mothers, partners, and women, they actively sought to re-establish their credentials and to justify their feeding behaviours. Thus moral repair work was just one more of the many challenges facing these new mothers.

Conclusion

In this chapter, we have looked at the 'problem of infant feeding' from a sociological perspective. We have examined the transformation of nutritional concerns into a problem of maternal behaviour. Issues of morality, risk, and individual responsibility have come to preoccupy both policy makers and mothers themselves. For policy

Elizabeth Murphy

makers and health practitioners, the problem may appear simple: babies should be breastfed, but too few mothers do so for long enough. Solutions proposed include educating supposedly ignorant mothers, but this approach has had limited success. I would argue that those developing policies to encourage breastfeeding must recognise that infant feeding is a moral as well as a nutritional matter, and that simply trying to change the knowledge or behaviour of individual women, without paying due attention to the broader cultural and material contexts in which they act, is likely to meet with limited success.

Acknowledgments

The empirical work discussed in this chapter was funded by the UK Economic and Social Research Council as part of the Nation's Diet Programme (L209252035). I am very grateful to the women and professionals who took part in this study, and to Dr Tony Avery and Lindsay Groom, of the Department of General Practice at the University of Nottingham, who gave me valuable assistance in locating and gaining access to the practices from which the sample was drawn. Special thanks are also due to Susan Parker and Christine Phipps, who carried out the interviews for this study and who made important contributions to an earlier version of this chapter.

SUMMARY OF MAIN POINTS

- Policy makers in most industrialised countries are concerned about low breastfeeding rates because of evidence of the health benefits of breastfeeding.
- Policy responses tend to individualise the problem, diverting attention from the social and economic conditions surrounding infant feeding decisions.
- Infant feeding has increasingly become an 'expert domain'. While experts cannot control mothers' feeding practices, they do set standards by which mothers are judged and judge themselves.
- Breastfeeding is a moral imperative and not breastfeeding leaves women vulnerable to the charge of being a 'poor mother'.
- Women have to combine breastfeeding with other moral imperatives including being a 'good partner' and a 'good woman'.

SOCIOLOGICAL REFLECTION

This chapter offers a sociological analysis of policy, practitioner and maternal engagement with the social problem of infant feeding. It shows how both historically and at the present time policy responses have individualised the failure of women to feed their babies in ways that fit with expert opinions about optimal nutrition. It shows infant feeding is located at the intersection of powerful discourses around risk, expertise and motherhood and how mothers resist attempts, grounded in these discourses, to constrain their feeding practices and deal with the threat to their moral identities created by failure to follow expert advice.

- In the light of what you have read in this chapter, do you think that current government initiatives around infant feeding, with their emphasis on individualising the problem of low breastfeeding rates, are appropriate?
- What are the consequences of treating infant feeding as a domain in which good practice is defined by professional experts?
- What problems do you see with the moralisation of infant feeding? What might be the unintended consequences of such approaches? What alternatives would you propose?

DISCUSSION QUESTIONS

1. Why are current trends in infant feeding in industrialised countries of concern to policy makers?
2. Can policy responses regarding infant feeding be seen as individualising a social problem?
3. Is infant feeding an example of medicalisation?
4. How do experts influence mothers' self-evaluations?
5. In what sense are expert discourses around infant feeding an example of the 'privatisation of risk'?
6. What does women's talk about feeding tell us about the ideology of motherhood?

Further investigation

1. The feeding of infants has increasingly become subject to processes of medicalisation. Discuss.
2. Trace the historical development of maternal ideologies with particular reference to infant feeding practices.

FURTHER READING AND WEB RESOURCES

Books

Arnup, K., Levesque, A. & Roach Pierson, R. 1990, *Delivering Motherhood: Maternal Ideologies and Practices in the 19th and 20th Centuries*, Routledge, London.

Blum, L. 1999, *At the Breast: Ideologies of Breastfeeding and Motherhood in the Contemporary United States*, Beacon Press, Boston.

Carter, P. 1995, *Feminism, Breasts and Breast Feeding*, Macmillan, Basingstoke, UK.

Elizabeth Murphy

Articles

Knaak, S. 2005, 'Breast-feeding, Bottle-feeding and Dr Spock: The Shifting Context of Choice', *Canadian Review of Sociology and Anthropology*, vol. 42, no. 2, pp. 197–216.

Murphy, E. 2000, 'Risk, Responsibility and Rhetoric in Infant Feeding', *Journal of Contemporary Ethnography*, vol. 29, pp. 291–325.

—— 2003, 'Expertise and Forms of Knowledge in the Government of Families', *The Sociological Review*, vol. 51, no. 4, pp. 433–62.

Websites

The Baby Friendly Initiative: www.babyfriendly.org.uk. A World Health Organization and United Nations' Children Fund (UNICEF) program to encourage breastfeeding and promote the International Code of Marketing of Breastmilk Substitutes

ChildInfo: www.childinfo.org. Provides access to statistical information collected by UNICEF.

Kellymom Breastfeeding & Parenting: http://kellymom.com. Provides evidence-based information on breastfeeding and parenting.

La Leche League International: www.lalecheleague.org. A global organisation that promotes breastfeeding and provides support and information for mothers.

REFERENCES

ABS—*see* Australian Bureau of Statistics.

American Academy of Pediatrics 2005, 'Breast Feeding and the Use of Human Milk', *Pediatrics*, vol. 115, no. 2, pp. 496–506.

Apple, R.D. 1987, *Mothers and Medicine: A Social History of Infant Feeding. 1890–1950*, University of Wisconsin Press, Wisconsin.

Arnup, K. 1990, 'Educating Mothers: Government Advice for Women in the Inter-War Years', in K. Arnup, A. Levesque & R. Roach Pierson (eds), *Delivering Motherhood: Maternal Ideologies and Practices in the 19th and 20th Centuries*, Routledge, London, pp. 190–210.

Australian Bureau of Statistics 2001, 'Breastfeeding in Australia', www.abs.gov.au/Ausstats [accessed 23/2/07].

Bailey, V.F. & Sherriff, J. 1993, 'Reasons for Early Cessation of Breastfeeding in Women from Lower Socio-economic Groups in Perth, Western Australia', *Breastfeeding Review*, vol. 11, pp. 390–3.

Bener, A., Denic, S. & Galadari, S. 2001, 'Longer Breast-feeding and Protection against Childhood Leukaemia and Lymphomas', *Eur J Cancer* vol. 37, pp. 234–8.

Blum, L. 1999, *At the Breast: Ideologies of Breastfeeding and Motherhood in the Contemporary United States*, Beacon Press, Boston.

British Paediatric Association 1994, 'Is Breastfeeding Beneficial in the UK? Statement of the Standing Committee on Nutrition', *Archives of the Disabled Child*, vol. 71, pp. 376–80.

Carter, P. 1995, *Feminism, Breasts and Breast Feeding*, Macmillan, Basingstoke, UK.

Carter, S. 1995, 'Boundaries of Danger and Uncertainty: An Analysis of the Technological Culture of Risk Assessment', in J. Gabe (ed.), *Medicine, Health and Risk*, Blackwell, Oxford, pp. 133–50.

CDCP—*see* Centers for Disease Control and Prevention.

Centers for Disease Control and Prevention 2006, 'Breastfeeding Practices—Results from the 2005 National Immunization Survey', www.cdc.gov/breastfeeding/data/NIS_data [accessed 23/2/2007].

Chulada, P.C., Arbes, S.J. Jr, Dunson, D. & Zeldin, D.C. 2003, 'Breast-feeding and the Prevalence of Asthma and Wheeze in Children: Analyses from the Third National Health and Nutrition Examination Survey, 1988–1994', *J Allergy Clin Immunol*, vol. 111, pp. 328–36.

Chunn, D. 1990, 'Boys Will Be Men, Girls Will Be Mothers', in P. Adler & P. Adler (eds), *Sociological Studies of Child Development*, JAI Press, Greenwich, Connecticut, pp. 87–110.

Davis, M.K., Savitz, D.A. & Graubard, B.L. 1988, 'Infant Feeding and Childhood Cancer', *Lancet* vol. 2(8607), pp. 365–8.

Department of Health 1994, *Weaning and the Weaning Diet: Report of the Working Group on the Weaning Diet of the Committee on Medical Aspects of Food Policy (no. 45)*, Her Majesty's Stationery Office, London.

—— 1999, *Saving Lives: Our Healthier Nation*, The Stationery Office, London.

—— 2003, 'Infant Feeding Recommendation', www.dh.gov.uk/assetRoot/04/09/69/99/04096999.pdf [accessed 23/2/2007].

—— 2004, *Choosing Health*, www.dh.gov.uk/PublicationsAndStatistics [accessed 23/2/2007].

DoH—*see* Department of Health.

Douglas, M. 1990, 'Risk as a Forensic Resource', *Daedalus*, Fall, pp. 1–16.

Fildes, V. 1992, 'Breast Feeding in London, 1905–19', *Journal of Biosocial Science*, vol. 24, pp. 53–70.

Ford, R.P.K., Taylor, B.J. & Mitchell, E.A. 1993, 'Breastfeeding and the Risk of Sudden Infant Death Syndrome', *International Journal of Epidemiology*, vol. 22, pp. 885–90.

Foster, F., Lader, D. & Cheesbrough, S. 1997, *Infant Feeding 1995*, The Stationery Office, London.

Giddens, A. 1991, *Modernity and Self-identity: Self and Society in the Late Modern Age*, Polity, Cambridge.

Gdalevich, M., Mimouni, D. & Mimouni, M. 2001, 'Breastfeeding and the Risk of Bronchial Asthma in Childhood: A Systematic Review and Meta-analysis of Prospective Studies', *J Pediatrics*, vol. 139, pp. 261–6.

Golding, J. 1993, *Breastfeeding and Sudden Infant Death Syndrome: Report of the Chief Medical Officer's Expert Group on the Sleeping Position of Infants and Cot Death*, Her Majesty's Stationery Office, London.

Greco, M. 1993, 'Psychomatic Subjects and the "Duty to be Well": Personal Agency within Medical Rationality', *Economy and Society*, vol. 22, 357–72.

Hamlyn, B., Brookner, S., Oleinikova, K. & Wands, S. 2002, *Infant Feeding 2000: A Survey Conducted on Behalf of the Department of Health*, The Scottish Executive, Social Services and Public Safety in Northern Ireland, & The Stationery Office, London.

Hartley, B. & O'Connor, M. 1996, 'Evaluation of the "Best-start" Breast Feeding Education Program', *Archives of Pediatric and Adolescent Medicine*, vol. 150, pp. 868–71.

Hays, S. 1998, *The Cultural Contradictions of Motherhood*, Yale University Press, New Haven CT.

Heinig, M.J. 2001, 'Host Defense Benefits of Breastfeeding for the Infant. Effect of Breastfeeding Duration and Exclusivity', *Pediatr Clin North Am*, vol. 48, pp. 105–23.

Hills-Bonczyk, S., Tromiczak, K., Avery, M., Potter, S., Savik, K. & Duckett, L. 1994, 'Women's Experiences of Breast Feeding Longer than 12 Months', *Birth*, vol. 21, pp. 206–12.

Howie, P.W., Forsyth, J.S., Ogsten, S.A., Clarke, A. & Florey, C. du V. 1990 'Protective Effect of Breast Feeding Against Infection', *British Medical Journal*, vol. 100, pp. 11–16.

Jamieson, L. & Toynbee, C. 1990, 'Shifting Patterns of Parental Authority, 1900–1980', in H. Corr & L. Jamieson (eds), *Politics of Everyday Life: Continuity and Change in Work and the Family*, Macmillan, London, pp. 86–113.

Jones, M., Swerdlow, A. et al. 1998, 'Pre-natal and Early Life Risk Factors for Childhood Onset Diabetes Mellitus: A Record Linkage Study', *Int J Epidemiol* vol. 27, pp. 444–9.

Kendall-Tackett, K. & Sugarman, M. 1995, 'The Social Consequences of Long-term Breast Feeding', *Journal of Human Lactation*, vol. 11, pp. 179–83.

Lawrence, R. 1995, 'The Clinician's Role in Teaching Proper Infant Feeding Techniques', *Journal of Pediatrics*, vol. 126 (supp.), pp. 112–17.

Knaak, S. 2005, 'Breast-feeding, Bottle-feeding and Dr Spock: The Shifting Context of Choice', *Canadian Review of Sociology and Anthropology*, vol. 42, no. 2, pp. 197–216.

Kukla, R. 2006, 'Ethics and Ideology in Breastfeeding Advocacy Campaigns', *Hypatia*, vol. 21, no. 1, pp. 157–80.

Lewis, J. 1990, '"Motherhood Issues" in Late Nineteenth and Twentieth Centuries', in K. Arnup, A. Levesque & R. Roach Pierson (eds), *Delivering Motherhood: Maternal Ideologies and Practices in the 19th and 20th Centuries*, Routledge, London, pp. 1–19.

Lopez-Alarcon, M., Villalpando, S. & Fajardo, A. 1997, 'Breast-feeding Lowers the Frequency and Duration of Acute Respiratory Infection and Diarrhea in Infants under Six Months of Age', *J Nutr*, vol. 127, pp. 436–43.

Lowe, T. 1993, 'Regional and Socio-economic Variations in the Duration of Breastfeeding in Victoria', *Breastfeeding Review*, vol. 2, pp. 312–15.

Lupton, D. 1993, 'Risk as Moral Danger: The Social and Political Functions of Risk Discourse in Public Health', *International Journal of Health Services*, vol. 23, pp. 425–35.

—— 1996, *Food, the Body and the Self*, Sage, London.

Maher, V. 1992, 'Breast Feeding in Cross-cultural Perspective: Paradoxes and Proposals', in V. Maher (ed.), *The Anthropology of Breast Feeding: Natural Law or Social Construct*, Berg, Oxford, pp. 1–36.

Marild, S., Hansson, S., Jodal, U., Oden, A. & Svedberg, K. 2004, 'Protective Effect of Breastfeeding Against Urinary Tract Infection', *Acta Paediatr*, vol. 93, pp. 164–8.

Marshall, H. 1991, 'The Social Construction of Motherhood: An Analysis of Childcare and Parenting Manuals', in A. Phoenix, A. Woollett & E. Lloyd (eds), *Motherhood: Meanings, Practices and Ideologies*, Sage, London, pp. 66–85.

Martin, J. & Monk, J. 1982, *Infant Feeding 1980*, Office of Population Censuses and Surveys, London.

McVea, K.L., Turner, P.D. & Peppler, D.K. 2000, 'The Role of Breastfeeding in Sudden Infant Death Syndrome', *J Hum Lact*, vol. 16, pp. 13 –20.

Mortensen, E.L., Michaelsen, K.F., Sanders, S.A. & Reinisch, J.M. 2002, 'The Association Between Duration of Breastfeeding and Adult Intelligence', *JAMA*, vol. 287, pp. 2365–71.

Murphy, E. 1999, '"Breast is Best": Infant Feeding Decisions and Maternal Deviance', *Sociology of Health and Illness*, vol. 21, pp. 187–208.

—— 2000, 'Risk, Responsibility and Rhetoric in Infant Feeding', *Journal of Contemporary Ethnography*, vol. 29, pp. 291–325.

—— 2003, 'Expertise and Forms of Knowledge in the Government of Families', *The Sociological Review*, vol. 51, no. 4, pp. 433–62.

—— 2004, 'Anticipatory Accounts', *Symbolic Interaction*, vol. 27, no. 2, pp. 129–54.

—— 2007, 'Images of Childhood in Mother's Accounts of Contemporary Childrearing', *Childhood*, vol. 14, no. 1, pp. 105–27.

——, Parker, S. & Phipps, C. 1998a, 'Competing Agendas in Infant Feeding', *British Food Journal*, vol. 100, no. 3, pp. 128–32.

Elizabeth Murphy

——, Parker, S. & Phipps, C. 1998b, 'Food Choices for Babies', in A. Murcott (ed.), *The Nation's Diet: The Social Science of Food Choice*, Addison Wesley Longman, London, pp. 250–66.

National Health and Medical Research Council 2003, *Dietary Guidelines for Children and Adolescents in Australia, Incorporating the Infant Feeding Guidelines for Health Workers*, AusInfo, Canberra.

Nettleton, S. 1997, 'Governing the Risky Self: How to Become Healthy, Wealthy and Wise', in A. Petersen & R. Bunton (eds), *Foucault, Health and Medicine*, Routledge, London, pp. 207–22.

Oakley, A. 1979, *Becoming a Mother*, Martin Robertson, Oxford.

Office on Women's Health 2001, *Breastfeeding*, www.4women.gov/Breastfeeding/.

Ogden, J. 1995, 'Psychosocial Theory and the Creation of the Risky Self', *Social Science and Medicine*, vol. 40, pp. 409–15.

Pessl, M. 1996, 'Are We Creating Our Own Breast Feeding Mythology?', *Journal of Human Lactation*, vol. 12, pp. 271–2.

Petersen, A. 1997, 'Risk, Governance and the New Public Health', in A. Petersen & R. Bunton (eds), *Foucault, Health and Medicine*, Routledge, London, pp. 189–206.

Phoenix, A. & Woollett, A. 1991, 'Motherhood: Social Construction, Politics and Psychology', in A. Phoenix, A. Woollett & E. Lloyd (eds), *Motherhood: Meanings, Practices and Ideologies*, Sage, London, pp. 13–27.

Piper, S. & Parks, P. 1996, 'Predicting the Duration of Lactation: Evidence from a National Survey', *Birth*, vol. 23, pp. 7–12.

Ribbens McCarthy, J., Edwards, R. & Gillies, V. 2000, *Parenting and Step-parenting: Contemporary Moral Tales*, Occasional paper, Centre for Family and Household Research, Issue 4.

Rose, N. 1996, 'Governing the Enterprising Self', in P. Heelas & P. Morris (eds), *The Values of the Enterprise Culture*, Routledge, London.

Ryan, A.S., Wenjun, Z. & Acosta, A. 2002, 'Breastfeeding Continues to Increase into the New Millennium', *Pediatrics*, vol. 110, pp. 1103–9.

Saarinen, U.M. & Kajosaari, M. 1995, 'Breast Feeding as Prophylaxis Against Atopic Disease: Prospective Follow-up Study until 17 Years Old', *Lancet*, vol. 346, pp. 1065–9.

Salt, M., Law, C., Bull, A. & Osmond, C. 1994, 'Determinants of Breast Feeding in Salisbury and Durham', *Journal of Public Health Medicine*, vol. 16, pp. 291–5.

Scott, M. & Lyman, S. 1963, 'Accounts', *American Sociological Review*, vol. 33, pp. 46–62.

UNICEF UK 2006, 'Breast Feeding', www.unicef.org.uk/unicefuk/policies [accessed 23/2/2007].

US Department of Health and Human Services 2000, *Healthy People 2010: Second Edition—Volume II*, US Department of Health and Human Services, Public

Health Service, Office of the Assistant Secretary for Health, Washington, DC, www.healthypeople.gov [accessed 23/2/2007].

Virtanen, S.M., Rasanen, L. & Aro, A. 1991,'Infant Feeding in Finnish Children 7Years of Age with Newly Diagnosed IDDM', *Diabetes Care*, vol. 13, pp. 415–17.

Wall, G. 2001, 'Moral Constructions of Motherhood in Breastfeeding Discourse', *Gender and Society*, vol. 15, no. 4, pp. 592–610.

Webb, B. & Stimson, G. 1976, 'People's Accounts of Medical Encounters', in M. Wadsworth & D. Robinson (eds), *Studies in Everyday Medical Life*, Martin Robertson, London.

White, A., Freeth, S. & O'Brien, M. 1992, *Infant Feeding 1990*, Her Majesty's Stationery Office, London.

WHO—*see* World Health Organization.

World Health Organization 2001,'Global strategy for infant and young child feeding. The optimal duration of exclusive breastfeeding', 54th World Health Assembly, Geneva.

CHAPTER 10

The Government of the Table: Nutrition Expertise and the Social Organisation of Family Food Habits

John Coveney

OVERVIEW

- How have changing social attitudes towards childhood affected nutrition advice about children's eating patterns?
- In what ways can nutrition advice be seen as a form of power?
- Does current child nutrition advice result in positive outcomes for children and parents?

In this chapter, the area of child nutrition is analysed in relation to changing views about family life in Australia over the past 60 years. I look at how the phenomenon of 'picky' or 'fussy' eaters—something largely absent from earlier discourses about the feeding of children— emerged as a problem for parents and professionals in the late twentieth century. I situate the changing attitudes towards the feeding of children in a wider context in which modern social views accord children the status of citizens with rights, responsibilities and autonomy. Indeed, the new social space that children occupy has been reproduced and reinforced in the advice of experts such as nutritionists. I also examine how the importance of 'food choice' in the eating habits of children is especially foregrounded in texts that advise parents on how to feed the family. Interviews with families are used to reveal the tensions that the new views of childhood—especially the notions of rights, independence and autonomy—bring to the process of feeding children. The chapter suggests that the feeding of children is made problematic by new social definitions of 'good' parenting that privilege independence for children, a belief that food and mealtimes should be enjoyable, and an imperative that food for children should be nutritious. This problematisation does not necessarily disempower parents. On the contrary, it provides them with yet more opportunities to establish codes of conduct, informed by expertise, for the management of children's feeding behaviour.

Key terms

ethics	Foucaultian perspective	normality
ethical responsibilities	government/governmentality	technologies of government

Introduction

The Australian National Health and Medical Research Council's guidelines on healthy diets for children (NHMRC 2003) represent the latest in a long line of advice from health and nutrition experts about the kinds of food that infants and children should eat. Indeed, expert advice on what children should eat has a long history, the Australian branch of which has been well documented by Nancy Hitchcock (1989a; 1989b). By contrast, expert recommendations about the management of children's social behaviour in relation to food—for example, how to cope with 'difficult' or 'fussy' eaters—has a much shorter history. To be sure, books, articles and papers on children's nutrition published early last century often contained sections in which these matters were briefly discussed. This advice, however, was quite different, in terms of both content and detail, from that provided today. Current manuals on parenting contain information designed to prepare parents for, and advise them about, what now appears to be an inevitable aspect of childhood: antisocial habits associated with food and feeding difficulties. This is not to say, of course, that children have only recently become so-called 'fussy' or 'picky' eaters. Rather, it is to say that the recognition of this phenomenon as a 'problem'—and its necessary management—has become part of expert advice to parents only quite recently.

The role of the expert in advising parents about the social management of children is not, of course, confined to feeding. According to Nikolas Rose (1990, p. 129), family life in general, and parenting in particular, has become governed by expertise. Expert advice now infuses and shapes the personal investments of parents, especially the ways in which they regulate and evaluate their actions and their goals. Through this process, expert opinion not only informs parents but also provides them with an index of what is considered to be the 'right' way of managing children. Expertise thus becomes the benchmark against which parental behaviour is judged by others and, importantly, by the parents themselves. In other words, parents know they are doing a 'good' job by reference to expert opinion. Expertise outlines and facilitates the production of '**normality**' in childhood, which, in the end, is what most parents aspire to for their children. The popularity of books, journals, articles and internet sites concerned with parenting skills is an indication of these aspirations. In trying to understand this popularity, we should not see parents as cultural or 'judgemental dopes' (Heritage 1987) who are beguiled by expert advice against their will or better nature. On the contrary, we should recognise that parents actively seek out this information in order to better handle the complex and often challenging process of bringing up children. And even when parents do not find expert advice especially useful, such advice is still recognised as having a certain validity. Comments like 'They say you should [do such and such], but I find that …' are frequently heard from parents, indicating the recognised authority with which experts speak.

John Coveney

It is the changing nature of 'doing it right', especially with regard to the feeding of children, that is the topic of this chapter and that demonstrates the emergence of the social management of eating, with its inherent problems in modern family settings. The subject is examined in a number of ways. First, expert advice on the feeding of children over the last century is compared with that available today. Second, this advice is situated within the larger context of the changes in Australian social life with respect to the family—especially attitudes to raising children—over the last 60 years. This comparison illustrates the new considerations that parents must take into account in relation to the feeding of children. Third, in order to ground the recognition of these changes—and the tensions they bring—in concrete experience, I examine interviews with families in which the feeding of children is discussed.

Setting an analytical context: Government and the family

The theoretical framework of the analysis presented here uses a **Foucaultian perspective** drawn from Michel Foucault, especially as his work has been used by Donzelot (1980) and Rose (1990). Briefly, this work acknowledges that the development of the 'modern family' (small, private, independent) began in the early part of the nineteenth century. This development culminated in the state making possible certain advantages and privileges for families that went beyond the provision of regulation and legislation. As Rose says, '"Familialization" was crucial to the means whereby personal capacities and conducts could be socialised, shaped and maximised in a manner that accorded with the moral and political principles of liberal societies' (1990, p. 126). One of the best ways of understanding this process is through the understanding of **governmentality** (Burchell et al. 1991; Dean & Hindess 1998). This understanding goes beyond the activities of state political power or authority. It is instead the 'conduct of conduct' or the **government** from a distance (Colebatch 2003). In other words the state should not necessarily be seen as a centralised bureaucracy from which power emanates. As Rose and Miller (1992) note, it is more productive to analyse political power from the point of view of government than of state apparatus. The difference is that government may be understood as a range of diffuse practices: 'tactics, strategies, techniques, programmes, dreams and aspirations of those authorities who shape the beliefs and conduct of the population' (Nettleton 1991, p. 99). As Rose and Miller point out, 'in Europe for many centuries economic activity was regulated, order was maintained, laws promulgated and enforced, assistance provided for the sick and needy, morality inculcated, if at all, through practices that had little to do with the state' (1992, p. 176). In other words, a range of organisations operating outside the apparatus and bureaucracy of the state have been, and still are, responsible for the **technologies of government**.

To give an example, much of the work in the early formation of the domesticated modern family was undertaken through philanthropic activity, especially that concerning health, welfare and hygiene (Donzelot 1980, p. 55). This assistance was almost always conditional upon families adopting 'good' moral principles, especially marriage, good housekeeping, sobriety and the moral supervision of children (Rose 1990, p. 127). As such, charitable organisations often worked more closely with families who had middle-class tendencies and aspirations. Even in the working classes, it was the 'deserving' families—those who, despite economic and social hardships, displayed certain moral principles—that were the main targets of middle-class philanthropy. Charitable organisations would not assist the 'undeserving' poor, whose plight was a product of 'drunkenness, laziness, roving dispositions, and dishonesty' (Finch 1993, p. 44).

Central to the technologies of government is knowledge—expertise or 'know-how'. This knowledge can be applied in programs that specify objects to be governed or managed and the uses to which these objects are to be put. By laying claim to certain bodies of knowledge, programs map out the problems that are to be addressed. Thus programs, through knowledge, become problematising activities that attempt to direct or control the behaviour of others. It is through such technologies of government that power is exercised. As Foucault says, 'power and knowledge directly imply one another; there is no power relationship without the correlative constitution of a field of knowledge, nor any knowledge that does not presuppose and constitute at the same time power relations' (Foucault 1979, p. 27). However, it is important to note that relationships of power are not necessarily negative. Foucault argued that power can be positive: 'It [power] needs to be considered as a productive network which runs through the whole social body, much more than as a negative instance whose function is to repress' (Foucault 1980, p. 119).

One aspect of the productive nature of power is the creation of socially desirable or ethical categories. We can see this in the development of family ideals during the last century, when expert advice from philanthropic organisations was available in the areas of health, hygiene and 'normality'. The latter quality was especially important for the promotion of happy, healthy family lives. 'Normal' families were those that had high standards of ethical conduct. Unsociable behaviour—debauchery, viciousness, masturbation, insanity and so on—was considered to be detrimental to the health and harmony of family life (Rose 1990, p. 128). But normality was not merely an observation; it was a valuation that defined a situation as 'that which should be', and the justification of which was increasingly made according to medical, psychological and other scientific knowledge. A number of proto-state services were established in this way. It was, for example, through the establishment of categories of 'normality' that child health and welfare services first made an appearance earlier in the twentieth century. In Australia, as in other countries, the early child welfare movement began as a philanthropic venture (Reiger 1986, p. 130). Attendance at the infant welfare clinic—then as now—became an exercise in examining children against a range of normal criteria for feeding, growth and development, and behaviour.

John Coveney

Today it is the reification of what is considered to be 'normal'—in family life in general, and childhood in particular—that imposes on parents an obligation (and fosters in them a commitment) to produce hygienic homes and to raise happy, healthy children. It is in the attainment of 'normality' that parents are judged by others and by themselves in terms of doing the 'right thing'. And it is the quest for the 'normal', especially in relation to child-rearing, which requires parents to seek out expert advice for reassurance or correction of parenting practices. It is important to stress again that it would be a mistake to view this analysis of the construction of the modern family as implying some kind of domination or repression on the part of the state. Quite the opposite: parents actively seek out expert advice about the 'proper way' of raising children, and they do not do so under any 'false consciousness'. They do it as a way of fulfilling their **ethical responsibilities** as parents. We should regard **ethics** as the body of obligations that individuals feel compelled to fulfil, especially in relation to moral codes defined by their social groups. Foucault sees the development of ethics as a 'process in which the individual delimits that part of himself [sic] that will form the object of his moral practice, defines his position relative to the precepts he will follow, and decides on a certain mode of being that will serve as his moral goal. And this requires him to act upon himself, to monitor, test, improve, and transform himself' (Foucault 1992, p. 28).

Moral conduct has, since the seventeenth century, become increasingly governed by expertise in the human sciences. We should thus understand the expert advice examined in this chapter as a form of 'control at a distance' (Rose & Miller 1992); it is a kind of control that requires families to be independent from, and yet cooperative with, the state. This control functions through the production and valorisation of specific forms of conduct, developed and outlined by experts, to which parents will want to aspire in order to recognise themselves as 'good', 'responsible' and 'committed' mothers and fathers, thus fulfilling their ethical responsibilities.

The changing nature of family life

Reporting on a survey of Australian family life undertaken in 1954, Harold Fallding noted that parents at this time saw themselves as pioneering a new era of child-rearing. This new form of parenting had four main elements (Fallding 1957, p. 71):

- a belief that one had to be equipped with knowledge in order to deal with children effectively, not simply repeat the methods used by one's own parents;
- a belief that one should be affectionate and companionable towards children, not the remote authorities that parents had been in previous generations;
- a desire to produce a self-regulated rather than an obedient child; and
- an aim to ensure the full development of the child's capacities rather than prepare him [sic] to be devoted to duty.

Fallding notes that, compared with the position of children in families before World War II, the status of post-war childhood had radically changed. Blind obedience was replaced by cooperation and negotiation between parents and children.

These changes in family life are very noticeable in the different obligations parents had before and after World War II in relation to the feeding of children. We can examine these changes by looking at the expert advice given to parents on the 'correct' ways of feeding children. In the early part of the twentieth century, advice for parents on feeding children focused almost exclusively on food rules and regimes. *The Australian Mothercraft Book* (Mothers and Babies' Health Association 1938), used by infant welfare nurses in the 1930s, lists the sequence in which foods should be introduced into a child's diet upon weaning. Also, special instructions are given on how to 'correctly' cook these foods and how to achieve the 'right' consistency. Specimen diets for older children are also provided, listing those foods that should be given and the times at which they should be offered. However, little is written about the ways in which parents should manage the social arrangement of mealtimes or about how to act if a meal is refused by a child. Another book of the day offering advice about the management of children in the nursery makes this suggestion:'As a rule it is wise not to coax an unwilling child to take its food … Faddiness about food should in no case be encouraged … The food provided should always be suitable and it should be *assumed that it will be eaten*' (Bennett & Isaacs 1931, italics added). Truby King's pre-war book *Feeding and Care of Baby* (1933), which was used extensively by infant welfare nurses in Australia, offers a range of timetables and menus, listing the foods that should be given, but it offers little guidance about the social management of feeding—that is, what to do if food is disliked and refused. King takes a rather 'no nonsense' approach, implicitly assuming that feeding children will be an unproblematic affair.

We should contrast this advice with that given in manuals written in the post-war period, when problems in feeding children started to surface. In his book *Baby and Child Care*, Ben Spock (1955) devotes almost a whole chapter to these feeding problems. Spock starts by noting that 'You don't see feeding problems in puppies or among young humans in places where mothers don't know enough about diet to worry' (1955, p. 448). He continues by stressing the importance of being patient, offering choices, and encouraging independence in eating. As a post-war text on child management, Spock's book stands in stark contrast to those written earlier in so far as feeding children is now a recognised problem. Another topic, that of fatness in children, which was not mentioned to any great degree in earlier texts, is also given special treatment by Spock. He provides advice on how to cope with fat children who 'crave large amounts of rich foods [cakes, biscuits, and pastry]' (p. 457). Obesity in children is now understood as a health problem requiring intervention by parents and doctors. Stressing the difficulties that beset the management of children's weight problems, Spock points out that 'A child has less will-power than an adult. If the mother serves the child less fattening foods it means either that the whole family must go without the richer dishes or that the fat child must be kept from eating the very things his heart craves while the rest of the family enjoy them. There are few fat children reasonable enough to think that's fair' (p. 459).

Note that Spock stresses children's ability to reason and implies that their views should be respected. According to Spock, if a child shows willingness to cooperate in dieting, then he or she should be encouraged to visit the doctor, preferably alone: 'Talking to the doctor, man to man, may give him a feeling of running his own life like a grown up' (p. 459). Essential to Spock's advice, then, is the assumption that reason, independence and self-regulation in children should be encouraged. Children should not be merely obedient.

The importance of fostering dietary freedom and independence in children becomes explicit in the recommendations of modern nutritionists. For example, in her book *The Complete Guide to Feeding Your Child*, Audrey Stewart-Turner (1986) points out that children should be given a choice of nutritious foods to encourage independence in eating. She puts children's capricious attitude to eating on the same footing as the food preferences of adults: 'remember that there are some foods [parents] like to eat more than others or feel like at certain times and not other times!' (p. 67). We are, then, invited to rationalise children's eating behaviours by comparing them with those of adults, who, presumably, know when they are hungry and when they are not and have recognisable and distinct food preferences.

A second example of modern advice is a book on child nutrition by Baker and Henry (1987), who recognise that many children are 'picky' eaters. In dealing with this problem, parents should show encouragement rather than use force. According to the authors, negative encounters with food should always be avoided and 'parents should respect children's food preferences and not try to dictate them' (p. 135). A more recent example is the nutrition book by Susan Thompson (1995), which points out that 'Finding the balance between self-expression and freedom on the part of your child, and meeting [parents'] ideas of a healthy diet can be difficult' (p. 14). Thompson paraphrases Ellen Satter—another child nutrition expert—who believes that 'The parent is responsible for what is presented to eat. The child is *responsible* for how much is eaten and even whether he eats' (Satter 1987, italics added). It is the recognition of the right—or responsibility—of children to make choices regarding their diet that is so apparent in modern texts. Such a recognition assumes that children will be accorded a degree of autonomy and social freedom, a notion that is utterly missing from earlier advice by experts.

Part of the rationale for encouraging self-expression and independence in children's food choices is the importance of harmony and happiness when eating. Parents are reminded that a child's happiness around food and eating should be preserved because unpleasant social experiences around food in childhood can lead to eating problems. As Thompson puts it, 'Studies have shown that if parents are rigid and authoritarian about food [amounts], children will lose their ability to control intake. There is a good chance that your child will become overweight, or even underweight if the battle becomes more important than eating' (1995, p. 70). The supposed scientific validity of this advice arises from quasi-experiments in child psychology, the social relevance of which has been questioned (Coveney 2002). However, the argument reaches something of an apogee in the work of Hirschmann and Zaphiropoulos, who, promoting a more child-centred approach to the management of eating, believe that 'by allowing the child to decide when to eat, what to eat, and how much to eat, we can strengthen her self-confidence, self-esteem, and sense of dignity and also avoid the kinds of eating difficulties that have plagued many of us for life' (1985, p. 13). Thus, the social organisation of the feeding of children, mostly taken for granted by experts of an earlier era, now becomes somewhat precarious. It requires sensitivity, so as to avoid rigidity and authoritarianism, the pathological consequences of which have now been established as scientific fact.

To summarise the discussion so far, in modern (that is, post–World War II) nutrition texts parents have new responsibilities concerning food that explicitly recognise and give importance to an emotional investment in eating. Coping with children's eating habits is now another opportunity for individuals to display prowess in the art of good parenting. This skill is 'in theory intellectually exciting, a test of personal capacities, virtually a profession in its own right; in practice [parenthood] is the site of a constant self-scrutiny and self-evaluation [by the parent] in relation to the norms of responsibility to one's child' (Rose 1990, p. 198). It is through this self-scrutiny of ethical conduct that parents recognise themselves as 'good' mothers and fathers.

However, the concept of children *choosing* food—especially nutritious food—is somewhat problematic, and encouraging self-expression and independence in children comes at a price. Commenting on this, Rosemary Stanton says that 'In Australia and New Zealand, we cannot assume that giving children a free choice of foods will produce an ideally balanced intake of nutrients' (1990, p. 6). Nevertheless, the idea that children should be given certain choices in relation to their diets endures. Stanton continues: 'Whatever your age it makes sense to follow the principles of a balanced diet. With this scheme, nothing is forbidden, but some foods are given a greater or lesser place than others' (p. 8). And yet, the issue of balancing diets and choice in eating is not easily managed. As we have seen, nutrition experts recognise this as 'difficult' because of the need to match the importance of encouraging the child's self-expression with the parent's responsibility to provide a healthy diet. The difficulty of managing this delicate balance has been readily recognised by the food industry, which often promotes certain foods to children as both 'nutritious' and 'enjoyable'. In reality, while many such foods are certainly enjoyable, they are not necessarily nutritious (Australian Consumers Association 1993, p. 21). Thus the freedom to choose—so much a part of the modern consumer ethos—becomes problematic because of the sheer variety of food in the marketplace, and because

John Coveney

many foods fall short of current nutritional guidelines. The responsibility now falls to parents, teachers and others, who are expected to instil in children the notion of 'correct' or 'incorrect' food choices.

Children as citizens

Modern attitudes to food choice did not, of course, arrive unannounced purely in the area of child nutrition. Instead, the recognition given to the new ways in which parents should interact with children can be seen as a manifestation of a new social view of childhood that emerged in the second half of the twentieth century. The growing importance of children in post-war families dramatically influenced their visibility and status. This new status can be seen in a number of developments. For example, in 1959 the United Nations unveiled a Declaration of the Rights of the Child (United Nations General Assembly 1960), which was reformulated and re-released in 1989 as the *United Nations International Convention for the Rights of the Child* (Greenwood 1993). Under this convention, the Australian government has to report to the United Nations every two years on how well it is complying with the convention's principles. The emergence of children's rights in the post-war period required that family life be opened up to closer scrutiny, to ensure that these rights were being respected. The granting of rights to children in effect extended to them a form of citizenship, not in the sense that they could participate in the execution of political power, but in the sense that they had the right to liberty and they had social rights (Rose 1990, p. 122). These rights provided for the exercising of choice by children.

Early-twentieth-century expert discourses on parenting emphasised the importance of avoiding 'molli-coddling' or 'spoiling' children. Frequent parent–child interactions, through play or even just cuddling, were believed to lead to overstimulation of the nervous system, which was thought to be detrimental to proper development (Reiger 1986, p. 148). However, with modern advances in understanding, especially in child psychology, attitudes towards parent–child interaction changed: emotional and cognitive development were to be strongly encouraged through play, discovery and frequent 'quality' interactions between adults and children. The home itself was believed to be the best place for these activities. The norms of good parenting were predicated less on the amount of discipline and control of children than on the extent to which parents maximised their children's learning and developmental potential: 'With the aid of books, games, toys, records, and other aids now made available for purchase, the intimate environment of the home was to be transformed into a veritable laboratory of cognitive growth' (Rose 1990, p. 196). We might note here that the recognition of children's choice and freedom went hand in hand with the greater economic and material possibilities of the so-called 'boom' after World War II. Choice and variety became not only possible but necessary in the modern consumerism.

On another level, children now had the right to be heard, and they had opinions that were to be taken seriously. The idea of choice and freedom for children in family life was played out in a number of regimes of new parenthood. As we have seen, the eating habits of children became an important site for encouraging the development of choice, self-expression and eventual independence of children. Thus the notion of choice for children became an important part of family food events. Indeed, the consequences of 'choice' and 'freedom', and the implications for children's eating habits, are now being questioned as part of the moral panic that accompanies the so-called childhood obesity 'epidemic' (Coveney 2006).

In the next section I will examine the experiences of individuals who are negotiating the role of parent. On the one hand, this role requires that they provide their children with foods they will enjoy and foods that allow them to display autonomy and self-expression. On the other hand, it requires that they provide a nutritious diet to their children. These possibilities carry obvious tensions, since most parents know that children will often prefer foods that are not the healthiest choices. But they are also aware of the problems that arise when healthy foods are forced on children and less healthy choices are restricted.

A study of family food experiences

This small study involved 12 families with young children from different parts of Adelaide, Australia. Although these families were randomly enlisted in the study, they are not presented here as representative of all families. They are, instead, used to illustrate examples of family life concerned with food. The material presented here was collected and compiled in the following way. In each family, the father and mother were interviewed—sometimes together, sometimes indi-vidually. An interview schedule was developed to guide the discussions with participants. The schedule consisted of open-ended questions about everyday routines concerning food preparation, shopping and other aspects of family food decision making. All the interviews were audio-taped (with permission) and transcribed. All transcriptions were reviewed and summarised with field notes, so that for each family an overall description of the couple's responses was produced. The interview transcripts were then 'thematised' using NUDIST (version 3.0.4, QSR Melbourne), a software package for handling qualitative data. Reported here are some of the themes that emerged—regarding the parents' food experiences during their own childhood compared with those of today, the management of social arrangements of family meals, and the obligations of parents in relation to nutrition and health.

The first extract discusses the differences between arrangements in family eating when the parents were children and those of today:

Angus: I think when I was a kid I was served meat and two veg …

Hilary: The same thing every night virtually.

Angus: And I was expected to pretty much eat it, and if I did not eat it I wouldn't get dessert. And that would be legit, like if I didn't eat it I wouldn't get dessert. Whereas these days … you serve meat and two veg or three veg and you say 'If you don't eat it you won't get dessert' and they don't eat it but they still get dessert. And it's not just us …

Hilary: But we're not strict like, we're just not strict.

Angus: It's not just us that are soft, I think it's just like everything shifts to the left, you know, society is just a bit more malleable whereas when I was a kid it was a bit more black and white.

These comments are typical; many respondents remembered childhood mealtimes to be more restricted than those of their own children. Many also remembered the hardships that their parents endured, with money often in short supply. This required that food be eaten and not wasted. The lack of mealtime rigidity that now exists for these families ('We are just not strict') may therefore result from a more affluent society, in which choice is not only desirable but a material possibility. In some cases, current family food arrangements were influenced by parents' own food experiences as children, as the following extracts indicate:

Greg: Well I think I quite often believe that a lot that I went through and was made to eat and whatever, that I don't believe you've got to … modern day children, or my children should not be forced to do that.

Wendy: OK, when I was growing up you ate whatever you got the first time, you didn't have to ask for seconds but you finished what was on your plate. Anyway my mother would serve this God-awful stuff, stewed tomatoes on toast with cheese, and it's nauseating … and we would have this I would say at least twice a month, and we had to eat it and I swore I would never do that to my children and I don't.

However, the different expectations parents have of mealtimes today are also the result of a change in parental attitudes; as Angus said, 'society is just a bit more malleable [today] whereas when I was a kid it was a bit more black and white'. Parents today are expected to be more flexible and to offer their children certain freedoms. The extent of the change may be judged by the influence children have over the family menu. This influence is brought out in the following extracts:

Stella: No. I had virtually no say in what meals went on the table as a child, whereas my kids do have a say in what does go on the table.

Greg: We [parents] try to I suppose change our own [food preferences] around to suit the children always.

Keeping the children happy and providing an enjoyable meal for them was a priority for many of these parents. Mealtimes together were expected to be occasions when the family came together to share not only food but also pleasant experiences. And respondents often justified the choice and freedom they gave to children by reference to a need to avoid unpleasant experiences:

Wendy: I don't see turning the mealtimes into a battleground anyway.

Diana: I always try to cook something that I know that [husband] is going to get a good meal and at least [son] will have something that he will like.

Sometimes, in order to ensure that mealtimes were positive occasions, parents specifically catered for the food preferences of children and prepared a separate meal for them, even if this meant extra work for the cook:

Alison: It's a nuisance. It's a great nuisance but I tend to do the things, when I'm cooking two separate things, I'll do things that I know the children will definitely eat. So at least I don't feel I've gone to all this trouble to do two separate things and find that they don't eat what I gave them anyway.

Jack: He [son] has been spoilt by his grandmother and [mother]; he quite often gets different things cooked for him because he doesn't like this and he doesn't like that.

For these families, then, the principles that informed meal preparation and presentation were based on the importance of providing children with a certain degree of choice and freedom. They were also informed by the need to provide a happy and harmonious environment in which the family can eat, thus avoiding a 'battleground' at mealtimes. A third obligation—that of providing nutritious foods—was often believed to be a necessary mealtime consideration. However, because this obligation often jeopardised harmony and choice, it was seen as problematic:

Rose: We try, I mean if you can get them to eat [healthy food]. Yeah, I would like them to eat meat and three vegetables every night, but they don't always.

Cassie: I mean, you go to the trouble of trying to prepare something different and something nutritious possibly, you know, and you sort of think 'God, this is a waste of time'.

Some parents took a broader view of the problems that confronted them in feeding the family. Below, Alison recognises the change in the status of children and the way that it has been cultivated in a number of institutions, especially school.

Alison: I've been trying to work out why [our children are difficult to feed], and I suspect that they seem to grow up a lot more quickly these days and I think partly because school encourages them to think a lot more for themselves and they are taught that they have rights as children and so they question what we tell them far more, and that includes things like what they're going to eat and what they're not going to eat and how they're going to eat it and where.

As Alison says, children's rights are dealt with explicitly at school, thereby providing children with notions of autonomy and choice. In the next extract, May, who had arrived in Australia from Vietnam 10 years earlier, contrasts the attitudes to children in Australia with those in Vietnam:

May: Maybe I [take notice of my children] because I think Vietnamese people you know, their children, when they upset about parent they don't want to say [anything] about them, only keep inside. Because now the children learn Australian school they have their opinion and I think I have to hear [pauses] listen to them, you know; in Vietnam parents very rarely listen to the children.

Interviewer: Is that right?

May: Yeah, the children only do what the parent say [and] they have to obey, or have to do anything that the parent wants them to do, you know, and now maybe my children is better than in Vietnam.

Children in Australia are thus constructed through discourses of freedom and choice, and May judged this preferable to the position of children (as she saw it) in Vietnam. She makes the point that children now have to be listened to; their views have to be considered. Autonomy and choice not only construct children as modern subjects, but also assist in the production of 'good parents'—ones who show the right ethical concern for their children's views. The relationship between views on the 'correct' way of feeding children and views on 'good' parenting was demonstrated in a study by Heather Morton and colleagues (1996). Mothers of two-year-olds considered themselves to be 'good' parents if, first, they gave their children the 'right' foods and, second, if the children ate with visible pleasure and enjoyment. Parental responsibilities concerning the provision of family foods are, then, informed by what is believed to be 'right'. Mealtimes and menus that are influenced by children's preferences should not therefore be seen as passive capitulation by parents. Instead, they should be considered as examples of parents actively seeking to do the 'right' thing by implementing child-rearing strategies based on negotiation and cooperation, which are designed to encourage autonomy and independence in children and promote happy and harmonious eating occasions.

Conclusion

This chapter set out to examine the way that nutrition advice has mirrored certain social expectations in family life over the course of the last century. It looked at the changing nature of expert advice on how to feed children over the last 60 years and has linked these changes to larger social trends in which the relationship between children and parents has undergone a profound change. The influence of expert knowledge has been granted an important role in this analysis, since changes in social attitudes have generally followed the standards and norms set by experts, whose knowledge is a 'technology of government'. Expert knowledge informs everyday ethical conduct by specifying what are the 'right' and the 'wrong' things to do: it provides the network—the power relationship—within which people act. The area of parenting, which is thoroughly imbued with the psychology of child development and family relationships, is a good example of this kind of power, and the examination of expert advice allows for an understanding of the way that specific acts are articulated so as to shape the desires and aspirations of parents. Of course, parents do not always do what experts say. What is suggested here is that expert discourse, often reified by science, becomes the moral fabric out of which 'normality' is fashioned. This is not to say, however, that expertise is wrong or ill-informed: this chapter has attempted to describe what is, not what should be. It is explanatory rather than critical or judgmental.

The interviews with families reported in this chapter highlighted a number of changes regarding what is considered 'normal' and the labile nature of social phenomena. Participants clearly articulated the changes in family eating habits and the increasing centrality of children. The rigid and often authoritarian family food practices that these parents experienced as children were entirely consistent with the expert advice of the time. Less well articulated—though still identifiable—were the parents' reasons for changing to a more flexible approach to family meals. Statements like 'We are just not strict' and phrases such as 'gone soft' highlight the way that parenting has undergone a change in direction. The new approach, which recognises the need for self-expression and freedom in childhood, assumes that children have autonomy and gives them responsibility for choosing to eat or not to eat. As shown earlier, this is either explicit or implicit in the advice of experts, who are both reflecting and reinforcing the new approaches to raising children. In reality, however, granting children some independence can often be problematic, since the training of children in proper dietary habits can be fraught with difficulties. It is especially difficult for parents to get their children to follow a healthy diet while still providing happy, positive mealtimes. The modern way out of this dilemma is not the traditional authoritarian approach, the pathological consequences of which have been outlined by experts. On the contrary, as in other areas of family difficulty, parents are encouraged to negotiate and reason with children. Such practices are, in fact, part of the role of today's 'good' parent: the listener, the reflective adviser, the 'sounding board' for children's thoughts, desires and beliefs (Gordon 1975).

The area of child nutrition, then, provides a way of understanding the process by which social priorities influence nutrition advice. The production of children as self-reflecting, self-regulating individuals is encouraged through allowing them to make some choices about their diets. But nutrition expertise can also be seen to inform cultural practice by virtue of the fact that it defines which foods are 'good'. Expertise—

John Coveney

in its many guises—thus produces 'good' parents: ones who can recognise themselves as having acquired the modern skills of parenting, in which enjoyment, health and, importantly, choice are central to the management of feeding the family. As this chapter has shown, this societal development is a relatively recent phenomenon, and can be understood through a cultural analysis of 'good food' and the 'good child'.

SUMMARY OF MAIN POINTS

- Social attitudes to childhood have changed over the last 60 years, such that children are now expected to have choice, autonomy and independence.
- The changing expectations of childhood are reflected in and reinforced by modern advice from nutrition experts about how children's eating habits should be managed.
- Expert advice on feeding the family can be analysed in terms of its government of daily conduct or ethics.
- Applying Foucault's ideas, we can regard expert knowledge on nutrition as a form of power.
- As an example of Foucaultian power, nutrition advice can be seen as positive and productive in that it outlines some of the ethical responsibilities of parents, or the proper and correct ways of behaving.

SOCIOLOGICAL REFLECTION

The current debates about who might be responsible for the so-called obesity 'epidemic' in children are useful to reflect upon. Many community and scientific groups are concerned about the role of food advertising of unhealthy products to children, the 'pester power' resulting from children being primed by advertising to want specific food opportunities (such as eating fast food) and the difficulty of parenting in the face of sophisticated commercialism. On the other hand, many politicians and parts of the food and advertising industry suggest that the responsibility lies with parents, who should merely police children's eating habits more carefully.

- What do you consider to be the main issues in this debate in terms of the responsibilities for influencing children's eating habits?

DISCUSSION QUESTIONS

1. What are the advantages of analysing the function of the state as 'technologies of government' rather than as a centralised bureaucratic power?
2. Apart from nutritionists, who may have been important in dispersing ideas to parents regarding the proper management of the feeding of children?

3. Brief mention was made in this chapter of the role of the food industry in the provision of food directed at children. Comment further on the sociological impact of the food industry's practices in this area.

4. What are the advantages and disadvantages of considering children as 'citizens', especially in terms of their having independence and autonomy?

5. Professional knowledge and expertise is often regarded as superior to lay knowledge, especially in areas like child-rearing. How might professionals be better informed than they currently are about what parents think about child nutrition?

6. What would be the benefits of understanding how parents view parenting practices?

Further investigation

1. Contrast Foucault's view of power, as described in this chapter, with that of a more traditional position in social theory (for example, a Marxist position). Highlight the implicit assumptions of each position. Comment on the explanatory possibilities that each position provides for the social actor.

2. Compare the information and advice provided by experts on the feeding of children before and after World War II. How might the greater material wealth of families have influenced attitudes to child-rearing?

3. This chapter has combined historical data and empirical data collected through interviews. Discuss the current debates about the collection of qualitative research data, in particular the 'crisis of representation' and the 'crisis of legitimation' (see Altheide & Johnson 1994). How are the solutions proposed expected to overcome some of the purported problems of qualitative research?

FURTHER READING AND WEB RESOURCES

Books

Charles, N. & Kerr, M. 1988, *Women, Food and Families*, Manchester University Press, Manchester.

Coveney, J. 2006, *Food, Morals and Meanings: The Pleasure and Anxiety of Eating*, 2nd edition, Routledge, London.

Donzelot, J. 1980, *The Policing of Families*, Hutchinson, London.

Rose, N. 1990, *Governing the Soul: The Shaping of the Private Self*, Routledge, London.

Articles

Altheide, D. & Johnson, J. 1994, 'Criteria for Assessing Interpretive Validity in Qualitative Research', in N. Denzin & Y. Lincoln (eds), *The Handbook of Qualitative Research*, Sage, Thousand Oaks, California.

Coveney, J. 2002, 'What does the Research on Families and Food Tell Us?', *Nutrition and Dietetics*, vol. 59, no. 2, pp. 113–19.

John Coveney

Nettleton, S. 1991,'Wisdom, Diligence and Teeth: Discursive Practice and the Creation of Mothers', *Sociology of Health and Illness*, vol. 13, pp. 98–111.

Rose, N. & Miller, P. 1992, 'Political Power Beyond the State: Problematics of Government', *British Journal of Sociology*, vol. 43, no. 2, pp. 173–205.

Websites

Foucault Info: www.foucault.info/

Governmentality.com: www.governmentality.com/

Michel Foucault Resources (by Clare O'Farrell): www.qut.edu.au/edu/cpol/foucault/

REFERENCES

Altheide, D. & Johnson, J. 1994, 'Criteria for Assessing Interpretive Validity in Qualitative Research', in N. Denzin & Y. Lincoln (eds), *The Handbook of Qualitative Research*, Sage, Thousand Oaks, California.

Australian Consumers Association 1993, 'Fruit Substitutes for Children', *Choice Magazine*, vol. 34, no. 3, pp. 21–3.

Baker, S. & Henry, R. 1987, *Parents' Guide to Nutrition: Healthy Eating from Birth through Adolescence*, Addison-Wesley, Reading, Massachusetts.

Bennett, V. & Isaacs, S. 1931, *Health and Education in the Nursery*, George Routledge & Sons, London.

Burchell, G., Gordon, C. & Miller, P. 1991, *The Foucault Effect: Studies in Governmentality*, Harvester/Wheatsheaf, Sydney.

Colebatch, H. 2003, *Policy*, Open University Press, Bucks, UK.

Coveney, J. 2002,'What does the Research on Families and Food Tell Us?', *Nutrition and Dietetics*, vol. 59, no. 2, pp. 113–19.

—— 2006, *Food, Morals and Meaning: The Pleasure and Anxiety of Eating*, 2nd edition, Routledge, London.

Dean, M. & Hindess, B. 1998, *Governing Australia: Studies in Contemporary Rationalities of Government*, Cambridge University Press, Melbourne.

Donzelot, J. 1980, *The Policing of Families*, Hutchinson, London.

Fallding, H. 1957,'Inside the Australian Family', in A. Elkin (ed.), *Marriage and the Family in Australia*, Angus & Robertson, Sydney.

Finch, L. 1993, *The Classing Gaze: Sexuality, Class and Surveillance*, Allen & Unwin, Sydney.

Foucault, M. 1979, *Discipline and Punish: The Birth of the Modern Prison*, Peregrine Books (Penguin), London.

—— 1980,'Truth and Power', in C. Gordon (ed.), *Power/Knowledge: Selected Interviews and Other Writings 1972–1977*, Pantheon Books, New York.

—— 1992, *The History of Sexuality: The Use of Pleasure*, vol. 2, Penguin Books, Harmondsworth.

Gordon, T. 1975, *Parent Effectiveness Training: The Tested New Way to Raise Responsible Children*, New American Library, New York.

Greenwood, A. 1993, *Children's Rights: The United Nations Convention on the Rights of the Child*, Australian Early Childhood Association, Canberra.

Heritage, J. 1987, 'Ethnomethodology', in A. Giddens & J. Turner (eds), *Social Action Today*, Stanford University Press, Stanford, California.

Hirschmann, J. & Zaphiropoulos, L. 1985, *Solve Your Child's Eating Problems*, Fawsett Columbine, New York.

Hitchcock, N. 1989a, 'Infant Feeding in Australia: An Historical Perspective Part 1: 1788–1900', *Australian Journal of Nutrition and Dietetics*, vol. 46, pp. 62–6.

—— 1989b, 'Infant Feeding in Australia: An Historical Perspective Part 2: 1900–1988', *Australian Journal of Nutrition and Dietetics*, vol. 46, pp. 102–8.

King, T. 1933, *Feeding and Care of Baby*, Macmillan & Co., London.

Morton, H., Santich, B. & Worsley, T. 1996, 'Mothers' Perception on the Eating Habits of Two-year-olds: A Pilot Study', *Australian Journal of Nutrition and Dietetics*, vol. 53, pp. 100–5.

Mothers and Babies' Health Association 1938, *The Australian Mothercraft Book*, Rigby, Adelaide.

National Health and Medical Research Council 2003, *Dietary Guidelines for Children and Adolescents in Australia, Incorporating the Infant Feeding Guidelines for Health Workers*, AusInfo, Canberra.

Nettleton, S. 1991, 'Wisdom, Diligence and Teeth: Discursive Practice and the Creation of Mothers', *Sociology of Health and Illness*, vol. 13, pp. 98–111.

NHMRC—*see* National Health and Medical Research Council.

Reiger, K. 1986, *Disenchantment of the Home: Modernising the Australian Family 1880–1940*, Oxford University Press, Melbourne.

Rose, N. 1990, *Governing the Soul: The Shaping of the Private Self*, Routledge, London.

—— & Miller, P. 1992, 'Political Power Beyond the State: Problematics of Government', *British Journal of Sociology*, vol. 43, no. 2, pp. 173–205.

Satter, E. 1987, *How to Get Your Child to Eat … But Not Too Much*, Bull Publishing Co., Palo Alto.

Spock, B. 1955, *Baby and Child Care*, Bodley Head, London.

Stanton, R. 1990, *Foods for Under Fives*, Allen & Unwin, Sydney.

Stewart-Turner, A. 1986, *The Complete Guide to Feeding Your Child*, Science Press, Sydney.

Thompson, S. 1995, *A Healthy Start for Kids: Building Good Eating Patterns for Life*, Simon & Schuster, Sydney.

United Nations General Assembly 1960, *Declaration of the Rights of the Child*, Her Majesty's Stationery Office, London.

PART 4

Food Consumption, Social Differentiation and Identity

Like cannibalism, a matter of taste.

G. K. Chesterton

The chapters in Part 4 are concerned with the role food consumption plays in the processes of social differentiation and personal identity. People can use their food habits, along with other consumption practices, to convey their membership of a particular social group. Food consumption can symbolise social status, class, ethnic heritage, religious beliefs or lifestyle choice, such as being a vegetarian. Each of the four chapters in this part exemplifies a different mode of such social differentiation:

- Chapter 11 discusses the role of food in social identity, exploring the traditions and changes occurring among the culinary cultures of Europe.
- Chapter 12 explores the continuing role that social class plays in shaping food habits.
- Chapter 13 discusses the rise of vegetarianism as both a way of defining the self and as a social movement.
- Chapter 14 examines the social impact of ageing on food habits, social interaction and self-identity.

CHAPTER 11

Culinary Cultures of Europe: Food, History, Health and Identity

Stephen Mennell

OVERVIEW

- What are culinary cultures?
- How do culinary cultures develop?
- What are some key trends affecting culinary cultures?

In 2005, the Council of Europe published a book entitled *Culinary Cultures of Europe: Identity, Diversity and Dialogue* (Goldstein & Merkle 2005), containing chapters about the food of nearly all the 46 member countries of the council. These chapters presented an aspect of each country's collective self-identity, and it is clear that what people see themselves as eating is important to them. Most countries dwelt lovingly on the traditions of the past. Yet it is clear not only that culinary cultures change, but also that they are changing at an accelerating pace. This chapter explores some of the reasons why that is true.

Key terms

class
fusion food
haute cuisine
social identity

Introduction

It used to be said that a society's taste in food was one of the most slowly changing, most conservative, aspects of its culture. This may still be true at a deep level of underlying attitudes to eating and its pleasures. But in recent decades, right across the world we have seen rapid changes in what people eat: food seems to have become part of the fashion industry. Australia is a vivid case in point: old cookery books depict a boring cuisine of almost exclusively British origin. Today, in line with the ethnic diversity of the population, one can eat in restaurants purveying fare from just about every country on the planet.

Much the same is true in Europe. It was only in 1964 that I ate my first Indian meal, in an Indian restaurant in Leeds, when Indian cuisine was unknown in my nearby home town of Huddersfield in the north of England; now there is an Indian restaurant in most large villages, not to mention towns, and a politician recently said that chicken tikka masala (rather than roast beef) was now the British national dish. Such trends were one reason why the Council of Europe, an intergovernmental organisation based in Strasbourg, France, published *Culinary Cultures of Europe*.

One reason why the study of culinary cultures and their history is so fascinating—indeed, I would say intellectually important—is that changes in the food people eat and the way they cook and enjoy it appear to serve as a highly sensitive marker for much broader social, political and economic changes in societies. The sheer social and historic diversity of the member states of the Council of Europe permitted glimpses of how food mirrors transitions of many kinds through which European societies have passed, in both the distant and the recent past—transitions which, moreover, are typical of many other parts of the world beyond Europe. Some of the most significant are discussed here.

The formation of local peasant cuisines and their gradual emancipation from climate and locality

The bedrock of culinary culture in most countries is a tradition of peasant food, the food of farmers—who grew and reared and ate their own products, which they traded locally but generally over no great distance. Many countries, in their contributions to *Culinary Cultures of Europe*, celebrate traditions of this kind that can be traced back over several centuries. The main common features of peasant cuisines are freshness and simplicity, derived from their dependence on locally grown or gathered produce. Dependence on the locality also meant dependence on climate and season. In consequence, despite underlying structural similarities, peasant cuisines differ greatly from each other in ingredients. In Lithuania mushrooms were important, in Bulgaria fruit. The hard conditions of survival in northerly latitudes, evident for example, in Estonia, Iceland and Norway, contrast strongly with the abundance recollected by those who lived in warmer climes—in Azerbaijan, Bulgaria, Slovakia and Ukraine, for example. And the further north one lived, the more rigorously did the seasons impose constraints on the rhythms of eating. Where the winters were long and freezing, stock had to be slaughtered and the meat salted down; and where the summers were short and their days long, the hours of labour and of meals were all the more determined by the rhythms of farm work.

Peasant traditions are easily romanticised. Yet other things—including climate—being equal, the smaller the locality on which a particular cuisine was dependent the greater the potential monotony of the peasant diet. True, people who had not experienced the vast diversity of modern eating may not have felt their diet to be boring. But to later observers it may appear so, with the prominence of staples such as grains, bread, milk and root vegetables. Over much of Europe, meat was not abundant for ordinary people, although it became more so in the period following the Black Death, when a third or more of Europe's population died.[1] Afterwards, the pace of change in the countryside reverted to its normal slow pace and, at least across much of Western Europe, the peasant diet appears to have remained virtually unaltered for centuries (Bloch 1970). In rural France the *pot au feu* permanently simmering in the peasant kitchen for many people provided *soupe* for breakfast, lunch and dinner; and the same went, *pari passu*, for much of the rest of Europe.

The monotony, more or less, of the peasant diet is easily forgotten. The cookery books of each nation tend to celebrate the great peasant dishes of the past. These were usually the exciting high spots of a generally unexciting diet, the special dishes for special occasions. Many of the chapters in *Culinary Cultures of Europe* mention the traditional feasts that in the past marked the year in agrarian societies, and which often continue today even in very different societies. But occasions for feasting originally stood out against the background of many periods of fasting. Sometimes the fasting was given a veneer of religious justification, but such religious rationalisations mostly helped people feel better about the pressing need to eke out stocks of food through frequent seasons and indeed whole years of dearth. It is not that 'rich peasant traditions' did not exist, but that the wonderful masterpieces served at Christmas, harvest or weddings were not eaten all the time. Nor were they all part of the repertoire across a vast area. So, for example, it has been said that the French peasant cuisine was 'invented' in the early twentieth century by Curnonsky and his circle (Curnonsky & De Croze 1933; Curnonsky & Rouff 1921–26), whose work was sponsored by tyre manufacturers interested in promoting tourism among the new generation of car-owners. What they actually did was to collect the gastronomic treasures of France in numerous volumes, with the consequence that these dishes became available more or less all the time and everywhere for those able to pay for them. It is perhaps a mark of France's distinctive place in the culinary history of Europe that these collectors of gastronomic folklore became quite so famous;

Stephen Mennell

but such initiatives were by no means confined to France. In Britain, for instance, Florence White (1932) explicitly modelled her English Folk Cookery Association on the more famous English Folk Song and Dance Association led by Cecil Sharp. It was in the same era that Béla Bartók[2] was collecting folk music in Hungary, and it seems probable that traditional recipes were being collected, even rescued, around the same time in many countries. We must not romanticise the past, nor imagine that a huge diversity of the best dishes were being eaten every day. Nor should we depict our forefathers as living in the Land of Cockaygne. Indeed the prevalence in European folklore of *mythes de ripaille*—roughly 'myths about having a good blowout'—is symptomatic of the dreams of people who frequently experienced the opposite, in times of scarcity.

Yet, at the same time, the recipes have been collected, and the dishes continue to be cooked, because the tastes and smells of a country's traditional table are the royal route to a part of its collective memory that is accessible to everyone. In a famous essay, Roland Barthes showed long ago how powerfully historical and rural themes are deployed in creating a sense of nostalgia that is a key part of the enjoyment of food in France (Barthes 1961). For a country like Britain, too, where manufactured food forms a large part of what people eat every day, and where people eat out upon a diversity of cuisines that reflect the ethnic diversity of society today, the entry in *Culinary Cultures of Europe* shows how the traditional dishes of the past are still cherished and celebrated. (The Poland chapter shows great realism in pointing out that its great traditional dishes may now be cooked more for visitors than for residents.)

One component of a definition of a peasant cuisine is its dependence on, its relatedness to, a 'locality'. But what is a 'locality'? Plainly it is an elastic concept. For one thing, self-sufficiency was always relative, and there would always have been some essential ingredients that had to be sought through trade beyond the local community. Salt is an example: the historic shortage of salt is mentioned in the case of Iceland, and Azerbaijan was the principal supplier of salt throughout the Caucasus region. Localities grow as trade grows, and as the distance over which trade takes place increases. The spreading web of trade in food in early modern Europe can be plotted quite precisely through the peaks and troughs of grain prices. As trade and transport improved, there was a diminution of the enormously high steeples of food prices when harvests failed in limited regions, and the risk of localised famine declined. The same spreading web of trade also tended to increase the diversity of ingredients, and thus of dishes, in a particular locality. Local differences do not necessarily disappear, of course: in Georgia 'food remains an important marker of cultural differences' among the five main subgroups of its population. Some countries were always situated on major trade routes, and this had a bearing on what they ate: that was true of Estonia, while in Croatia both local traditions and the intermingling of traditions in the ethnic cockpit of the Balkans played their part. In its chapter

Croatia introduced a brave note into the often-cosy world of food history: that the intermingling of food traditions results from war as well as from peaceful trade.

Lest cosiness also permeate a picture of inevitable progress from localised and restricted peasant cuisines, through the development of trade to the modern diversity of eating, it must be remembered that there have been bad times in which the trend was reversed. War again, most obviously, has occasioned reversions in the direction of self-sufficiency. Several of the new member countries of the Council of Europe also mention the hard times they experienced under the former communist regimes. In Poland, 'under authoritarian rule, tradition is … used for political purposes, to compensate for privileges lost to the people. But cuisine usually loses in this process …'. In the 1980s, as the communist economy began to collapse, Poles resorted to something that might be called 'emergency peasantisation', when town-dwellers went out into the countryside to strike deals, sometimes bartering, with farmers—returning home perhaps with the whole carcass of a pig that would be shared among a few families.

The stratification of cuisines: Courts, aristocrats and bourgeois

Peasant farmers constituted the great majority of the European population in the past—the more remote past in some parts of the continent than in others. Yet eating was always socially stratified. We know, for instance, that before the Black Death nutrition was very unequally distributed among members of the various estates—and that was especially true of meat, with the peasantry's diet dominated by vegetable and dairy products. The upper strata may have been less likely to go hungry in times of dearth, but it would appear that even the warrior aristocracy ate essentially the seasonal produce of their own land, and did not generally have it cooked by means much more elaborate than roasting and boiling. To generalise, when the social divisions between strata are very deep and the interdependence between them is very unequal—when the power that they have over each other is very asymmetrical—then the power and status of the upper strata is more likely to find expression in quantity rather than quality, in periodical displays of indiscriminate heaps of food at ceremonial banquets, for instance, rather than through the quality and labour-intensiveness that are among the marks of a true *haute cuisine* (Mennell 1996).

It is true that the manuscript recipes from a very few major courts towards the end of the Middle Ages—the *Forme of Cury* (a manuscript from the late fourteenth-century court of King Richard II of England; see Pegge 1780) and Taillevent (a similar manuscript from the late-medieval court of France; see Taillevent c.1380), for example—show something more complicated, characterised by the use of spices and flavourings that could have reached these courts only via very long trade routes. But,

Stephen Mennell

significantly, there is an old debate about whether this late medieval *haute cuisine* for the very few represents a debased form, a remote echo, of the cuisine of ancient Rome, when the chains of social and economic interdependence were indeed longer and denser than they were for many centuries afterwards. In any case, this *haute cuisine* appears to have been confined to a few major European princely courts and – from relatively scanty documentary sources – does not seem to have changed rapidly at all in response to fashion, as later *hautes cuisines* were to do.

A large body of modern research on European food history suggests that the rate of change in 'taste' accelerates when the strata of society become more closely and more equally interdependent, and when social competition becomes more intense. Thus, as far as we can tell, courtly cuisine did not change very quickly when an only partially pacified warrior nobility's reference groups were other courts at a great distance. *Hautes cuisines*—which can be defined by their typical dishes requiring complex sequences of stages, considerable division of labour among kitchen staff, and thus by their costliness—have tended to emerge in court societies from Ancient Egypt onwards. That appears to be true to varying degrees of several of the national traditions that are now influential throughout the world: those of China and India, and from Europe, of France, Italy and Turkey.

The case of France is especially significant, because from the late seventeenth century onwards, and especially in the nineteenth century, French cuisine 'conquered the world', in the sense that it came to set the models and standards for upper-class eating throughout much of Europe and beyond, for instance in North America (Mennell 1996; Ferguson 2004). The rapid elaboration of French cookery was connected with the consolidation of the absolutist monarchy of the *ancien régime*, in the course of which the court aristocracy became a 'two-front stratum', defunctionalised and squeezed between the monarchy and the 'pressure from below' of an expanding merchant and professional bourgeois **class**.[3] Their whole **social identity** became bound up with virtuoso display, in their manners, clothes, houses, pastimes and eating. Although some of the same trends were present in Britain, there were subtle differences. The development of royal absolutism in England was nipped in the bud a century and half before the Revolution in France, and English nobility and gentry retained more of their old social functions—including their ties and influence in the provinces where they still lived for much of the year on their country estates—so that virtuoso consumption became less essential to their social identity and the marks of rural life endured more clearly in their tastes.

In both Austria and Turkey there is a clear culinary legacy from the imperial courts and the nobility—Habsburg and Ottoman respectively. Courtly cuisine is of course always essentially an urban phenomenon, because the elaboration of a great variety of dishes requires a great variety of ingredients, which are brought together in the markets of the great cities, not in the countryside. In Turkey the great Spice Road brought ingredients from afar, but a courtly elite cuisine also affected the food of the peasants in the countryside by skimming off the finest produce: the best fish, for instance, found its way from the Black Sea directly to Istanbul. Where a great royal court was associated with an empire, its tastes in food could be a model over great distances. Azerbaijan, Bulgaria and Serbia–Montenegro were all influenced in their culinary traditions by once having belonged to the Ottoman Empire. Greek and Turkish cuisines show broad similarities, although the two countries are also proud of their differences. In its contribution to *Culinary Cultures of Europe*, Austria takes a wry pride in contending that Wiener schnitzel is not distinctively Viennese at all, but derives from Byzantium via Italy; on the other hand, Austrian influence is seen in Croatia, Poland and again Serbia–Montenegro, and Habsburg influence is no doubt evident in other former provinces of the empire such as Slovenia, despite its not being explicitly stated. Spain, the home of Europe's other great Habsburg court, drew a large variety of new ingredients from its vast overseas empire—after all, how would a Spanish omelette be possible if potatoes had never been discovered in South America?—but courtly influence is not much stressed, either in the entry in *Culinary Cultures of Europe* or in Spanish cookery books. If the Spanish aristocracy did not have so great a modelling influence on Spanish cookery as did their counterparts in France on French cuisine, it may be because of the greater social distance between the nobility and the bourgeoisie, and the weakness of any pressure from below on the part of an aspirant upwardly mobile middle class in eighteenth- and nineteenth-century Spain. In some countries—Norway and the Netherlands, for example—food has been shaped by the *absence* of a royal and aristocratic court society.[4] Norwegians are proud of a good—*but not great*—cuisine, while the Dutch are characteristically modest about the plainness of their food.

Although courts historically laid the foundations of *grandes cuisines*, the pace of culinary change accelerated markedly when, for whatever reason, the competitive virtuoso consumption among courtiers was supplanted by the commercial competition that takes place among restaurateurs using product differentiation to attract customers. In the culinary history of Western Europe we tend to point to the proliferation of restaurants in Paris after the French Revolution as a decisive step in this process. An important part of the story of how culinary innovations and fashions in taste spread from the high-class restaurants to the less prestigious establishments and into the domestic kitchen can broadly be described as the 'trickle down' model. Aron (1973) depicted in some detail the culinary ladder linking the high and the low in nineteenth-century Paris. Not every country was like France, however. Even though the London taverns served as models for the first Paris restaurants in the eighteenth century, Britain later fell far behind France in the abundance and variety of its eating places, and 'eating out' remained an exceptional experience for all but the fairly well-to-do until roughly the last four decades. Several other countries mention that the mass of the people have been attracted only quite recently to eat frequently in what is now the great variety of restaurants in all parts of Europe.

Stephen Mennell

National culinary integration

In some countries, regional variations persist strongly within their borders, while in others there is an overall national style of cookery. In fact these are not necessarily incompatible: it is partly a matter of the focal length of the lens through which one is looking. There are always local variants on a national style where that exists. Not just in a large country like Germany, but in small countries like Croatia, Serbia, Montenegro and Slovakia there are many regional variants. In Croatia and Serbia–Montenegro can be seen the culinary influences of ethnic minorities at one of the cultural crossroads of Europe, something to celebrate in view of the difficult and complex history of the Balkans. In Germany there are Polish influences, such as *pirogi* (dumplings) in its north-eastern border areas, but there is also a more important *kleindeutsch* inheritance (from the mass of tiny principalities that composed Germany to its north until the second half of the nineteenth century). Late national unification is probably correlated with the strength of distinctive regional dishes, which one can observe everywhere in Germany. The same is probably true of Italy, which like Germany was unified only in the second half of the nineteenth century. Most people would agree that both in Germany and Italy, the regional specialities belong within a broad national style.

National culinary styles do not necessarily change abruptly when one walks across an international border in Europe. Transitions are often more gradual, just as linguistic transitions used to be more gradual than they are today. In Strasbourg, home of the Council of Europe, one hears French; in Kehl, a stroll across the bridge over the Rhine, one hears German. True, if one listens carefully, one can still hear the Alsatian dialect, but it is less common than it was. But in the restaurant alternatively known as *Aux armes de Strasbourg* or *Stadtwappe*, the food shows both German and French traits. Elsewhere the culinary transitions are still more gradual, with strong similarities, for example, among the various Slavic countries. Poland has its eastern 'borderlands' with Lithuania, Belarus and Ukraine, associated with a 'joint supper', consumed by many peoples. For the Poles, culinary traditions played their part (along with Catholicism) in preserving the strong sense of national pride and identity through the tribulations of Polish history. Three times at the end of the eighteenth century the national territory was partitioned between the three neighbouring great powers of Prussia, Austria and Russia, a partition that endured until 1918, when the Polish state was resurrected, only to undergo radical changes in its boundaries, immense movements of population, and subsumption into the Soviet empire after World War II (Davis 1981).

One of the most encouraging conclusions from the story of Poland, and many other countries too, is that however much food and culinary tradition can serve as a badge of national pride and identity, they do not necessarily have to serve an exclusionary function. A history as complex as Poland's has promoted culinary diversity, and continuing influence from neighbouring countries—east as well as west—is welcomed.

The industrialisation of eating

In *Culinary Cultures of Europe*, Finland states the unvarnished truth that its people have today been transformed from food producers into food consumers. That is the outcome of the industrialisation of eating, which is now evident everywhere. It impinges even on traditional food production: Georgia, listing some of its local specialities, casually mentions 'beer locally made from barley … *in plastic bottles'*. But industrialisation of food production is not a particularly new process. Its roots lie back in the nineteenth century, and the effects of industrial production of food are not easy to separate from the effects of industrialisation more generally. Sweden mentions the impact of canals, railways and later asphalt roads upon the country's food culture. In what is perhaps an implicit allusion to what Benedict Anderson (1983) called 'print capitalism' and to the role that it played in the construction of 'imagined communities', in Sweden, as part of processes of nation building in the nineteenth century, novel culinary ideals were spread with the help of newspapers, and the food culture of the bourgeoisie became the model for the aspirations of the new working and middle classes. The new urban foods were what migrants from the countryside wanted to eat too. A century later, industrialisation had a very similar effect in reducing the contrasts between the diets of the people of the lowlands and uplands in Slovakia. It is as well to remember that the industrialisation of eating has had beneficial effects, for (despite the low-quality industrial food found in eastern Europe under communism), it is too easy to dwell upon the aesthetic downside of mass-produced food. It is again necessary not to romanticise the past. When judged by the finest culinary creations once consumed by a tiny privileged minority, the chilled and frozen foods from the supermarket and the hamburgers and pizzas from the chain eating places may look like decline. When viewed from the perspective of the often-monotonous diets of poor people in the past, such food may seem a veritable cornucopia.

Eating as a problem: The beginnings of dietary advice and food policy

A cornucopia gives rise to its own problems. In Turkey, health problems have arisen with the transformation of its traditional diet, which from a nutritional point of view had many virtues. Where food has become so much more diverse and abundant—and also more secure and regular—as it has across most of Europe, control of the appetite has become problematic in a way that it rarely was in the past. Farm labourers often wolfed down prodigious quantities of food at harvest suppers. Their way of life was extremely strenuous, and they often went hungry, so why worry when the opportunity came for a blow-out? Very often, being plump was a source of prestige, and that attitude has not entirely disappeared from Europe today: the Austria entry in *Culinary Cultures of Europe* somewhat gloatingly dwelt upon its people's perception of themselves as 'informed by unbridled gluttony, the preference for being *gourmand* rather than *gourmet*, and the partiality for large quantities of food of the fatty or sugar-laden variety', a point of view that would be regarded as politically incorrect in many other countries. Iceland could easily have gone in the same direction, had not poverty and taxation prevented it: instead it went down the route of very heavy consumption of sugar—something else that is not exactly in line with modern dietetic opinion. In fact, that route of adaptation was not unique to Iceland; it was common among working-class people in the late nineteenth and early twentieth centuries, the age of bread and jam (Mintz 1985). From the same period in several countries—Britain, the Netherlands, Scandinavia, and also the United States of America—came middle-class initiatives to provide cookery lessons for housewives, and cookery schools for domestic servants. While welfare was one motive, it is clear that another was, *de haut en bas*—to 'improve', to 'refine', and to 'civilise' the 'lower orders'; in other words, the teachers' mixed motives often included the satisfaction of manifesting their own social superiority (Mennell 1996, pp. 226–8). Cookery lessons also found their way into the curriculum for schoolgirls. Interestingly, such initiatives were far less evident in France, where it seems to have been taken more for granted that an interest in food and some skill in its preparation would be encountered within the home.

It is significant that, again a little more than a century ago, what are now called 'eating disorders' first became a concern, mainly in the better-off ranks of society where food was never in short supply (Mennell 1987). It was then that anorexia nervosa was first described and named by clinicians, and that cookery books began to have sections on how to cope with obesity. The two disorders, apparently opposites, in fact have something in common in their aetiology—both represent the failure of a steady and even self-control over appetite capable of maintaining a normally healthy body weight. The fear of fatness is now widespread, both on the part of individuals and governments. People are, in many countries, on average becoming steadily plumper, yet the cultural ideal of the sexually attractive body is becoming steadily slimmer. So for individuals, being fat causes anxieties about attractiveness as well as healthiness. For governments, the increasing prevalence of fatness is a public health and even an economic problem. Campaigns to persuade people to take more exercise, as well as to eat more sensibly, are prevalent—although their effectiveness is debatable.[5]

Globalisation and multicultural eating

Today, the diversity of ethnic influences found in the cooking and taste of all the richer countries of the world, enmeshed as they are in worldwide food chains, makes it more difficult of speak of separate national culinary cultures. In one way we may even have reverted to a pattern reminiscent of the medieval world. The separate strata are now at a global level, with the rich countries looking towards each other to make sure that they are not too far out of step, while a huge gap divides them from the large part of the world's people who form the nutritional underclass. Those are people who often go hungry or, even when they are not hungry, live somewhat monotonously off the product of their own labours; they are (sadly) irrelevant to the culinary cultural consciousness of the West and of Europe.

One consequence of this pattern of global stratification is that we are living through a second great age of the migration of peoples,[6] which dwarfs in scale those of the previous two millennia. There is nothing new in the principle of ethnic migrations and diasporas. Over much of Europe, but especially in Central and Eastern Europe, cuisine was significantly enriched by the traditions of the Jews. This is especially clear in Poland, to which the Jews were invited as an oppressed minority by the enlightened Casimir the Great,[7] many centuries before Poland under the Nazis became a 'Jewish cemetery'. The Roma, or Gypsies as they are more familiarly known, are also represented in the lexicon of European cookery: many dishes are described as being *in der Zigeuner Art* (although whether real Roma would recognise them is another question—like all recipes, those of minorities change over time and are adapted by host communities).

But the scale of mass migration since the second half of the twentieth century is unprecedented; it has had, and is continuing to have, huge effects on how people eat in most of the countries of Europe. Of course, the impact of migration is centuries old; and ethnic diversity does has no absolute beginning. In Sweden the impact of that its recent immigrants have had on its food can be seen for instance in the difference between recipes for meatballs in 1938 and 1999. Yet old traditions are typically not overwhelmed by new ethnic influences; in Sweden, for new migrants 'eating Swedish' is one important means of assimilation to Swedish society. There are many puzzles concerning which new culinary influences are adopted and which old traditions stand their ground. It is curious that the Dutch dominated world trade for a century and a half in and after their Golden Age,[8] yet their one contribution to world cuisine (they wryly note) was the doughnut. That is all the more puzzling when, having lost its empire and suffered surprisingly little collective trauma through its loss, the Netherlands now has a strikingly multicultural eating scene. There is much here that merits further investigation and reflection.

There is an overall trend towards 'diminishing contrasts, increasing varieties' (Mennell 1996, pp. 318–32). Economic inequality has not disappeared—indeed, in many Western societies it has increased over the last quarter of a century—but old-style class inequalities cross-cut with ethnicity to an extent inconceivable in Europe half a century ago. Above all, they cross-cut with many different kinds of status groups that are defined as much by their patterns of consumption and taste as by their disposable income. This has led to a culinary pluralism that is the counterpart of something that is more familiar in the arts: the loss of a single dominant style. Styles

Stephen Mennell

like the Baroque and Rococo enjoyed virtually unchallenged dominance in their age, more unchallenged indeed than the aristocratic upper classes with which they were associated. In a more problematic way so did Romanticism dominate an age and spread across the range of the arts. During the last hundred years or more, however, this stylistic unity has been lost. There is a greater diversity of tastes coexisting and competing at one time—competing more equally, again like classes and interests in society. There is a rapid succession of fashions in artistic styles. And the mixture of elements deriving from several styles is common: the label *Kitsch*, often applied to incongruous mixtures of style in other aspects of culture, can also be used about the domain of food (Elias 1996 [1935]).

One such mixture is the modern so-called '**fusion food**'. In 1988 in the Netherlands I was served *kipfilet* (chicken breast) surmounted by a slice of Brie, accompanied by sauerkraut mixed with mangoes and lychees. Similar mixtures are evident in Australia (I am tempted to caricature the Australian national dish as meat pies with lemongrass). Such a mixing of traditions is made possible not only by long chains of interdependence, but also by a loosening of the model-setting centres for taste that would previously have judged such a combination to be incongruous. But I would also add that the sheer pace of change itself probably means that incongruity appears and disappears before the arbiters of taste—such as they still are—have a chance to label it incongruous. We shall never again see the codification of high culinary taste in coherent systems such as those represented by, say, Carême, Escoffier[9] or (to a lesser extent) the *nouvelle cuisiniers*[10] of the 1960s (Mennell 1996), which is not to say that there will not be fashions that spread internationally and last for a longer or shorter period. One example of the last decade or so is the fashion adopted by many restaurants for the *tian*, in which the fish or meat is piled on top of vegetables and potatoes in the middle of the plate, surrounded by sauce.

The democratisation of eating

Three decades ago the Council of Europe sponsored an intense discussion of the rival merits of the notions of the 'democratisation of culture' on the one hand and 'cultural democracy' on the other (Mennell 1976). The first phrase was used to denote traditional attempts to spread knowledge and enjoyment of 'elite culture'—whether drama, music, literature or art—to the masses, those who by reason of socioeconomic condition or lack of education had not had access to it. In the wake of *les événements de mai* 1968 (the student protests of May 1968 in Paris) a certain loss of nerve was apparent. At any rate, there was no denying *le refus ouvrier* ('working class rejection'): the workers, or most of them, did not much care for Sophocles, Shakespeare or Schoenberg. The ideology of 'cultural democracy' was a response to that, and meant that equal value should be accorded to the 'cultural expression' of all social groups. Since it was unclear how 'cultural democracy' was to be distinguished from the mass culture provided by the mass media (which commercial interests justify by saying that they are giving people 'what they want', even though 'the people' may still have little knowledge of or access to anything different) one could be sceptical about whether this conceptual dichotomy represented real policy alternatives (Mennell 1979).

These issues play themselves out in curious ways in the specific field of food culture. The democratisation of eating has been underway for a long time. It can be seen two centuries ago, with the shifting of the locus of culinary innovation and leadership from the kitchens of great houses to the restaurants where cooks competed for the favour of the eating public. Also associated in France with the aftermath of the Revolution was the emergence of the knowledgeable gastronome, men like Grimod de la Reynière[11] and Brillat-Savarin[12], who wrote the precursors of the restaurant guides—*Michelin, Gault Millau,*[13] the *Good Food Guide*—and of the cookery columns in newspapers and magazines (Mennell 1996). At first glance they, and their successors, can appear to be snobbishly decreeing for the ignorant populace what their betters consider to be good and bad food. But in broader perspective they can also be seen to have democratised good eating, working along with cooks to educate the palates of diners, spreading knowledge over great distances through print and later the electronic media.

Still, the democratisation of eating does not involve only the trickle *down* of tastes and dishes that once may have been known only to the wealthy, privileged and well travelled. 'Trickle *up*' also occurs, when tastes and dishes that once belonged to the lower strata of society are adopted by higher strata. The activities of collectors of old recipes and promoters of the romantic image of peasant cuisines have already been mentioned. Also active in effecting the upward social mobility of simple farmers' fare, however, have been some of the most famous chefs. Elizabeth David (1964) described what she called the 'butterisation' of simple Provençal recipes by the great Escoffier himself; he might take a dish of artichokes and potatoes baked in olive oil and transform it by adding truffles (very expensive) and using this as the bed on which to serve a choice cut of lamb to his rich customers. That would represent long-range upward social mobility for the humble vegetarian dish from Provence, and probably— as in the social ascent of people—the upward social mobility of foods is more likely to be over a shorter than a longer range. Examples abound: cases include both the humble pizza and eating with the fingers in the street. Across much of Europe today, the eating scene is reminiscent of Peter Burke's (1978) description of popular culture in the late Middle Ages. Then, all ranks of society participated in popular culture, and it was only with printing and more widespread literacy that the upper classes withdrew into a more exclusive high culture. Today, one might argue that all ranks participate in the fast food and manufactured food cultures, even if only the better off come to sample elite cuisines and search for new ways of distinguishing themselves (Bourdieu 1979/1984; Finkelstein 1989). The use they make of food and eating to symbolise their styles of life is now well recognised. Above all, however, interest in

Stephen Mennell

and the *enjoyment* of food—and, moreover, the *opportunity* to enjoy it—appears to be spread more widely through the ranks of society than it ever was before.

Conclusion

Can any conclusions and recommendations be drawn from a book like *Culinary Cultures of Europe*, for governments, local authorities and people at large? Perhaps. As noted at the beginning of this chapter, it used to be a truism that people's tastes in food were among the most conservative aspects of cultures, the most resistant to change. And yet today it is probably the speed of change and the burgeoning diversity of eating across the world that most strikes the reader. The two statements may not be so incompatible as they appear at first glance. Undoubtedly, the development of food manufacturing, transport and distribution since World War II has filled the supermarket shelves with an abundance of new products and exotic flavours which must occasionally tempt even the most conservative shopper. Can we now imagine life without the supermarkets, even though they have spread widely only since about the 1960s? Can we remember that in northern Europe most people in the 1960s had never seen a pepper (capsicum) or aubergine (eggplant)? That mangos became a familiar fruit far more recently than that? Or, indeed, that bananas were almost unobtainable in parts of Eastern Europe in the 1980s? At the same time, it is too simple to say that the old conservatism has vanished. People in most countries still enjoy, celebrate and take pride in their traditional foods and recipes. But it does not prevent them from enjoying a change. This facet of modern European culinary culture may be seen as one manifestation of what has been called a 'quest for excitement' that is characteristic of modern society (Elias & Dunning 1986). People do not need just to 'relax' from the strains and stresses of work; they need the pleasurable arousal and excitement, and the pleasurable catharsis that follows, from playing a hard-fought game of tennis, watching a fast-moving game of soccer, reading a thriller or great literature, being in the audience at a good play or concert. Or eating out, perhaps sampling food from an unfamiliar country or culture.

It follows that sampling other people's foods is one of the simplest and most direct ways to promote multicultural understanding. It should not, however, be promoted heavy-handedly. There is a certain tension—albeit an often pleasurable and exciting tension—for most people between their attachment to the old ways of eating in their country and their interest in the new foods they encounter when travelling abroad, or in new ethnic restaurants or among newcomers in their own country. It would most likely be disastrous were officials to decree that 'Thou *shalt* enjoy rogan josh/moussaka/baklava/pirozhki/bryndza' (delete as appropriate). That would obviously provoke the reaction 'Why shouldn't we just carry on eating our fish and chips/Bratkartoffeln/lasagne/paella' (or whatever). If adventurous eating is encouraged with a gentle touch from schooldays onwards, however, what more directly enjoyable way is there of coming to know, to understand, and to *like* other cultures?

Acknowledgment

This chapter is adapted from the conclusion ('Culinary Transitions in Europe: An Overview', pp. 469–88) that I wrote for Darra Goldstein and Kathrin Merkle (eds), 2005, *Culinary Cultures of Europe: Identity, Diversity and Dialogue*, Strasbourg, Council of Europe; and was written during research leave in 2006–07 at St Catharine's College, Cambridge, with the support of a Government of Ireland Senior Research Fellowship awarded by the Irish Research Council for the Humanities and Social Sciences.

SUMMARY OF MAIN POINTS

- The book *Culinary Cultures of Europe* contains chapters from 46 European countries, depicting for the most part what they are most proud of in their traditions of cooking and eating.
- Old self-sufficient 'peasant' traditions are easy to romanticise. When people had to rely on what they grew and reared in their own neighbourhoods, their diets were often very monotonous by modern standards. The 'great festival dishes', often celebrated today, were few and far between.
- In long-term perspective, cuisine has become less socially stratified. Styles of cookery that originated in the most elite circles—royal and noble courts—have trickled down over the centuries to influence what ordinary people eat. National styles emerged, but now an internationalisation of eating is evident, partly through the 'industrialisation of eating'.
- Eating as a social problem and as a matter of public policy—worries about anorexia on the one hand and obesity on the other—are recent developments.
- The present phase is one of the 'democratisation of eating', marked by 'trickle up' as well as 'trickle down', with people of all social strata participating in the popular culture of burgers and so on.

SOCIOLOGICAL REFLECTION

- How would you describe your own country's culinary cuisine?
- What are some iconic examples of national dishes, ingredients and modes of cooking or consuming food that reflect your national culture?
- How much are your own food habits a reflection of regional, national and/or global influences?

Stephen Mennell

DISCUSSION QUESTIONS

1. What are some of the main reasons that distinctive culinary cuisines developed?
2. What role did social stratification play in the development of culinary cuisines?
3. How have the processes of industrialisation and globalisation impacted upon culinary cuisines?
4. What are some examples of, and reasons for, the rise of fusion food in your country?
5. What are some contemporary examples of 'diminishing contrasts and increasing varieties' in the culinary cuisine of your country?
6. In what ways has eating become 'democratised' in your country?

Further investigation

1. The increasing availability of national cuisines across the globe reflects the rise of cosmopolitanism and cultural tolerance. Discuss.
2. Food habits are not simply a matter a personal taste, but reflect regional, national and global influences. Discuss.

FURTHER READING AND WEB RESOURCES

Books

Elias, N. 1996 [originally 1935], 'The Kitsch Style and the Age of Kitsch', pp. 26–35, in Johan Goudsblom & Stephen Mennell (eds), *The Norbert Elias Reader*, Blackwell, Oxford.

Goldstein, D. & Merkle, D. (eds) 2005, *Culinary Cultures of Europe: Identity, Diversity and Dialogue*, Council of Europe, Strasbourg.

Mennell, S. 1987, 'On the Civilising of Appetite', *Theory, Culture and Society*, vol. 4, nos 2–3, pp. 373–403.

—— 1996, *All Manners of Food: Eating and Taste in England France from the Middle Ages to the Present*, Revised edition, University of Illinois Press, Champaign, IL.

Websites

Ethnic and Cultural Resources (USDA): http://fnic.nal.usda.gov/nal_display/index. php?info_center=4&tax_level=2&tax_subject=270&topic_id=1339

Gastronomica: The Journal of Food and Culture: www.gastronomica.org/

Research Centre for the History of Food and Drink (University of Adelaide, Australia): www.arts.adelaide.edu.au/centrefooddrink/

World Food Habits Bibliography: http://lilt.ilstu.edu/rtdirks/

Films and documentaries

Babette's Feast (1987): Nordisk Film/Danish Film Institute, 109 minutes with English subtitles.

Chocolat (2000): France, film directed by Lasse Hallstrom, 121 minutes.

Eat, Drink, Man, Woman (1994): Taiwan, 123 minutes with English subtitles.

Like Water for Chocolate (1993): Mexico, 113 minutes with English subtitles.

The Wedding Banquet (1993): Taiwan, 111 minutes with English subtitles.

NOTES

1   The Black Death was the most devastating pandemic in human history, spreading from south-western Asia to Europe by the late 1340s, killing an estimated minimum of 75 million people worldwide.

2   Béla Bartók (1881–1945), Hungarian composer and collector of Eastern European folk music, one of the founders of the field of ethnomusicology.

3   'Two-front stratum' is a concept from Georg Simmel's *Soziologie* (1908); the idea was developed in Norbert Elias's idea of 'pressure from below', in *The Civilising Process* (2000).

4   Strictly speaking, there was a court society around the Stadhouder—who became King only after 1815—at Den Haag (with a subsidiary branch at Leeuwarden), but the political and economic power, and thus most of the cultural model-setting power, rested with the mercantile Regenten elite in the commercial towns of the Randstad (Amsterdam, Haarlem, Rotterdam and Utrecht).

5   For more than 30 years, the Council of Europe has promoted exercise under its slogan of 'Sport for All'; it is less easy to think of such a straightforward and effective slogan for promoting sensible eating. The message would have to cut two ways: too many people in the world are still going hungry, while others are eating far too much.

6   The term 'age of the great migrations of peoples' was originally applied to the movements across the Eurasian landmass during the first millennium ad.

7   Casimir III, King of Poland 1333–70.

8   The seventeenth century, in which Dutch trade, science and art were among the most acclaimed in the world.

9   Antonin Carême (1784–1833) and Georges Auguste Escoffier (1846–1935) were the most famous French chefs of their respective ages, and both of them codified French cuisine in major cookery books that had great influence on upper-class eating throughout the Western world.

10   The term *nouvelle cuisine* was applied to a new style of French cuisine that was simpler and lighter, and dispensed with the heavy sauces of the Escoffier era. It was developed in the 1960s and 1970s by such French cooks as Jean and Pierre Troisgros, Paul Bocuse and Michel Guerard.

11   Alexandre Balthazar Grimod de la Reynière (1758–1838), author of the *Almanach des Gourmands*, a pioneering gastronomic guide to Paris, which appeared in annual editions for about a decade from 1803 onwards.

12   Jean Anthelme Brillat-Savarin (1755–1826), author of *Physiologie du Goût* (1826).

13   *Gault Millau* is one of the most famous contemporary restaurant guides in France, taking its name from its editors, Henri Gault and Christian Millau, who are credited with inventing the term *nouvelle cuisine*.

REFERENCES

Anderson, B. 1983, *Imagined Communities: Reflections on the Origin and Spread of Nationalism*, Verso, London.

Aron, J-P. 1973, *Le Mangeur du 19e siècle*, Laffont, Paris.

Barthes, R. 1961 'Pour une psychosociologie de l'alimentation contemporaine', *Annales E-S-C*, vol. 16, no. pp. 977–86. [English translation: 'Toward a Psycho-sociology of Contemporary Food Consumption', pp. 166–73 in R. Forster & O. Ranum (eds), *Food and Drink in History*, Johns Hopkins University Press, Baltimore, MD, 1979].

Bloch, M. 1970, 'Les aliments de l'ancienne France', in J.J. Hémardinquer (ed.), *Pour une histoire de l'alimentation*, A. Colin, Paris, pp. 231–5.

Bourdieu, P. 1979, *La Distinction*, Le Minuit, Paris.

Burke, P. 1978, *Popular Culture in Early Modern Europe*, Temple Smith, London.

Curnonsky (pseud. of Maurice-Edmond Sailland) and de Croze, A. 1933, *Le Trésor gastronomique de France*, Librairie Delagrave, Paris.

—— & Rouff, M. 1921–26, *La France gastronomique: Guide des merveilleuses culinaires et des bonnes auberges françaises*, F. Rouff, Paris.

Elias, N. 1996 [originally 1935], 'The Kitsch Style and the Age of Kitsch', pp. 26–35 in Johan Goudsblom and Stephen Mennell (eds), *The Norbert Elias Reader*, Blackwell, Oxford.

—— & Dunning, E. 1986, *Quest for Excitement: Sport and Leisure in the Civilising Process*, Blackwell, Oxford.

David, E. 1964, 'French Provincial Cooking', *Wine and Food*, vol. 121, pp. 28–31.

Davis, N. 1981, *God's Playground: A History of Poland. 2 vols*, Oxford University Press, Oxford.

Ferguson, P.P. 2004, *Accounting for Taste: The Triumph of French Cuisine*, University of Chicago Press, Chicago.

Finkelstein, J. 1989, *Eating Out: A Sociology of Modern Manners*, Polity Press, Cambridge.

Goldstein, D. & Merkle, K. (eds) 2005, *Culinary Cultures of Europe: Identity, Diversity and Dialogue*, Council of Europe, Strasbourg.

Lévi-Strauss, C. 1969, *The Raw and the Cooked*, Jonathan Cape, London.

Mennell, S. 1976, *Cultural Policy in Towns*, Council of Europe, Strasbourg.

—— 1987, 'On the Civilising of Appetite', *Theory, Culture and Society*, vol. 4, nos 2–3, pp. 373–403.

—— 1979, 'Theoretical Considerations on the Study of Cultural "Needs"', *Sociology*, vol. 13, no. 2, pp. 235–57.

—— 1996, *All Manners of Food: Eating and Taste in England and France from the Middle Ages to the Present*, Revised edition, University of Illinois Press, Champaign, IL. [First edition published 1985, by Blackwell, Oxford.]

Mintz, S. 1985, *Sweetness and Power: The Place of Sugar in Modern History*, Viking, New York.

Pegge, S. (ed.) 1780, *The Forme of Cury*, J. Nichols, printer to the Society of Antiquaries, London.

Taillevent, G. Tirel dit, 1992 [c. 1380], *The Cookery Book*, D. Atkinson, Oxford.

White, F. 1932, *Good Things in England*, Jonathan Cape, London.

Stephen Mennell

CHAPTER 12

Food, Class and Identity

John Germov

OVERVIEW

- How is social class related to food habits?
- Are class differences in food habits diminishing?
- Do working-class food habits result in nutrition-related health problems?

Class-based food consumption provides a classic example of the social appetite. Food is one of the most basic necessities of life and its inequitable distribution may be as old as human society itself. Public anxiety about diet-related health in developed countries has renewed the interest in class-based differences in food habits. As this chapter shows, class differences in nutritional intake and food choice have diminished in a number of countries. Nevertheless, class patterns in food consumption persist, fuelling a public discourse that blames the 'poor diets of the poor' for working-class health problems. Yet the relationship between class, food and health is much more complex, particularly given the connections between food habits and class identity. Concerns by nutrition experts about working-class diets may have more to do with social differentiation than with nutrition-related health inequality. Drawing on a range of social research, this chapter examines the relationship between class and food. In particular, insights gained from Pierre Bourdieu's concepts of 'habitus' and 'cultural capital', and recent work on individualisation and cosmopolitanism, are discussed.

Key terms

class	fusion food	McDonaldisation
conspicuous consumption	globalisation	reflexive modernity
cosmopolitanism	habitus	social differentiation
cultural capital	life chances	structure/agency debate
food insecurity	life choices	

Introduction

Class has long been associated with food consumption, exemplified by the alleged 'good taste' and 'good manners' of the upper classes compared to the working class. Such pejorative views with moralistic overtones are still evident today. Hallmarks of the class–food nexus exist in exclusive and expensive restaurants, gourmet food and wine, glossy food magazines and TV shows that exalt novel ingredients and cuisines, and laud celebrity chefs, with an emphasis on the artistry of cooking and the etiquette of eating. The privileges that money brings to the upper classes have often been displayed through their consumption practices—and food habits have been one of the social markers used to reinforce class distinctions—what Thorstein Veblen (1899/1975) referred to as **conspicuous consumption**.

Increased understanding of the link between diet and health has been accompanied by popular and scientific assumptions that the 'poor diets of the poor' are partially responsible for the persistence of health inequalities between classes. The diet of the working class is often viewed as uniformly 'unhealthy', while the upper classes are often assumed to be consistently 'healthier'—yet the available evidence does not support such an oversimplified view of class-based food habits. Moreover, a number of commentators suggest that the influence of class on people's lifestyles, including food consumption, is diminishing. This chapter seeks to clarify the association between class and food in contemporary developed societies (see Chapter 2 for a discussion of world hunger in less developed countries). In doing so, it assesses the extent to which class-based food habits impact on health outcomes or reflect the prejudices of privilege (see Box 12.1).

A brief history of class and food

'Please, sir, I want some more.'

Charles Dickens, *Oliver Twist* (1837–39)

The famous line from *Oliver Twist* evokes images of a bygone era of rigid class structures, poverty, and **food insecurity**. Until the Industrial Revolution, subsistence economies and limited means of transportation and storage left European populations susceptible to famine. As Stephen Mennell (1996) notes, food scarcity meant that even the wealthy ate frugally, though they could afford to eat considerably more than the poor, who subsisted mostly on cereals, pulses, potatoes, some milk, and very small quantities of meat (mostly pork, which was considered of low status and was less expensive). Social status in times of food scarcity was often conveyed by a person's girth—that is, a large body was a sign of wealth and of the ability to overconsume when food was available (Mennell 1996). At this time, the 'fat ideal'

John Germov

BOX 12.1

Conceptualising class

Class is a central topic of research and debate in sociology. Due to the differences in theoretical perspectives and research methodologies used by sociologists, the terminology used to signify social inequality varies. For example, it is common to find the terms class and socioeconomic status (SES) or socioeconomic position (SEP) used interchangeably, though they are quite different concepts.

Class refers to a system of social inequality based on an unequal distribution of wealth, status and power. Classes, such as the working, middle and upper classes, refer to real groups of people who share common class-based values, interests and lifestyles. The concept of SES/SEP refers to a statistical grouping of people into high, medium and low groups according to certain criteria (usually a composite index of income, occupation and education). In fact, much of the empirical study of class uses the concept of SES because it is perceived as less controversial and easier to operationalise. It is common for education, income or occupation to be used as an individual surrogate indicator of SES/SEP, and while each overlaps to an extent, they represent 'a different underlying social process and hence they are not interchangeable; they do not serve as adequate proxies for one another' (Turrell et al. 2003, p. 191).

SES/SEP figures can indicate levels of social inequality, but it should be remembered that they are abstract categorisations used for statistical analysis (Connell 1977). For example, very few people identify themselves as a member of a middle SES group! Therefore, SES/SEP should not be automatically substituted for class, because class is meant to refer to actual groups of people with identifiable class-based identities (see Connell 1977; 1983; Crompton 1998).

While some authors have proclaimed 'class is dead', or at least less influential today than it was in the past (Pakulski & Waters 1996), it is important to note that class is not the only basis of **social differentiation** or social inequality. Social research has found a range of demographic factors other than class as useful for explaining social differences, such as gender, ethnicity, age and the presence of children in the household.

was the symbol of beauty, as represented in the famous paintings of voluptuous women by Renoir and Bertolucci, among others. Only the very wealthy could afford to host feasts and banquets, the 'gastro-orgies' of endless dishes and hearty servings that, though rare, reflected the chasm in living standards between the rich and poor (Mennell 1996).

The working class had poor access to food in terms of both quantity and quality. As Friedrich Engels noted in *The Condition of the Working Class in England* (1845/1958,

p. 103), 'the working-people, to whom a couple of farthings are important … cannot afford to inquire too closely into the quality of their purchase … to their share fall all the adulterated, poisoned provisions'. For example, in the 1800s it was a widespread practice to adulterate milk by watering it down by at least 25 per cent, and then adding flour for thickening, chalk for whitening, the juice of boiled carrots for sweetening, and even lamb brains for froth. Bread was commonly whitened with chalk, while clay and sawdust were often used to add weight to a loaf (Atkins 1991; Murcott 1999). The adulteration of food was commonplace in Australia as well, so much so that some of the earliest public health laws in the world were introduced to address this problem—for example, the *Adulteration of Bread Act 1838* (NSW) and the *Act to Prevent the Adulteration of Articles of Food and Drink 1863* (Vic.) (Commonwealth of Australia 2001). In Britain, enormous differences between the diets of the working class and upper classes persisted well into the early twentieth century, and the poorest 10 per cent of the population 'barely subsisted' on a diet of tea, butter, bread, potatoes, and a small amount of meat (Nelson 1993). The situation was somewhat different in Australia and the United States of America, where food scarcity was rare and those who had employment could afford meat regularly (Symons 1982; Levenstein 1988). Nonetheless, the continued existence of food aid programs such as food stamps, soup kitchens, food banks and food cooperatives is evidence of the persistence of food insecurity in developed countries (Riches 1997; 2003).

Theorising food and class: Habitus, cultural capital and identity

Pierre Bourdieu (1930–2002) has had a considerable influence on sociological studies of class and food, particularly through his book *Distinction*. In this book, Bourdieu (1979/1984) examined how the upper classes used particular lifestyles and taste preferences as modes of distinction to symbolically express their domination over the working class. In studying the consumption practices of the French, Bourdieu argued that distinct class-related 'tastes' in art, film, literature, fashion and food were the major means through which class differences were produced and reproduced. According to Bourdieu, in terms of food consumption the working class had 'a taste for the heavy, the fat and the coarse', while the upper classes preferred 'the light, the refined and the delicate' (1979/1984, p. 185). In an age of food abundance, the upper classes were concerned with health and refinement, eating exotic ingredients and 'foreign foods' and valuing the artistry, aesthetics and novelty of food and its preparation. The working class was distinctly different, and in 'the face of the new ethic of sobriety for the sake of slimness … industrial workers maintain an ethic of convivial indulgence' (p. 179). Thus food habits serve as clear social markers of class identity.

The upper and middle classes use food consumption, among other things, as a symbolic way of differentiating themselves from the working class through an

John Germov

appreciation of etiquette, modest serves and aesthetic factors, as reflected in common notions of 'good' and 'bad' taste. Bourdieu sought to explain how such class distinctions were formed and reproduced through the concepts of **habitus** and **cultural capital**. 'Habitus', an expansion of the notion of habit, refers to 'a disposition that generates meaningful practices and meaning-giving perceptions' (p. 170). In particular, Bourdieu conceptualised it as the internalised and taken-for-granted personal dispositions we all possess—such as our accent, gestures and preferences in food, fashion and entertainment—which convey status and class background. 'Cultural capital' refers to a particular set of values and knowledge, possessed by the upper classes, upon which social hierarchies are formed. In this sense, cultural capital is similar to an economic asset in that it confers privilege and high social status.

Bourdieu's conceptual schema attempts to transcend the **structure/agency debate** by presupposing that 'social reality exists both inside and outside of individuals, both in our minds and in things' (Swartz 1997, p. 96). Thus people act according to their class dispositions (habitus), which ultimately leads to the reproduction of class lifestyles (Swartz 1997). Class-based food habits become a routine part of daily life and are not necessarily the result of conscious decisions, but rather an expression of the underlying class logic of a person's habitus. In this way, Bourdieu binds **life choices** with **life chances** so that personal experiences of particular living and working conditions shape beliefs about diet, health and illness (Williams 1995). By adding a cultural dimension to class analysis, he identified the importance of consumption practices in the production and reproduction of social differentiation.

Bourdieu's insights provide a theoretical explanation of why class-based food habits persist. As he states, 'Tastes in food also depend on the idea each class has of the body and of the effects of food on the body, that is, on its strength, health and beauty … some of which may be important for one class and ignored by another, and which the different classes may rank in very different ways' (1979/1984, p. 190). Those who have more cultural capital—that is, those groups who are better able to create notions of 'good taste'—can legitimate forms of consumption to which they have more access. They are able to define their bodies, their lifestyles and their preferred food habits as superior (Williams 1995). Thus Indian and Thai takeaway are better than McDonald's hamburgers and fish and chips from the corner store; what is more, they are chosen by better-educated and better-paid people. Yet class-based food habits are not fixed or immutable, and their gradual emulation by lower classes results in a continuous reinvention of class distinction; witnessed by the working class now commonly consuming multicultural cuisines such as Indian, Thai, Mexican, Chinese and Italian.

Class-based food habits do not necessarily lead to problematic nutritional intake among the working class. As we shall see later in the chapter, the available evidence suggests that the nutritional intakes of the working class differ little from the upper classes. Nevertheless, this does not mean they do not experience deprivation due to a lack of access to highly valued foods, the preferred amount of food, or consistent amounts of food. A study from the United Kingdom of low-income families found food budgets were often elastic, so that when money was scarce (due to unexpected bills), the quality and quantity of food was often sacrificed (Dobson et al. 1994). In such situations, food shopping was done more frequently to avoid a build-up of food supplies that may be consumed too quickly and cause a food shortage later in the week. A lack of experimentation with novel ingredients and meals was also common, because experimentation carried the risk of wastage if family members found new foods unpalatable (see Charles & Kerr 1988; DeVault 1991). Food poverty was generally well hidden by families, by avoiding guests for dinner or specially saving for such events; and in the case of children being visited by their friends, only once their mothers had saved money to provide brand-name snacks. In one instance, a mother filled an empty Coca-Cola bottle with low-cost cola to serve her son's friends, to 'save face' and effectively hide their food poverty (Dobson et al. 1994; Beardsworth & Keil 1997, pp. 93–4).

While Bourdieu's ideas are insightful, they should not be adopted uncritically. The ideas presented in *Distinction* were based on a study of French society at a particular time; the data was collected in the 1960s. Bourdieu himself acknowledged that all theorising is culturally and historically contingent. Therefore, the extent to which his ideas apply today, particularly in countries such as Australia, the USA, Canada and the UK, requires empirical investigation. Despite his attempt to provide an explanation that integrated structure and agency, Bourdieu appears to accord habitus a particularly deterministic quality that belies the internal differentiation among the working class, not to mention the influence of other identity-forming characteristics, such as ethnicity and gender (Mennell 1996; Swartz 1997). Indeed, a number of authors suggest that class is diminishing in importance; it may well be that a person's habitus today reflects a much wider range of dispositions than in the past.

Are class-based food habits diminishing?

In *All Manners of Food*, Mennell (1996) suggests that **globalisation** and industrialis-ation processes have precipitated a decline in class-based food habits. Since the mid 1800s, the mass production of food has continued unabated; canned food, in particular, played a significant role early on in making food relatively cheap and widely accessible (Levenstein 1988; Burnett 1989). Food shortages and rationing during the Depression and World War II further lessened class differences in food habits (Hollingsworth 1985; Braybon & Summerfield 1987). This period is sometimes seen as a time when dietary restrictions made affluent diets 'healthier', and contributed to lower rates of some diseases (such as diabetes). It is at least as plausible that the diets of the poorest sections of the population were improved by wartime organisation of the food supply, which ensured that what was available was distributed with reasonable equity. While those with more resources always had more options, the homogenising influence on diets across classes was considerable (Mennell 1996).

John Germov

Post-war affluence in developed countries had a further homogenising influence on food habits, with post-war migration and international trade resulting in the exchange of foods between cultures, as foods from the USA and Europe began to be widely introduced in countries such as Australia. By the 1990s, the standardising influence exerted by the food industry was such that George Ritzer (1993) developed the concept of **McDonaldisation** to describe it. According to Mennell, 'If commercial interests make people's tastes more standardised than they conceivably could be in the past, they impose far less strict limits than did the physical constraints to which most people's diet was subject … the main trend has been towards *diminishing contrasts* and *increasing varieties* in food habits and culinary taste' (1996, pp. 321–2, italics in original). In an age of plenty, significant class-based differences in food consumption become difficult to sustain. The mass production of food has increased the consumption choices available to people through the greater number of food products and outlets, and the greater access to cuisines from across the globe. According to Alan Warde (1997) though, Mennell 'overestimates the extent of class decline and the erosion of social differentiation' (p. 29), suggesting that what 'best explains Mennell's description of the 20th century is commodification' (p. 171).

Some authors have gone as far as suggesting that a new form of **cosmopolitanism** has emerged (Beck 2000), referring to the worldwide hybridisation of cultures, tastes and cuisines, which has left class distinctions as somewhat antiquated and peripheral to people's everyday lives. Globalisation, particularly via the media, international trade and travel, has resulted in a cosmopolitanisation of food (Tomlinson 1999). People have greater access to, and openness towards, cultures other than their own and, particularly in terms of food, are able to incorporate multicultural aspects into their lifestyle. Cosmopolitanism does not imply an overarching trend towards uniformity and homogeneity, but rather a plurality of lifestyles—irrespective of class, people now partake in multiple ethnic cuisines and **fusion food**. The work of Anthony Giddens and Ulrich Beck suggests that such developments are characteristic of the contemporary age, which they describe as **reflexive modernity** (Beck et al. 1994). According to Giddens, our exposure to information and other cultures makes us open to reflection and change, so that 'lifestyle choice is increasingly important in the constitution of self-identity and daily activity' (1991, p. 5). Processes of individualisation have undermined collective identities and lifestyles (Bottero 2004), so that class-based food habits now function via a hierarchy of tastes that are influenced by a range of contextual social factors. A number of studies have documented the complexity of influences on food habits, whereby class/SES differences are mediated by other social factors such as gender, age, education, occupation and presence of children in the household (Tomlinson & Warde 1993; Gerhardy et al. 1995; Devine et al. 2003). Therefore, a person's life course may play a significant role in influencing their dietary patterns. Such findings show the complexity of attempting to measure and identify class-related food habits and lend credence to the 'diminishing contrasts' thesis.

The curious case of class-based food habits and nutritional intake

Empirical studies from developed countries have documented class differences in food habits (Crotty et al. 1992; Prattala et al. 1992; Nelson 1993; Popkin et al. 1996; Turrell 1996; James et al. 1997; Dobson et al. 1997; Hulshof et al. 2003; Turrell et al. 2003; Turrell et al. 2004; Inglis et al. 2005; Turrell & Kavanagh 2006; Lallukka et al. 2007; Roos et al. 2007). Using a range of SES indicators, such as area-based measures, income, education and occupation, these studies generally find that the food habits of higher SES groups tend to be closer to dietary recommendations (see Chapter 6), but that 'differences were more evident on the food level than on the nutrient level' (Hulshof et al. 2003, p. 135).

In Australia, it was the pioneering work of Pat Crotty and colleagues (1992) that highlighted the need to adopt a nuanced approach to the study of low-income diets, given their finding of negligible differences between low-income and affluent Australians. While these findings were supported by Gavin Turrell's study (1996), he additionally found that those on low incomes who were also welfare recipients had distinctly different food habits from all other SES groups. Turrell notes that welfare recipients are often under-represented in studies examining SES and food, suggesting that this may disguise important dietary differences within low SES groups. This study also examined the proposition that healthy food was more expensive, which some commentators have assumed is an explanation for the 'poor diets of the poor'. However, in Australia at least, cost and access to fresh fruit and vegetables, and meat, does not appear to be a major barrier to a healthy diet (Turrell 1996; Worsley et al. 2003; Turrell et al. 2004). Despite this, a subsequent Australian study found that low SES participants cited the cost of healthy food as a barrier to healthy eating, suggesting that subjective perceptions regarding healthy food do not tally with the objective cost (Turrell & Kavanagh 2006). Once again, this highlights the importance of cultural practices among different class groups first noted by Bourdieu.

A qualitative study of food habits and shopping patterns among low-income earners in Britain (Hitchman et al. 2002) found a tendency to purchase highly processed, low-cost, energy-dense foods that provided 'cheap calories' (p. 22), with food choices highly influenced by special offers and promotional discounts, and possession of instrumental views of food in terms of energy and satiety. A preference for energy-dense (and processed) foods by low SES groups may be a rational response to managing a limited budget (see Giskes et al. 2002; Drewnowski & Specter 2004). This may particularly be the case in limiting loss due to spoilage, especially if refrigeration is not available. A number of studies have found that low SES suburbs tend to have higher concentrations of fast-food outlets, suggesting an obesogenic effect in the way in which local environments can impact on food habits and possibly health outcomes (Cummins et al. 2005; Macdonald et al. 2007).

John Germov

The most comprehensive study to date in this field is the *Low Income Diet and Nutrition Survey* (LIDNS), produced by the Food Standards Agency in the UK. Using a nationally representative sample of 3728 people, it provides significant data on the food habits, nutritional status and health of the low-income population (the bottom 15 per cent). The study collected information via face-to-face interviews, a self-completed survey, four 24-hour diet recalls per person, as well as collecting physical measurements on weight, height, waist and hip circumference, mid-upper arm circumference, blood pressure and a blood sample. The study took place between November 2003 and January 2005, with results published in 2007 (Nelson et al. 2007a; 2007b).

The study found that the overall nutritional intakes for people on a low income were similar to the general population (Nelson et al. 2007a). The study notes that: 'Contrary to expectations fewer differences were seen between the low income and the general population in terms of mean nutrient intake as a percentage of the Estimated Average Requirement (EAR) or Reference Nutrient Intake (RNI) and percentage of food energy from nutrients'. However, there were differences in foods consumed. When compared to the general population, adults aged 19–64 in the low-income group:

- consumed less breakfast cereals, wholemeal bread, fruit and vegetables, and low fat milk
- ate more fat spreads and oils, non-diet soft drinks, meat (beef, veal, lamb and pork) and processed meats, table sugar and whole milk
- drank less alcohol overall (lower mean daily intakes and fewer consumers), but had higher mean daily intakes among those who did consume alcohol
- had lower levels of physical activity and significantly higher rates of smoking (45 per cent and 40 per cent of adult men and women respectively) (Nelson et al. 2007a; 2007b).

Interestingly, mean daily energy intakes were similar between the low income and general population (with low income men having slightly lower intakes) and there were negligible differences in the intakes of carbohydrate, protein and total fat. A striking finding of the UK study was the high level of food insecurity reported, with:

- 29 per cent of the low-income group reporting that access to food had been limited (due to lack of money, storage or transport) at some time during the previous 12 months
- 22 per cent reporting they had missed or reduced meals
- 5 per cent reporting they had experienced times when they had not eaten at all for a day due to a lack of money to purchase food (Nelson et al. 2007b, p. 339).

There are parallels between the UK study and the data from the *1995 Australian National Nutrition Survey* (NNS) (ABS 1997). A major analysis of the Australian

NNS data using an index of relative disadvantage for geographical areas, the Socio-Economic Index for Areas (SEIFA), has allowed a comparison of the diets of those in the most disadvantaged quintile (quintile 1, the poorest 20 per cent of the population) with the diets of those in the upper four quintiles (Wood et al. 2000a; 2000b; see also Baghurst 2003 for a good summary of the data). The sample for the study consisted of 2052 people in quintile 1 and 9203 people in quintiles 2–5. The main findings are summarised in Table 12.1.

Table 12.1 1995 Australian NNS results: Comparison of most disadvantaged areas (quintile 1) with all other areas (quintiles 2–5)

Measure	Quintile 1 (most disadvantaged)	Quintile 2–5
Median intake of all food and beverages	2541 grams per day	2672 grams per day
Reported running out of food over past 12 months	8.9%	4.1%
Eat cereals and cereal products	93.0%	95.1%
Consume milk products/dishes	91.7%	94.0%
Eat seed and nut products/dishes	10.0%	12.8%
Use fats and oils	74.2%	76.2%
Usually eat less than two serves of fruit a day	49.7%	45.2%
Use whole milk	41.9%	37.6%
Trim fat off meat	69.6%	73.8%
Consume alcohol	27.0%	34.3%
Median consumption of alcoholic beverages	571 grams per day	393 grams per day

In the most disadvantaged areas, people were found to have a lower median intake of all food and beverages (2541g for quintile 1 versus 2672g for the upper four quintiles). Furthermore, 8.9 per cent of people in quintile 1 reported 'running out of food and having no money to buy more at some time during the last 12 months', compared to 4.1 per cent for the other quintiles, indicating that food insecurity is a significant problem in Australia (affecting around 5 per cent of the total Australian population) (Wood et al. 2000a, p. 8). People living in the most disadvantaged areas tend to consume slightly lesser amounts of cereals, milk products, seed and nut products, fats and oils, and fruit and vegetables. They are also less likely to trim fat off meat or use low-fat milk. While fewer quintile 1 people consume alcohol overall, those who do consume have a median alcohol intake that is considerably higher than people in higher quintiles. However, in terms of overall food intake, the differences between people living in the most disadvantaged areas compared to all other areas are relatively small and unlikely to account for class-based health inequalities. It is also important to note that like many studies, the NNS data under-represents the most disadvantaged members of society because of the use of a broad geographic indicator of SES. Nonetheless, the results from both the UK and Australian national surveys suggest that food insecurity—poverty rather than class—may be a better indicator of nutritional inequality.

Conclusion

The literature on developed countries suggests that class-based food habits and nutrient intakes, however measured, have diminished without disappearing altogether. To what extent the remaining differences explain health differentials remains the subject of conjecture. Aside from various subgroups that experience food insecurity due to poverty, concerns about working-class diets appear misplaced in terms of nutrient intake. Following Bourdieu's insights, a sociological analysis of class-based food habits exposes the role of symbolic consumption as a key feature of social differentiation.

Acknowledgment

In the previous edition, this chapter was co-authored with Pat Crotty, who also wrote the original chapter in the first edition. Some of the material from the previous editions is reproduced here with permission. I thank Pat for her work on the previous editions and for her influence on my thinking on this topic.

SUMMARY OF MAIN POINTS

- In developed countries, there is mounting evidence that differentials in diet between the upper and working classes are diminishing and that those that persist are not great.
- The common assumption that the 'poor diets of the poor' (that is, the food habits of the working class) are responsible for health inequalities is ill-informed.
- The Australian data suggest there are likely to be subgroups within the population that experience poverty and have diets very different from those of other groups due to food insecurity, and this is where nutrition interventions may need to be targeted.
- There may be differences in food habits that are not class-related but are related to other socio-demographic factors, such as region, age, ethnicity, gender and presence of children in the household; these factors may have good explanatory power for understanding food habits.
- The idea of creating distinction helps us to improve on simplistic interpretations of the links between food habits, health and class; the available data suggest that the relationships are more complex than is usually assumed.

SOCIOLOGICAL REFLECTION

- Describe some class differences in food consumption in your community.
- Do your food habits reflect class?
- The working class generally experiences higher-than average rates of diet-related illness and death. What are some of the reasons for this?

DISCUSSION QUESTIONS

1. What are some examples of class-based food habits in your community?
2. What are some other forms of food consumption by which class distinctions or social differentiation can be observed?
3. What are the implications for public policy of the fact that those households most likely to benefit from improved diets are the least able to respond to current dietary guidelines?
4. People who use the services of welfare agencies are probably the most at risk of having limited food choices, insufficient food and nutritionally inadequate diets. What groups in society may be represented in this category?
5. How might life chances and life choices converge to produce healthy food habits and diets among low-income groups?
6. How can Bourdieu's concepts of cultural capital and habitus help to explain class differences in food consumption? In light of the arguments of Mennell, are Bourdieu's ideas relevant to your society?

Further investigation

1. The higher morbidity and mortality rates of the working class are due to the 'poor diets of the poor'. Discuss.
2. Class differences in food consumption are diminishing as a result of food abundance and cosmopolitanism. Discuss.
3. One of the major differences in expenditure on food between the working class and the upper classes is the amount of money spent on food eaten away from home. Discuss.

FURTHER READING AND WEB RESOURCES

Books

Baghurst, K. 2003, 'Appendix B: Social Status, Nutrition and the Cost of Healthy Eating', in *National Health and Medical Research Council, Dietary Guidelines for Australian Adults*, AusInfo, Canberra. Available online at: www.nhmrc.gov.au/publications/synopses/dietsyn.htm.

John Germov

Hitchman, C., Christie, I., Harrison, M. & Lang, T. 2002, *Inconvenience Food: The Struggle to Eat Well on a Low Income*, Demos, London. Available online at: www.demos.co.uk/files/inconveniencefood.pdf.

Mennell, S. 1996, *All Manners of Food: Eating and Taste in England and France from the Middle Ages to the Present*, Revised edition, University of Illinois Press, Chicago.

Warde, A. 1997, *Consumption, Food and Taste: Culinary Antinomies and Commodity Culture*, Sage, London.

Websites

Low Income Diet and Nutrition Survey (LIDNS): www.food.gov.uk/science/dietarysurveys/lidnsbranch/. Research commissioned by the UK Food Standards Agency.

Sustain (UK): www.sustainweb.org/. Contains information on a range of food campaigns for the promotion of sustainable food production and healthy eating.

VicHealth—Healthy Eating (Australia): www.vichealth.vic.gov.au/Content.aspx?topic ID=18. Website of Victorian Health Promotion Foundation, established by the Victorian government in Australia, provides access to a range of resources and research reports on food insecurity and social determinants and interventions related to food and health.

WHO Global Strategy on Diet, Physical Activity and Health: www.who.int/diet physicalactivity/en/. A World Health Organization (WHO) website that provides access to reports, research and policy statements.

REFERENCES

ABS—*see* Australian Bureau of Statistics.

Atkins, P.J. 1991, 'Sophistication Detected or, the Adulteration of the Milk Supply, 1850–1914', *Social History*, vol. 16, no. 3, pp. 317–39.

Australian Bureau of Statistics 1997, *1995 National Nutrition Survey: Summary of Results*, Australian Bureau of Statistics, Canberra.

—— 1999, National Nutrition Survey: Foods Eaten, Australia 1995, Australian Bureau of Statistics, Canberra.

Baghurst, K. 2003, 'Appendix B: Social Status, Nutrition and the Cost of Healthy Eating', in National Health and Medical Research Council, *Dietary Guidelines for Australian Adults*, AusInfo, Canberra.

Beardsworth, A. & Keil, T. 1997, *Sociology on the Menu*, Routledge, London.

Beck, U. 2000, 'The Cosmopolitan Perspective: On the Sociology of the Second Age of Modernity', *British Journal of Sociology*, vol. 51, pp. 79–106.

——, Giddens, A. & Lash, S. 1994, *Reflexive Modernization: Politics, Tradition and Aesthetics in the Modern Social Order*, Polity Press and Blackwell Publishers, Cambridge.

Bottero, W. 2004, 'Class Identities and the Identity of Class', *Sociology*, vol. 38, no. 5, pp. 985–1003.

Bourdieu, P. 1979/1984, *Distinction: A Social Critique of the Judgement of Taste*, Routledge, London.

Braybon, G. & Summerfield, P. 1987, *Out of the Cage: Women's Experiences in Two World Wars*, Pandora, London.

Burnett, J. 1989, *Plenty and Want: A Social History of Food in England from 1815 to the Present Day*, 3rd edition, Routledge, London.

Charles, N. & Kerr, M. 1988, *Women, Food and Families*, Manchester University Press, Manchester.

Commonwealth of Australia 2001, *Food Regulation in Australia: A Chronology*, Department of the Parliamentary Library, Canberra.

Connell, R.W. 1977, *Ruling Class, Ruling Culture*, Cambridge University Press, Cambridge.

—— 1983, *Which Way is Up? Essays on Sex, Class and Culture*, Allen & Unwin, Sydney.

Crompton, R. 1998, *Class and Stratification: An Introduction to Current Debates*, 2nd edition, Polity Press, Cambridge.

Crotty, P.A., Rutishauser, I.H.E. & Cahill, M. 1992, 'Food in Low–income Families', *Australian Journal of Public Health*, vol. 16, no. 2, pp. 168–74.

Cummins, S.C.J., McKay, L. & MacIntyre, S. 2005, 'McDonald's Restaurants and Neighborhood Deprivation in Scotland and England', *American Journal of Preventive Medicine*, vol. 29, no. 4, pp. 308–10.

DeVault, M.L. 1991, *Feeding the Family: The Social Organization of Caring as Gendered Work*, University of Chicago Press, Chicago.

Devine, C.M., Connors, M.M., Sobal, J. & Bisogni, C.A. 2003, 'Sandwiching it in: Spillover of Work onto Food Choices and Family Roles in Low- and Moderate-income Urban Households', *Social Science and Medicine*, vol. 56, pp. 617–30.

Dobson, A., Porteous, J., McElduff, P. & Alexander, H. 1997, 'Whose Diet has Changed?', *Australian and New Zealand Journal of Public Health*, vol. 21, no. 2, pp. 147–54.

Dobson, B., Beardsworth, A., Keil, T. & Walker, R. 1994, *Diet, Choice and Poverty: Social, Cultural and Nutritional Aspects of Food Consumption among Low-income Families*, Family Policy Studies Centre and Joseph Rowntree Foundation, London.

Drewnowski, A. & Specter, S. 2004, 'Poverty and Obesity: The Role of Energy Density and Energy Costs', *American Journal of Clinical Nutrition*, vol. 79, pp. 6–16.

Engels, F. 1845/1958, *The Condition of the Working Class in England*, Basil Blackwell, Oxford.

Gerhardy, H., Hutchins, R.K. & Marshall, D.W. 1995, 'Socio-economic Criteria and Food Choice Across Meals', *British Food Journal*, vol. 97, no. 10, pp. 24–8.

Giddens, A. 1991, *Modernity and Self-Identity: Self and Society in the Late Modern Age*, Stanford University Press, Stanford, California.

Giskes, K., Turrell, G., Patterson, C. & Newman, B. 2002, 'Socioeconomic Differences among Australian Adults in Consumption of Fruit and Vegetables and Intakes of Vitamins A, C and Folate', *Journal of Human Nutrition and Dietetics*, vol. 15, pp. 375–85.

Hitchman, C., Christie, I., Harrison, M. & Lang, T. 2002, *Inconvenience Food: The Struggle to Eat Well on a Low Income*, Demos, London.

Hollingsworth, D. 1985, 'Rationing and Economic Constraints on Food Consumption in Britain since the Second World War', in D.J. Oddy & D.S. Miller (eds), *Diet and Health in Modern Britain*, Croom Helm, Kent, pp. 255–73.

Hulshof, K.F.A.M., Brussaard, J.H., Kruizinga, A.G., Telman, J. & Löwik, M.R.H. 2003, 'Socio-economic Status, Dietary Intake and 10 y Trends: The Dutch National Food Consumption Survey', *European Journal of Clinical Nutrition*, vol. 57, pp. 128–37.

James, W.P.T., Nelson, M., Ralph, A. & Leather, S. 1997, 'Socioeconomic Determinants of Health: The Contribution of Nutrition to Inequalities in Health', *British Medical Journal*, vol. 314, pp. 1545–9.

Inglis, V., Ball, K. & Crawford, D. 2005, 'Why do Women of Low Socioeconomic Status have Poorer Dietary Behaviours than Women of Higher Socioeconomic Status? A Qualitative Exploration', *Appetite*, vol. 45, pp. 334–43.

Lallukka, T., Laaksonen, M., Rahkonen, O., Roos, E. & Lahelma, E. 2007, 'Multiple Socio-economic Circumstances and Healthy Food Habits', *European Journal of Clinical Nutrition*, vol. 61, pp. 701–10.

Levenstein, H.A. 1988, Revolution at the Table: The Transformation of the American Diet, Oxford University Press, New York.

Macdonald, L., Cummins, S. & MacIntyre, S. 2007, 'Neighbourhood Fast Food Environment and Area Deprivation—Substitution or Concentration?', *Appetite*, vol. 49, pp. 251–4.

Mennell, S. 1996, *All Manners of Food: Eating and Taste in England and France from the Middle Ages to the Present*, Revised edition, University of Illinois Press, Chicago.

Murcott, A. 1999, 'Scarcity in Abundance: Food and Non-food', *Social Research*, vol. 66, no. 1, pp. 305–39.

National Health and Medical Research Council 1992, *Dietary Guidelines for Australians*, Australian Government Publishing Service, Canberra.

—— 2003, Dietary Guidelines for Australian Adults, AusInfo, Canberra.

Nelson, M. 1993, 'Social Class Trends in British Diet, 1860–1980', in C. Geissler & D. Oddy (eds), *Food, Diet and Economic Change Past and Present*, Leicester University Press, Leicester, pp. 101–20.

Nelson, M., Erens, B., Bates, B., Church, S. & Boshier, T. 2007a, *Low Income Diet and Nutrition Survey: Summary of Key Findings*, The Stationery Office, Norwich.

—— 2007b, *Low Income Diet and Nutrition Survey: Volume 2—Food Consumption and Nutrient Intake*, The Stationery Office, Norwich.

NHMRC—*see* National Health and Medical Research Council.

Pakulski, J. & Waters, M. 1996, *The Death of Class*, Sage, London.

Popkin, B.M., Siega-Riz, A.M. & Haines, P. 1996, 'A Comparison of Dietary Trends Among Racial and Socioeconomic Groups in the United States', *New England Journal of Medicine*, vol. 335, pp. 716–20.

Prattala, R., Berg, M.A. & Puska, P. 1992, 'Diminishing or Increasing Contrasts? Social Class Variation in Finnish Food Consumption Patterns', *European Journal of Clinical Nutrition*, vol. 46, pp. 279–87.

Riches, G. (ed.) 1997, *First World Hunger*, Macmillan, London.

—— 2003, 'Food Banks and Food Security: Welfare Reform, Human Rights and Social Policy. Lessons from Canada?', in E. Dowler & C.J. Finer (eds), *The Welfare of Food: Rights and Responsibilities in a Changing World*, Blackwell, Oxford, pp. 91–105.

Ritzer, G. 1993, *The McDonaldization of Society*, Pine Forge Press, Thousand Oaks, California.

Roos, E., Talala, K., Laaksonen, M., Helakorpi, S., Rahkonen, O., Uutela, A. & Prättälä, R. 2007, 'Trends of Socioeconomic Differences in Daily Vegetable Consumption, 1979–2002', *European Journal of Clinical Nutrition*, advance online publication, 23 May 2007.

Symons, M. 1982, *One Continuous Picnic: A History of Eating in Australia*, Duck Press, Adelaide.

Swartz, D. 1997, *Culture & Power: The Sociology of Pierre Bourdieu*, University of Chicago Press, Chicago.

Tomlinson, J. 1999, *Globalization and Culture*, Polity, Cambridge.

Tomlinson, M. & Warde, A. 1993, 'Social Class and Change in Eating Habits', *British Food Journal*, vol. 95, no. 1, pp. 3–10.

Turrell, G. 1996, 'Structural, Material and Economic Influences on the Food Purchasing Choices of Socioeconomic Groups', *Australian and New Zealand Journal of Public Health*, vol. 20, no. 6, pp. 611–17.

——, Blakely, T., Patterson, C. & Oldenburg, B. 2004, 'A Multilevel Analysis of Socio-economic (small area) Differences in Household Food Purchasing Behaviour', *Journal of Epidemiology and Community Health*, vol. 58, no. 3, pp. 208–15.

——, Hewitt, B., Patterson, C. & Oldenburg, B. 2003, 'Measuring Socio-economic Position in Dietary Research: Is Choice of Socio-economic Indicator Important?', *Public Health Nutrition*, vol. 6, no. 2, pp. 191–200.

—— & Kavanagh, A.M. 2006, 'Socio-economic Pathways to Diet: Modelling the Association between Socio-economic Position and Food Purchasing Behaviour', *Public Health Nutrition*, vol. 9, no. 3, pp. 375–83.

John Germov

Veblen, T. 1899/1975, *The Theory of the Leisure Class*, Allen & Unwin, London.

Warde, A. 1997, Consumption, Food and Taste: Culinary Antinomies and Commodity Culture, Sage, London.

Williams, S.J. 1995, 'Theorising Class, Health and Lifestyles: Can Bourdieu Help Us?', *Sociology of Health and Illness*, vol. 17, no. 5, pp. 577–604.

Wood B., Wattanapenpaiboon, N., Ross, K. & Kouris–Blazos, A. 2000a, 1995 National Nutrition Survey: Data for Persons 16 Years and Over Grouped by Socio-economic Disadvantaged Area. Executive Summary of the SEIFA Report, Healthy Eating Healthy Living Program, Monash University, Melbourne.

—— 2000b, 1995 National Nutrition Survey: Data for Persons 16 Years and Over Grouped by Socio-economic Disadvantaged Area. The SEIFA Report, Healthy Eating Healthy Living Program, Monash University, Melbourne.

Worsley, A., Blasche, R., Ball, K. & Crawford, D. 2003, 'Income Differences in Food Consumption in the 1995 Australian National Nutrition Survey', *European Journal of Clinical Nutrition*, vol. 57, pp. 1198–211.

CHAPTER 13

Humans, Food and Other Animals: The Vegetarian Option

Deidre Wicks

OVERVIEW

- Why are large numbers of people voluntarily removing meat from their diets?
- What are some of the processes that operate to separate 'meat' from the living animal from which it came?
- What concepts derived from sociology can enhance our understanding of vegetarianism?

This chapter reviews the recent sociological literature on vegetarianism. The focus is on the voluntary rejection of meat, which is explored in relation to theories of oppression and liberation, cultural denial, ecology, aesthetics and health. Vegetarianism is sociologically significant because it links the 'natural' (hunger, food and eating) with the 'social' (what we eat, how, when and why). It also links the 'personal' (choice, belief and preference) with institutions and wider social structures (the food industry and state policy). The chapter examines Elias's notion of the 'civilising process' and Giddens' concept of 'life politics' as useful ways for understanding vegetarianism in late modernity. It concludes by exploring the contradictory forces at work that are influencing the survival and possible growth of vegetarianism into the future.

Key terms

anti-vivisection	*haute cuisine*	socialism
biological determinism	globalisation	speciesism
civilising process	life politics	unproblematised
emancipatory politics	modernity	vegetarianism
epidemiology	pacifism	

Introduction

Eating is a highly personal act. At the same time, for most people, it is a social act. When we eat, how we eat and, more particularly, what we eat are, for those of us not experiencing genuine scarcity, decisions that are driven by complex motives. While these motives include the 'natural' or the biological—such as hunger—they also include social factors, such as taste, manners, expectations and obligations. In this way, the act of eating becomes imbued with social meaning. The connections between nature, culture, eating and the meaning of food become even more complex when we examine the choice to include certain foods, such as meat, in the diet, or to exclude them. For this very reason, such an examination ought to hold great interest for students of human behaviour and of social movements and social change.

For the purposes of this chapter, we can divide people who do not eat meat into two categories. First, there are those who are forced to exclude meat from their diet. These include people compelled to take this course of action for either economic or environmental reasons, or a combination of both. Second, there are those who voluntarily exclude meat. This group can itself be divided into people who exclude meat for religious reasons and those who do so for a variety of other reasons, such as philosophical and ethical, political or health motives. It is this second group with which we will be primarily concerned in this chapter, not because they are the most important but because they hold the most interest sociologically. These people are at the nexus of the natural and the social, the private and the public. In what follows, I will examine the key issues that underlie the decision of a growing number of people to voluntarily forgo a nourishing and pleasure-giving food. I will then attempt to interpret these decisions within a framework of recent sociological theory.

Vegetarianism and the social sciences

Despite the potential for rich social observation and analysis, there has been little research and writing on **vegetarianism** from the perspective of the social sciences, although, as we shall see, there have recently been some very useful exceptions. Why this long period of neglect within a discipline that is always on the 'look out' for new areas of social analysis? It can partly be explained by the social sciences' more general neglect of the whole area of food consumption (Murcott 1983). This in itself is interesting and relates to the more specific reasons for the neglect (or avoidance) of the subject of vegetarianism by social scientists. It is fair to say that sociologists are uncomfortable and suspicious of theoretically focusing on 'the natural' or 'the biological' for analysis of social issues, social patterns of behaviour or social change. There are good reasons for this. In a very real sense, sociology is constructed around opposition to the notion that the social can be reduced to our biological origins and destiny (**biological determinism**). Over several decades, sociologists have successfully challenged biologically determinist accounts and rationalisations of inequality in the areas of class, gender and ethnicity. Clearly these challenges have been confined neither to the pages of books nor to debates within universities, but have had profound effects on social attitudes and social policy worldwide.

Yet while behaviour and attitudes concerning discrimination based on class, gender and ethnicity are regarded as socially constructed and therefore socially amenable to change, the issue of what we eat—and therefore our relationship with other living creatures—has remained strangely **unproblematised** and therefore implicitly regarded as natural. When searching for reasons for this blind spot in social analysis, it is impossible to ignore the bedrock of Judaeo-Christian teachings, which conveniently mesh with a sociological view of humans as having distinct and unique characteristics that mark them out as superior to all other living creatures. In so doing, sociologists have reinforced the tendency to deny the *animal* in humans as well as the *social* in animals (Noske 1997). Social scientists have, on the whole, been content to leave the study of animals to the natural scientists and to criticise their subject–object approach only if it is applied to humans (Noske 1997, p. 78). Whatever the reasons for the past neglect, social scientists are now turning their attentions to the area of food in general and diet choice in particular for research and analysis.

Historical overview

While vegetarianism is a relatively modern phenomenon, it is informed and underpinned by a collection of rich and varied historical antecedents. Alan Beardsworth and Teresa Keil (1997) provide a useful account of the historical and cultural background of meat-rejection, as does Colin Spencer (1995). Suffice to say that one of the earliest coherent philosophies of meat rejection was put forward by the Greek philosopher and mathematician, Pythagoras (born approximately 580 BC). The Pythagorean doctrine was based on the belief of the transmigration of souls, which implied a kindred relationship and a common fate for all living creatures. The document also embodied what would now be called environmental or ecological concerns (Beardsworth & Keil 1997, p. 220). This theme, concerning the connection and relatedness of all creatures (including humans), has surfaced many times throughout the history of Western thought and has been a constant in many Eastern religions as well as the belief systems of many indigenous peoples. It is encapsulated in the words of Della Porta: 'When one part suffers, the rest also suffer with it' (as quoted in Merchant 1980, p. 104).

Another historical theme that has emerged at various times and places has been concerned with the connection between the rejection of meat and the health of individuals and societies. In Italy in 1558, in England in the seventeenth century, and in Germany, Britain and the United States of America in the nineteenth century, various theorists have posited the connection between vegetarianism and a long and healthy life (Spencer 1995, p. 274). In the 1830s in the USA, a Presbyterian preacher named Sylvester Graham (of Graham Cracker fame, makers of a wholemeal biscuit) preached that vegetarianism was the natural diet and that meat was probably not included in the food of the 'first family and the first generations of mankind' (as quoted in Fieldhouse 1995, p. 155). These theories were enhanced by the 'conversion' of prominent individuals, such as the co-founder of Methodism, John Wesley, and literary figures such as Percy Bysshe Shelley, Leo Tolstoy and George Bernard Shaw. Spencer (1995) makes the important point that, as well as the emphasis on health, the vegetarian movement has historically maintained long-standing links with movements such as ethical **socialism**, animal rights, **anti-vivisection** and **pacifism**. There were also many links with the anti-slavery movement (Phillips 2003). Links with other, kindred social movements are still apparent within modern vegetarianism.

What is a vegetarian?

Before studying the extent of modern vegetarianism and the reasons for its voluntary adoption, we must first be clear on what we mean by vegetarianism, which is a surprisingly 'broader church' than is commonly thought. Technically speaking, a vegetarian is a person who eats no flesh. There are further subcategories, such as lacto-vegetarians and ovo-vegetarians, who eat no flesh but who eat some of the products of animals—in this case milk and eggs respectively. A vegan, on the other hand, not only refuses flesh, but also abstains from eating (and sometimes wearing) all animal products. Vegans argue that animal products cannot be separated from animal mistreatment. They point, for instance, to the connection between eating eggs and the keeping of hens in 'battery' cages, and between drinking milk and the breeding and slaughter of 'veal' calves which are necessary to keep dairy cows in milk (Singer 1975, p. 179–80; Marcus 2001, p. 128–32). For this reason, many vegans also refuse to wear or use products based on animal material—for example, soap, wool and leather. They make the point that it would be incongruous to be entertained by a vegetarian on a leather lounge. Other variations are vegetarians who will eat free-range eggs but refuse milk, and others who will eat fish but refuse the flesh of other animals.

How many vegetarians are there?

Notwithstanding problems of definition, there have been several attempts to calculate the extent of vegetarianism across a number of countries. Overall, around one billion people are estimated to be either vegetarian or almost vegetarian (Gold 2004, p. 66). These figures would also include those who adopt a vegetarian diet for religious reasons. Beardsworth and Keil (1997) make the point that the data available for countries such as the United Kingdom and USA are sparse and fragmentary. On the basis of conflicting surveys, they estimate the proportion of self-defined vegetarians in the UK to be between 4 and 6 per cent and conclude that this proportion is steadily rising. Spencer (1995, p. 338) has calculated that the number of people who avoid red meat in the UK has increased from around 2.2 million in 1984 to 8.2 million in 1991, which is 16 per cent of the population. He notes that, 'Historically, of course, in the West, this is the greatest number of vegetarians ever to exist within a meat eating society who are not part of any one idealistic or religious group, who have abstained from meat for a variety of different reasons, though they broadly share the same view of society itself' (1995, p. 338).

According to *Time Magazine* (quoted in Pollan 2006, p. 313) the number of vegetarians in the USA can be calculated at 10 million. This does not necessarily mean that all these individuals refrain from eating exactly the same food. It does mean that a very large and ever-increasing number of people have adopted a vegetarian identity and make a conscious effort to remove animal products from their diet, or at least to restrict them. The Australian situation appears to be similar, as indicated by the *1995 National Nutrition Survey* (1997) (McLennan & Podger 1997). In this case, 14 000 respondents were asked to self-report on their type of diet. In the category 'Special Diet', respondents were given the options of: 'vegetarian', 'weight-reduction', 'diabetic', 'fat-modified' and 'other(s)'. The highest numbers of self-reported vegetarians occurred in the 19–24 years category, with males at 2.4 per cent and females at 6.2 per cent. More generally, there were 2.6 per cent of males and 4.9 per cent of females aged 19 years and over who classified themselves as vegetarian. It is, however, important to note that a further 10.3 per cent of males and 11.8 per cent of females over 19 years placed their diets in the non-specific 'other(s)' category of 'special diet'. As there were no categories for 'partly vegetarian' or 'vegan', it is reasonable to assume that some of these diets were included in the category of 'other(s)' and so the numbers for different types and degrees of vegetarian diets may well be under-reported (McLennan & Podger 1997). Certainly, the survey categories and the associated findings can be criticised for being wide and inexact. Yet these figures, like those for the UK and the USA, point to the fact that vegetarianism in the West is no longer the territory of a few 'cranks', but has become something approaching a mass movement, with millions of adherents worldwide.

Why become vegetarian?

There are many reasons for the voluntary abstinence from meat, and sociology has provided concepts and theories as well as in-depth studies that help us to more fully understand this phenomenon. These will be dealt with in the next section. The decision to stop eating meat is inevitably tied up with questions such as: Who am I? Why am I here? What is my place in relation to others on the planet? These are the important, difficult questions that organised religion and secular philosophy

Deidre Wicks

have attempted to answer since the beginning of human time. For those of us with a Judaeo-Christian heritage, they are tied up with interpretations from the Old Testament concerning the place of humans in relation to other species. The pivotal passage comes from Genesis, where we are told:

> And God blessed them, and God said unto them, Be fruitful, and multiply, and replenish the earth, and subdue it; and have dominion over the fish of the sea, and over the fowl of the air, and over every living thing that moveth upon the earth (Gen. 1:24–8).

The Jewish and Christian religions have, on the whole, chosen to interpret 'dominion' as the right to have power over, to control and to use all other species for the benefit of the human species. These religious traditions are so pervasive in the West that they constitute the bedrock of morality for the majority of people, including those who do not ostensibly adhere to organised religions. We are brought up to believe that eating meat is not wrong or, more commonly, that we are not even required to question whether it is right or wrong. This is not to say that individuals and sects of Jews and Christians have not questioned the morality of the killing and eating of animals, but they have usually been treated as outsiders at best and, at worst, as heretics (Singer 1975; Spencer 1995; Patterson 2002). These individuals and sects have often come to another interpretation of 'dominion', one that emphasises the responsibilities of care and nurture that inhere to humans in relation to other species on the planet. This interpretation has had a profound influence on the animal rights movement, as well as on the environmental and ecological movements more generally.

Sociological theories of power, oppression and liberation

There have also been attempts to develop philosophies of animal rights within secular traditions. Probably the best known is 'animal liberation', a philosophy and a social and political movement developed and championed by the Australian philosopher Peter Singer. Though a philosophy, the concept of animal liberation developed by Singer owes a debt to the liberation sociology of the 1960s when concepts such as racism and sexism were developed, analysed and applied to situations of race and gender oppression. These are concepts that permit an understanding of inequality that does not rely on the supposed inferior characteristics of a particular social group, but that focuses on the ability of the dominant group to accrue unequal benefits by using their power to define the 'other' as inferior and to institutionalise these attitudes in social institutions and practices. Fundamental to this process is an assumption that the interests of the dominant group are more important than the interests of the oppressed group. This understanding of the operation of power paved the way for theories and strategies of liberation for oppressed groups. Singer invokes the analogy of the oppression of women and people of colour and asks us to see attitudes to non-humans as a form of prejudice and an abuse of power no less objectionable as racism or sexism. The key point for Singer when determining the issue of 'rights' is not the degree of intelligence, wealth, beauty or status held by any living creature but rather the degree to which it is capable of suffering (Singer 2000, p. 35). Like the British philosopher, Jeremy Bentham, before him, Singer argues that the capacity of animals to experience suffering and pleasure implies that they have their own interests that ought not to be violated. When humans allow the interests of their own species to justify causing pain and suffering to another species the pattern is identical to that of racism and sexism: Singer calls this **speciesism**.

In his book *Animal Liberation* (1975), and more recently his co-authored book *The Ethics of What We Eat* (2006), Singer details the shocking litany of mistreatment inflicted on animals through animal experimentation and meat production and slaughter, particularly those associated with modern, intensive farming methods. *Animal Liberation* was one of the first public exposés of, for instance, the fact that chickens, 'battery hens', spend their entire lives in cages no larger than the area of an A4 page and that the lights in the battery sheds are left on over a 24-hour period so that their bodies are tricked into producing two eggs instead of one. More recent publications make it clear that little has changed in the egg industry except that the practice of packing hens into tiny cages has spread more extensively throughout the world. Animal behaviourists are now well aware that in these cramped conditions, birds are unable to spread their wings or fulfil any of their natural behaviours, such as nesting, dust-bathing, socialising and pecking the ground. These impoverished conditions can also lead to aggressive and frustrated behaviour such as feather picking and cannibalism. In order to prevent birds from pecking each other, the ends of beaks are routinely cut off. The cramped conditions also lead to health problems such as brittle and broken bones caused by lack of exercise and damage to feet such as when they grow around and into the wire floor of the cage (Gold 2004, p. 49).

In his most recent co-authored publication, Singer makes the point that chickens raised for meat or 'broilers' endure a different kind of misery (Singer & Mason 2006). The question, which provides the *raison d être* for, the industry is: 'What is the least amount of floor space necessary per bird to produce the greatest return on investment?' (quoted in Singer & Mason 2006, p. 21). An already crowded broiler shed is made worse by the fact that chickens have been selectively bred over decades so that they now achieve maximum growth in the shortest amount of time. It is routine for each broiler shed to contain up to 40 000 birds at densities of 18–19 per square metre. By the end of their short lives these birds are huge and their bone growth has been outpaced by the growth of their muscles and fat. Overcrowding is a problem and many lame birds are unable to reach food or water and so are crushed or die of hunger or thirst. Mortality rates (the number that die before they are six weeks old) level out at around 6 per cent, that is 48 million per annum in the UK alone (Gold 2004, p. 48).

Deidre Wicks

Birds who squat in the litter to relieve the pressure on their legs frequently contract burns on their hocks and breasts due to the high concentrations of ammonia present in their excrement-filled litter. These abnormal levels of ammonia also cause sore eyes, blindness and chronic respiratory disease. At the end of six weeks, the birds are caught, crammed into cages and then driven to the slaughterhouse, a journey that can take many hours. A typical killing line now moves at 90 birds a minute and speeds can be as high as 120 birds a minute (Singer & Mason 2006, p. 24). At such speeds some birds miss either the electrified water bath or having their throat cut and so go into the scalding tank fully conscious. In other words, they are boiled alive. Documents obtained under the US *Freedom of Information Act* (1966) indicate that this could be the fate of up to three million birds a year in the USA alone (Singer & Mason 2006, p. 24). This may be sobering reading for those who like to order chicken caesar salad for lunch at their favourite café. While on the subject of caesar salad, what about that lovely, crisp bacon sitting on the top?

Singer and Mason point to just some of the documented research that demonstrates, contrary to popular opinion that pigs are 'stupid', that in fact pigs are affectionate and inquisitive animals (2006, p. 41). They are easily trained and learn quickly to perform the kinds of tasks normally associated with dogs. Yet it would be regarded as cruel and unacceptable to keep a dog locked up for life in a cage that is too narrow to turn around in or to walk more than one or two steps back or forwards in. These are the conditions in which breeding sows live out their short lives. (Breeding sows are the pigs that give birth to piglets that are fattened for pork, ham and bacon.) They are kept indoors on concrete floors through repeated pregnancies either tethered or in 'sow stalls' where they are unable to lie down comfortably, turn around, take more than one step forwards or back or nuzzle their young when they are born. Sow stalls have now been banned in the UK and Sweden and are due for phasing out in the European Union (EU) from 2013. They are also banned in the state of Florida in the USA and, in addition, the two biggest commercial producers (Smithfield and Maple Leaf) in the USA and Canada have stated that the restrictive stalls are no longer needed. Yet, while the rest of the developed world has begun the process of ethically re-evaluating and phasing out this cruel practice, in 2007 Australia decided to extend the practice of confining breeding sows in these stalls for another 10 years. After this 10-year period, Australian pig farmers will have to reduce the maximum amount of time they keep sows in stalls from 16 weeks to six weeks. Under the new code, stall length will be increased by 20 centimetres and will remain 60 centimetres wide (Lee 2007).

After giving birth to the litter, piglets are taken away at three to four weeks. Such early weaning allows the sows to produce five litters in two years. At that point they are usually sent to slaughter for processed meat. The piglets (which are bred for rapid growth) are then fattened for around six months. While conditions vary, bare, cold, overcrowded concrete or slatted pens are the norm. These frustrate instinctive digging behaviour and cause lameness. Overcrowded conditions lead to fighting and tail biting so that teeth clipping and tail docking are carried out routinely, without anaesthetic. The same transport and slaughter problems described in relation to chickens also apply to pigs. Globally, 1.2 billion pigs are slaughtered for meat every year (Gold 2004, p. 50).

It was the uncovering of conditions such as these that led Singer to describe such treatment as speciesism. It can be argued that no creature would willingly subject itself to such treatment; therefore, the relationship must be seen as one which involves oppression and exploitation. This led Singer to the conclusion that for reasons of intellectual and theoretical consistency alone (not to mention compassion) we must become vegetarian. However, as Matt Cartmill points out in his wonderful book (1993, p. 224), most humans prize consistency less highly than sausage.

Gender and ethnicity

Another contribution that helps us understand vegetarianism through socio-logical concepts is Carol Adams' *The Sexual Politics of Meat* (2002), which makes the connection between the objectification and oppression of women and the treatment of animals. At the beginning of her book, Adams refers to the work of noted anthropologist Mary Douglas, who suggests in her essay 'Deciphering a Meal' that the order in which we serve foods, and the foods that we insist be present at a meal, reflects and reinforces our larger culture (Adams 2002, p. 47). Adams makes the point that to remove meat is to threaten the structure of the larger patriarchal culture. She goes on to give numerous examples of the way that meat is seen as a symbol of masculinity and that the refusal of women to serve meat is frequently perceived as a hostile act and one that can lead to domestic violence.

Adams develops her argument through the aid of a concept she terms the 'absent referent' (2002, p. 53). Adams explains that through the act of butchering, animals become absent referents by the fact that in name and body they are made absent as animals so that meat can exist. It is not possible to eat meat without the death of an animal. Live animals are therefore the absent referents in the concept of meat. As well as their literal absence as live animals they are also absent in language. When people eat animals they change the way they talk about them. For instance, they do not use the term baby animal but rather, lamb or veal (2002, p. 51). After they have been butchered new names are used to disguise the fact that these were once animals. Cows become beef, steak and mince; pigs become rashers, bacon, ham, lardoons; lamb becomes cutlets, chops, crown roast. Adams develops a unified theory that incorporates sexual violence against women and the butchering of animals through an analysis of the social and political processes of objectification, fragmentation and consumption (2002, p. 58). She ends by providing the building blocks for a feminist-vegetarian critical theory (2002, p. 178).

Deidre Wicks

A more recent contribution to our quest for a sociological understanding of vegetarianism that also lies within the tradition of power/oppression/liberation is the work of Charles Patterson (2002), whose project is to understand and elucidate the connection between racism and the treatment of non-human animals. Patterson makes the key point that the construction of a great divide between humans and animals provided a standard by which to judge other people: 'If the essence of humanity was defined as consisting of a specific quality or set of qualities, such as reason, intelligible language, religion, culture, or manners, it followed that anyone who did not fully possess those qualities was "subhuman"' (2002, p. 25). This then opened up the possibility of those judged as less than human being turned into slaves, beasts of burden, internees in 'hospitals', prisons, vermin to be eradicated, specimens to be experimented on, or food to be eaten.

Patterson then goes on to describe in disturbing detail the way that the practice of vilifying people by designating them as animals serves as a prelude to their persecution, exploitation and murder (2002, pp. 27–50). Equally disturbing though illuminating is his exposition on the origins of the technology of institutionalised violence against animals and the mass slaughter of Jews in concentration camps. He traces a direct line between the design of assembly-line killing at the Chicago slaughterhouse to Henry Ford's application of the same principles in the industrial manufacture of automobiles and to Nazi Germany's assembly-line mass murder of Jews at the death camps (2002, p. 71). Ford himself acknowledged that the inspiration for assembly-line production came from a visit to a Chicago slaughterhouse as a young man (Ford, quoted in Patterson 2002, p. 72). While Patterson provides the most comprehensive and detailed analysis of the interconnections between animal and human mistreatment, he is not the only one to do so. Indeed, he quotes Theodor Adorno, one of the founders of modern critical sociology, who noted: 'Auschwitz begins wherever someone looks at a slaughterhouse and thinks: they're only animals' (quoted in Patterson 2002, p. 51).

Understandably, there has been debate and disagreement about this analogy and it appears that Peter Singer himself takes some issue with it (see Coetzee 2001; Gaita 2002; and Singer in Coetzee 2001, p. 86). Singer, however, makes the point that a comparison (between the Nazi death camps and industrial animal slaughter) is not necessarily an equation. He argues that the people who have made the connection (such as novelists Isaac Bashevis Singer and J.M. Coetzee) are making at least two points. The first is that while both crimes are not equally evil, both are based on the principle that might is right, and the strong can do what they please with those who are in their power. The second point concerns the way that so many people prefer not to think too much about what is being done to those outside the sphere of the favoured group, how 'we avoid things that might disturb us and look the other way while evil is being done' (Singer in Coetzee 2001, p. 86). I will examine this in more detail in the section below.

'Sociology of denial'

Through their analyses of the interconnectedness of abuses of power through speciesism, sexism and racism, sociologists have provided us with ways to understand why individuals have made conscious decisions to become vegetarian. The question is: given the evidence presented above, why are there so few vegetarians? Here also, sociology provides us with tools to assist our understanding. In addition to general concepts such as discourse and ideology, which could be used to elucidate the process of silencing knowledge and language about the suffering of animals involved in their killing for food, we have a recent development in the *sociology of denial* which looks specifically at the process used by individuals and groups to 'not see' the pain and terror experienced by others (Cohen 2001).

While written with a sole focus on human atrocities and suffering, the concepts presented in Cohen's book are equally applicable to the way we deny and ignore the daily realities of animal suffering when live animals are turned into meat. Cohen defines denial as 'the maintenance of social worlds in which an undesirable situation (event, condition, phenomenon) is unrecognised, ignored or made to seem normal' (2001, p. 51). He looks first at different types or levels of denial that he names as: personal, official and cultural. Cultural denial, which is of most interest to us in this context, is neither wholly private nor officially organised by the state. According to Cohen, whole societies may slip into collective denial without either public sanctions or overt methods of control. Without being told what to think, societies arrive at unwritten agreements about what can be known, remembered and said (2001, p. 11). Denial and 'normalisation' reflect both personal and collective states where suffering is not acknowledged. Normalisation happens through: routinisation, tolerance, accommodation, collusion and cover up. Cohen uses the example of domestic violence against women to illustrate the social process of cultural denial and the journey towards acknowledgment through political and social action (2001, p. 51). He points out that in the denial phase domestic violence was hidden, normalised, contained and covered up. It was designated as private and therefore nobody else's business. It relied on people turning a blind eye to women's bruises, with a shared vocabulary of such stock in trade expressions as 'she deserved it' and 'he loses his temper a bit sometimes'. Indeed, Cohen makes the point that cultural denial must draw on shared cultural vocabularies if it is to be credible. These shared vocabularies represent a commitment between people (couples, families or entire populations) to support and collude in each other's denials (2001, p. 64).

Without conscious negotiation, people know which facts are better not noticed and what trouble spots to avoid. For instance, people do not consciously repress references to slaughterhouses when they are guests at a barbecue or dinner party where meat is being served. There is, however, an unspoken, indeed unconscious agreement that such references would be bad manners or bad taste. This is why the mere presence of a vegetarian at a dinner table can make people uncomfortable. Their presence raises into consciousness all those ideas and images so carefully 'not known' and 'not seen'. The discomfort felt by others at the table can lead to either aggression or self-justification directed to the vegetarian. However, *this* is not seen as a breach of good taste or good manners, because the vegetarian is the outsider, the threat to social cohesion. The existence of a self-declared vegetarian at the table punctures the carefully constructed edifice of personal and cultural denial concerning the suffering of animals, which is necessary to produce the meat being eaten.

The edifice of cultural denial surrounding meat eating, while still pervasive, is less secure and monolithic than it once was due to the efforts of animal rights activists, who have increased awareness and changed the behaviour of enough individuals to make vegetarianism a social movement. The work of animal rights activists has exposed forms of cruelty that have either been hidden from view or 'normalised', promoting an alternative discourse that eventually leads to new laws based on revised concepts of what is normal and acceptable.

Environmental sociology

Meat production is an inefficient and energy-intensive process, especially when intensive farming methods are involved. Grain, which could be used to feed people, is instead fed to cattle, pigs and fowl, and in the process of converting grain to meat, a large amount of food energy is wasted. There are two dimensions to the environmental consequences of this process. These entail the effects on both human and non-human life forms. In terms of human consequences, it is clear that the high meat consumption within affluent countries has an adverse impact on people in developing countries. This is illustrated by the fact that the EU is the largest buyer of animal feed in the world, and 60 per cent of this imported grain comes from developing countries. These countries grow the cereals as cash crops (for desperately needed foreign exchange) when they could instead grow crops for food to halt malnutrition among their own people (Spencer 1995, p. 341).

Jonathon Porritt has argued that when we read that the global meat demand is expected to grow from 209 million tons in 1997 to around 327 million tons in 2020, we must consider all the extra hectares of land required, all the extra water to be consumed, the extra energy to be burned and the extra chemicals needed simply to grow the requisite amount of grain and grass in order to produce that 327 million tons of meat (Porritt, Foreword in Gold 2004, p. 5). It is surely only a matter of time until there are firm calculations as to the contribution of industrial meat production to global warming and it is interesting, sociologically, to note that thus far there has been complete silence on this most obvious contributing factor to the warming of the planet.

Jeremy Rifkin (1993) describes beef as an inefficient food. It requires 5455 litres of water to produce one 250-gram boneless steak in California. In US feedlots (where cattle are kept in small holding areas for their entire lives and fed solely on grain and processed food), this intensive feeding results in a 10-fold loss of energy. In fact, it takes 8–10 kilograms of grain to produce 1 kilogram of meat. Rifkin claims that cattle production is destroying Central American rainforests and North American rangelands, and is polluting lakes and waterways. The problem of waste is even more dramatic in countries with small acreage and highly developed farming, such as the Netherlands. Dutch farms produce 94 million tonnes of manure every year, the problem being that their soil can only absorb 50 million tonnes (Spencer 1995, p. 331). Even a country with a vast landmass such as Australia experiences serious problems with animal waste run-off, with riverways and bore water sites badly polluted. The rise in pollution is attributed to run-off and leakages from piggeries, animal feedlots, dairies and septic and sewerage systems (see Lawrence et al. 1992).

The relationship between meat production and environmental degradation can be seen with pristine clarity when we focus on hamburger production. Hamburger chains such as McDonald's make billions of dollars worldwide each year through manipulative and aggressive marketing. This marketing successfully presents their hamburgers as an integral and fun-filled part of today's busy lifestyles. The reality is that the production and consumption of these hamburgers is having a catastrophic effect on the surviving rainforests of the planet. It has been calculated that, after rainforest clearing for cattle grazing, the cost of a hamburger produced in the first year is approximately half a tonne of mature forest, since such forest naturally supports about 800 000 kilograms of plants and animals per hectare. This same area under pasture will yield around 1600 hamburgers. This means that the real price of a hamburger is around 9 square metres of rich, highly diversified and irreplaceable rainforest (Spencer 1995, p. 331).

Pollution due to meat production is not limited to land-based animals. Increased consumption of fish, combined with overfishing, has encouraged the intensive farming of many varieties of fish, including Atlantic salmon, rainbow trout and Atlantic cod (Purvis 2003). The environmental problems caused by fish farms are now very serious. For instance, the fish imprisoned in fish cages are an easy target for sea lice that bore through the skin and feast on their flesh. When the fish dies, the lice that have multiplied 10-fold move on and attack other fish, including exhausted wild salmon returning from their spawning ground. Norway's Institute of Marine Research (2005) has calculated that 86 per cent of young wild salmon are eaten alive or fatally infected with viral anaemia by sea lice. The situation is similar in Scotland and Ireland where lice have gone close to wiping out the wild sea trout. Another hazard concerns salmon escaped from the cages. Not only do escapees compete for spawning sites, but they also debase the wild species by interbreeding. Because farmed fish do not originate from a home river, they have no instinct to return to one in order to breed. Instead, they swim aimlessly about in fjords, sea lochs and estuaries. Norwegian scientists have calculated that the degree of genetic distinction between farmed and wild fish is being halved every 3.3 generations. The inevitable consequence is that the wild population will eventually be composed entirely of descendents from farmed fish (*Sunday Times*, September 30, 2001).

Health sociology

Epidemiological surveys in public health allow for the analysis of disease patterns and the risk factors associated with the development and distribution of specific diseases. The information gathered from these large-scale studies is then disseminated, first, to other researchers and academics, and then to the general public through the mass media. This constant flow of information regarding health risks has made many people highly conscious of the links between eating behaviour and potential illness, resulting in many people changing their diets to minimise the risk of various chronic and acute diseases. In a UK Gallop survey, adults gave the main reason for becoming vegetarian as health (76 per cent), although other reasons such as animal welfare followed closely (cited in Spencer 1995, p. 338). Fears about food revolve around issues concerning contamination from additives (chemicals, antibiotics and hormones) as well as those concerned with bacterial contamination. There is evidence to indicate that both of these motivations are valid.

In terms of the positive motivation to improve health, there are at least two major studies worth noting. The 'China Study' began in 1983 and its results were published in 1990. It involved a survey of 6500 Chinese who contributed 367 facts about their diet. In general terms, the study found that the fewer animal products eaten, the lower the incidence of disease and death (Berriman 1996, p. 54). More specifically, the study found that in those regions of China where meat consumption has begun to increase, it has been closely followed by an increase in the 'diseases of affluence', such as cardiovascular disease (up to 50 times the rate for a more traditional Chinese diet), cancer and diabetes (Spencer 1995, p. 339). The larger 'Oxford Study' echoed these findings. In this study of 11 000 people, half were maintained on their traditional meat-based diet, while the other half consumed either vegetarian or near vegetarian diets. It was found that the latter group had nearly 40 per cent less cancer, 30 per cent less heart disease and were 20 per cent less likely to die up to the age of 80 years. These figures were adjusted for factors such as smoking and alcohol consumption (Berriman 1996, p. 54). This study was followed in the mid 1990s by a comprehensive study from the World Cancer Research Fund (WCRF) and the American Institute for Cancer Research, which appointed a panel of leading international experts to collate all existing research. The study concluded that 'diets containing substantial amounts of red meat probably increase the risk of colorectal cancer' as well as 'possibly increasing the risk of pancreatic, breast, prostate and renal cancers' (quoted in Gold 2004, p. 17). Summarising the comprehensive study, the Director of Science at the

WCRF advised that to protect from cancer we should 'choose predominantly plant-based diets rich in a variety of vegetables and fruits, pulses (legumes) and minimally processed starchy staple foods' (quoted in Gold 2004, p. 17).

More recent reports have, however, used a more cautious tone. In the 2002 WHO/FAO draft paper that summarised the most recent evidence from around the world, the authors emphasised the difficulties involved with isolating diet from other lifestyle factors and argued that the connection between diet and cancer may be lower than the 30 per cent previously suggested. They do, nevertheless, uphold the view that there is a 'probable' increased risk of colorectal cancer associated with red meat and preserved meats (quoted in Gold 2004, p. 17). Two recent studies have published results that link the consumption of red meat with breast cancer in women. The first, a study of more than 90 600 pre-menopausal nurses over eight years, was published in the *Archives of Internal Medicine* (Cho et al. 2006). The study found that women who eat red meat more than once a day double their risk of getting the most common form of breast cancer. This risk for hormone sensitive cancers was further pronounced if the meat eaten was of the processed kind, such as hamburgers, salami and sausages. A study published in the *British Journal of Cancer* (Taylor et al. 2007) found that eating even small amounts of red meat can increase a woman's risk of breast cancer. The researchers found that post-menopausal women who ate more than 103g of processed meat a day could be 64 per cent more likely to suffer the disease, while as little as 57g of beef, pork or lamb a day showed an effect. These are dramatic findings and it is certainly worthy of note that they attracted little publicity when first announced and, for sociologists, must beg questions concerning the operation of power and the ability of vested interest groups in keeping threatening and de-stabilising research and opinions off the political agenda (see Lukes 1974, pp. 21–6).

Food safety

Public fears over contamination of meat have grown as more information concerning practices associated with intense 'factory farming' have filtered into public awareness. The problem of overuse of drugs on farms is now a global problem. In particular, antibiotics are given to animals both to combat infections but also as growth promoters, which is a side effect of their intended use (Gold 2004). Together with foreign travel, increased use of antibiotics in farm animals has been cited as a major cause of antibiotic resistant infections in humans (Gold 2004, p. 45). In the USA, almost half of the 23 000 tonnes of antibiotics sold are fed to animals. In the UK, 30 per cent of 1200 tonnes of antibiotics go to animals. In 1997, the WHO called for a worldwide ban on the routine use of antibiotics as growth promoters in livestock, but no ban has taken place. In the UK, which claims to have among the strictest laws in the world, it was revealed in 1996 that 62 different antibiotics were licensed for use in feed and water for dairy cows and other lactating animals (Gold 2004, p. 45).

Another area of concern in relation to drug use in farm animals concerns the use of growth-promoting hormones. While these have been banned by the EU since 1988, in the USA cattle are still routinely implanted with sex hormones in order to promote rapid weight gain. The USA is making every attempt to overturn this European ban including taking a legal case under the World Trade Organization's (WTO) GATT agreement. The WTO ruled in favour of the USA and ordered that the EU should pay US$150 million per annum compensation for the US loss of profit. These challenges are ongoing and demonstrate how current free trade rules make it difficult to restrict imports on grounds of health, compassion or sustainability (Gold 2004, p. 46). Despite US protestations concerning the safety of growth hormones, reports to the contrary continue to surface. One of the most recent was an article in the journal *Human Reproduction* (Swan et al. 2007), which reported on a study of 387 partners of pregnant women in five US cities. It found that sons born to women in North America who ate a lot of beef during their pregnancy had a sperm count 25 per cent below normal and three times the normal risk of fertility problems. In the editorial accompanying the article, it was stated that these same hormones could also alter the incidence of polycystic ovarian syndrome, the age of puberty onset and postnatal growth rate. Six growth-promoting hormones are used in cattle fattening in the USA and Canada. Not all of these hormones have been metabolised by the time of slaughter. A spokesperson for Meat and Livestock Australia stated that the use of hormones was widespread in some sections of the Australian beef industry, but claimed that the products were 'totally safe' for human consumption (*Sydney Morning Herald*, 29 March 2007).

Health sociologists have long pointed to the way industrialised methods of food production are placing a heavy burden on both the public health and the public purse. It has been estimated that 10 000 Britons suffer from food poisoning each week, while 100 people die from it each year. More than 95 per cent of these cases originate in animal or poultry products (Spencer 1995, p. 335). In the UK, it is estimated that 10 per cent of the population, around 6 million people, have a case of food poisoning each year (BBC News 2006). The British Medical Association issued a public warning to treat all raw meat as infected, a claim dismissed by the Meat and Livestock Commission as 'scare mongering' (*Guardian Weekly*, 18 January 1998). In Australia, outbreaks of food poisoning occur regularly, the most recent being in March 2007 when 10 people were hospitalised and another 30 treated for gastroenteritis after eating chicken and pork buns from a hot bread shop in Homebush in Sydney (*Sydney Morning Herald*, 28 March 2007).

Everyday in the USA, approximately 200 000 people are made sick by a food-borne disease, 900 are hospitalised and 14 die (Schlosser 2001, p. 195). According to the US Centers for Disease Control and Prevention (CDC), more than a quarter of the US population suffers from a bout of food poisoning each year (Schlosser 2001). Over the past decade, scientists have discovered more than a dozen new food-borne pathogens; however, the CDC estimates that more than three-quarters of food-related illnesses and deaths in the USA are caused by pathogens not yet identified. Eric Schlosser argues that it is the rise of huge feedlots, slaughterhouses and hamburger grinders that have provided the means for pathogens to become widely distributed into the nation's food supply. He contends that the meat-packing system that arose to supply the fast-food chains—a system moulded to provide massive amounts of uniform ground beef—has proved to be an extremely efficient system for spreading disease. Schlosser makes the further point that the enormous power of the giant meat-packing firms, sustained by their close ties and large donations to the Republican Party, has allowed them to successfully oppose any further regulation of their food safety practices (2001, p. 196). It is most likely that meat becomes tainted through contact with an infected animal's stomach contents or faeces during slaughter or processing. A national study published in 1996 found that '7.5 per cent of the ground beef samples taken at processing plants were contaminated with *Salmonella*, 11.7 per cent were contaminated with *Listeria monocytogenes*, 30 per cent with *Staph. Aureus* and 53.3 per cent with *Clostridium perfringens*' (Schlosser 2001, p. 197). All of these pathogens cause illness and can be fatal in some cases.

The major food scare and scandal of the last decade has concerned bovine spongiform encephalopathy (BSE) or 'mad cow' disease. This disease causes the development of holes in the cow's brain and is exactly the same symptom that affects sheep suffering from the disease called scrapie. Most experts now concede that it was the feeding of feed-lot cows with the scrapie-infected sheep meat plus the feeding of calves with contaminated milk substitutes and pellet meal that caused the disease to occur in cattle (Berriman 1996, p. 47). It is now known that this disease can manifest itself in humans who have consumed infected meat as the brain-destroying Creutzfeld-Jakob Disease (CJD). While the numbers of human fatalities have been relatively small (129 deaths to date), it is not possible, due to the very long incubation period of up to 20 years, to say that the number of human fatalities has peaked. Millions of cattle have been destroyed in the UK, Republic of Ireland and elsewhere in Europe, yet it is clear that the disease is still present in some stock. In Ireland, despite banning the feeding of cattle with meat and bone meal since 1989, there was a peak of 333 BSE cases in 2002, but these had steadily declined to 41 cases by 2006 (Department of Agriculture, Fisheries & Food 2007).

In Britain, 180 000 BSE cases were recorded up to January 2003 (*Financial Times*, 31 January 2003), and there are also fears that more people than expected may have contracted the human form of BSE. These fears have been raised by the discovery of the infectious agent in a random screening program of tonsils and appendixes that were removed in routine surgery between 1995 and 1999. If this were to hold true for the whole of the population it would indicate an infection rate of approximately 6000 people (*Financial Times*, 20 September 2002). Meanwhile, the WHO has warned that countries outside the EU, especially in Central and Eastern Europe and South-

Deidre Wicks

east Asia were not doing enough to prevent another epidemic of BSE. While most of the 2790 non-UK BSE cases have been in Western Europe, BSE has been reported in Japan and Israel (see WHO 2007). In France, where four people have died from CJD and where imports of British beef were banned between 1996 and 2006, the French population was alarmed to discover that not only had the food chain Buffalo Grill been illegally importing British beef, but that two of the French BSE fatalities had dined there regularly over many years.

As the facts emerged, ordinary people in many countries were disgusted to learn that recycled waste from intensive farming—the excreta, feathers, soiled straw and remains of dead birds and animals—was being pasteurised and processed into pellets and fed to domestic and farm animals, including the naturally herbivorous cow (Spencer 1995, p. 335). While the BSE scare has been focused on the UK, it is important to note that until recently many intensively reared animals in Australia were fed a diet that included between 4–10 per cent animal protein, most commonly a rendering of bone, fat and blood. Not unrelated to this practice was the outbreak of botulism, which occurred in two cattle feed-lots in Queensland in 1990 after chicken litter, including carcasses, were used in the feed—a practice now banned (Berriman 1996, p. 47). In the USA, about 75 per cent of cattle were routinely fed the rendered remains of dead sheep and cattle until August 1997. They were also fed millions of dead cats and dogs every year, purchased from animal shelters, a practice no longer allowed. Current regulations, however, permit dead pigs, horses and poultry to be rendered into cattle feed. The regulations also allow dead cattle to be fed to poultry (Schlosser 2001, p. 202). The image of an endless recycling of infected animal matter, which is able to infect humans, is a powerful reminder of the 'danger' of meat eating in the late modern era. According to Spencer (1995, p. 336), there can be little doubt that the image of, and increasing knowledge about, the realities of factory farming has increased the number of vegetarians.

'The civilising process'

Norbert Elias's opus, *The Civilizing Process*, holds two particular points of interest in the context of vegetarianism. The first is his theoretical exposition of historical change, which is based on linking the long-term structural development of societies with changes in people's behaviour. The second is connected to the first in that Elias attempts to understand the process of historical change, primarily in Western Europe, through a detailed, historical analysis of changes in personal habits to do with such 'natural' functions as eating, washing, spitting, urinating and defecating (Elias 2000, first published in English in 1978). While these might appear trivial behaviours on which to focus, it is precisely the unavoidable necessity of the tasks that makes any changes in the way they are performed visible as social changes. It is Elias's detailed study of changing daily habits in the preparation and consumption of food that is of immediate interest for our sociological understanding of vegetarianism. Elias points out that delicacy and a heightened sense of beauty and ugliness may prompt the refusal of meat.

Through the lens provided by Elias, it is possible to see vegetarianism as a logical development in the **civilising process**, which entails a strong and conscious effort to remove the distasteful from the sight of society. This process has resulted in activities such as urination, vomiting and defecation being removed from the public sphere and located in the private sphere. In relation to meat-eating, it has entailed the removal of the obvious signs of the living and dead animal from public view (2000, p. 102). Where once a whole carcass would be carved at table, it is now likely to be hidden from view, with the diner being presented with a dainty portion of meat often surrounded and hidden by vegetables and salad. In the same way, from the 1960s onwards, butchers carved the animal carcass at the back of the shop and began to remove pigs' and calves' heads from the window. There was a discernible move towards buying meat cut, sealed and packaged and a shift towards buying it in a supermarket rather than from the more confronting (and more honest) butcher's shop (Spencer 1995, p. 327).

By following Elias' theory it is possible to see that the rejection of meat altogether is the next logical step on this civilising curve. Those who are repulsed by the sight and taste of meat have a 'threshold of repugnance' that is in advance of current civilised standards in general. He argues that while their contemporaries may consider vegetarians abnormal, they are in fact at the vanguard of a larger social movement of the type that has produced social change in the past (Elias 2000, p. 102). These sentiments are echoed in the statement of an interviewee in Willetts' study, a teacher who commented on the large number of his students who were vegetarian: 'I have a prediction that in about a hundred years eating meat will be seen as something you don't mention, something obscene. It might not be outlawed, but you'd have to go to special restaurants to eat it' (as quoted in Willetts 1997, p. 125). Then again, George Bernard Shaw said something similar over one hundred years ago when he made the statement: 'A hundred years hence a cultivated man [sic] will no more dream of eating flesh or smoking than he now does of living, as Pepys' contemporaries did, in a house with a cesspool under it' (as quoted in Smith 1997). Clearly the civilising process is not linear in its progression and occurs through reaction to action in a complex and uneven way.

Just before Christmas 2000, the top three-star Michelin chef, Alan Passard, announced he was going to serve only vegetarian food at his famous Paris restaurant, L'Arpege. At the time Passard said: 'I can no longer stand the idea that we humans have turned herbivore ruminants into carnivores. Personally, it is many years since I have eaten meat'. Later in the same interview he added: 'I can't get excited about a

Deidre Wicks

lump of barbecue meat. Vegetables are so much more colourful, more perfumed. You can play with the harmony of colours, everything is luminous. And it has been some time since I have been able to find any culinary inspiration in animal products. I want to become the first three-star chef to use only vegetables, a driving force in the field of vegetable and flower cuisine' (quoted in Jeffries 2001). There appears to be growing support for **haute cuisine** vegetarian restaurants worldwide. Joia, run by chef Pietro Leemann in Milan, is another. This restaurant has also produced a glossy cookbook of the same name in which Leemann states: 'Death in cuisine is associated above all with the animal world. In spite of the fact that death accompanies us throughout our life… [m]y cuisine is a hymn to life and to nature' (Leemann 2000).

While these are trends at the top end of the market, it does seem that more people in Western, developed countries are eating less meat and more meatless dishes. Among these 'voluntary abstainers', the class composition of vegetarianism appears to also be changing. Research undertaken in 1988 and 1990 showed that the converts were from the lower middle classes and lower-income groups. No longer just a movement of middle-class radicals, converts are growing across the class structure, with the numbers of converts thinnest among the top-income groups (Spencer 1995, p. 337). At the same time, the gender balance remains strongly in favour of women. In the UK, the 1995 Realeat Survey indicated that women were showing twice the rate of vegetarianism as men (cited in Beardsworth & Keil 1997, p. 224). Australian data, as noted earlier, also show clear gender differences. More recently, a UK poll of more than 1000 people showed that one in three people bought meat-substitute meals during the period while half of those asked said that they would consider a meat-substitute at a barbecue this summer (*Financial Times*, 24 May 2003).

Life politics and emancipatory politics

Do these trends indicate a real and long-lasting shift in eating behaviour? There are times in history when whole groups en masse begin to embrace an attitude and forms of behaviour that are significantly different from what has been considered the social norm. One social theorist who is interested in this phenomenon and who has clearly been influenced by Norbert Elias is Anthony Giddens, whose recent work has explored changes in the ways that people think and act in their daily lives within the period that he calls 'high' or 'late modernism' (the late twentieth and early twenty-first centuries). This work also has some useful insights and concepts for understanding the emergence of vegetarianism in the late modern age (Giddens 1991). In particular, Giddens is interested in the emergence of what he calls **life politics**, which is a politics of lifestyle in the sense that it involves a politics of life decisions or life choices (1991, p. 215). The decisions that are involved in life politics concern those questions that philosophical thought has always been concerned with: Who am I?

What am I here for? How should I live? In the deepest sense, the decisions involved in life politics affect self-identity itself (1991, p. 215). Giddens, however, sees this as a reflexive process, one in which self-identity is constructed out of the debates and contestations that derive from the dynamic between the ongoing formation of identity and the changing context of external life circumstances.

Before making connections between life politics and the growth of vegetarianism, it is important to grasp another concept that is related to the idea of life politics. Giddens argues that in order for people to be in a position to make life choices, they must have attained a certain level of autonomy of action (1991, p. 214). People are only able to make choices when they are in a material and political position to make them. Giddens goes on to argue that the ability to make such choices is unique to the period of high **modernity** and it is built on the political orientations and achievements of the modern period—orientations in which **emancipatory politics** were of central concern. Giddens defines emancipatory politics as 'a generic outlook concerned above all with liberating individuals and groups from constraints which adversely affect their life chances' (1991, p. 210). He goes on to say that emancipatory politics is concerned to reduce or eliminate exploitation, inequality and oppression. In all cases, the objective is either to 'release under-privileged groups from their unhappy condition, or to eliminate the relative differences between them' (1991, p. 211). The aim of liberating people from exploitation is predicated on the adoption of moral values, and indeed these values are often expressed within a framework of justice ('social justice', for example). It is possible, then, according to Giddens, to see emancipatory politics as a politics concerned with the conditions that liberate us in order to make choices. So, while emancipatory politics is a politics of life chances, life politics is a politics of choice (1991, p. 214).

It is possible to see the adoption of a vegetarian diet as a choice that is part of the life politics of late modernity. It is also possible to regard it as a choice that involves the application and extension of the emancipatory politics of the modern period beyond the human species. In the modern period, the concepts of oppression and emancipation extended to apply to all humans, regardless of race or gender. It may be that the conditions of late modernity are conducive to the extension of the concept of emancipation to the animal world. This, of course, is precisely what philosophers such as Singer (1975) have been attempting to achieve. What Giddens shows is that this attempt can be seen in a social and political context as part of a great social movement—in fact, a 'remoralising' of social life. This gives us a sociological framework for understanding the growing awareness of animal rights and the voluntary adoption, by growing numbers of people, of a meatless diet for reasons connected with animal welfare. If Giddens is correct when he states that 'the concerns of life politics presage future changes of a far-reaching sort: essentially, the development of forms of social order "on the other side" of modernity itself', then it may well be that the growing numbers of voluntary vegetarians are indicative of a real change in social attitudes and behaviour towards animals (Giddens 1991, p. 214).

Conclusion: The future of vegetarianism

While Giddens provides us with a theoretical framework for understanding the emergence of life politics—which, I suggest, includes for many the choice to abstain from meat—it by no means enables us to predict the future of vegetarianism as a social movement in Western developed countries. While the data are too fragmentary to generate any predictive certainty (Beardsworth & Keil 1997, p. 240), there are, as we have seen, indications that voluntary vegetarianism is on the increase. It is also true to say, however, that late modernity produces contradictory pressures on individuals and groups. On the one hand, late modernity has produced a level of personal autonomy for many in the developed world, particularly the educated middle class. Yet, on the other hand, for many of these same people, late modernity has also provided more rushed and busy lives with little time for the promised leisure and pleasure. In this environment, life choices may become pragmatic, based more on expediency and survival than on principle. It may be that a remoralising of social life and a heightened sensitivity to personal and political issues results in an 'I should but ...' attitude, with associated guilt and neurosis becoming a defining feature of the construction of the self in late modernity.

At a less individual and personal level, social, economic and environmental pressures regarding meat consumption are also contradictory. On the one hand, there are the increasing numbers of people in Western societies who, for health or ethical reasons, are eating less meat. On the other hand, the trend for meat production from industrialised systems, which grew more than six times as fast as from grazing systems in the period 1983–93, continues to accelerate. The developed world's model of food production—rapid growth in meat consumption fuelled by grain and soya fed animals—is already being imitated in the developing world (Garces 2002). Demand for grain to feed livestock in developing nations is projected to double in the period 1993–2020. Taking one example among many, China's consumption of meat products rose by 85 per cent between 1995 and 2001 and is forecast to be responsible for 40 per cent of the total world increase up to 2020. This development has helped to transform China from a net exporter of grain to the second-largest importer in the world (Gold 2004, p. 28).

It is clear that the twenty-first century will be marked by economic pressures towards increased productivity and an expanded market share for meat-based products. This strategy must inevitably entail a continuation and expansion of intensive farming methods. At the same time, the growth of ecological and animal rights movements, concerns about health and a move towards the 'remoralising' of private and public life, will mean that these economic strategies will come under great pressure from social movements within the political arena.

At the start of the chapter it was noted that vegetarianism was at the nexus of the natural and the social. It is now apparent that the issues of meat-eating and vegetarianism are also positioned at the nexus of **globalisation** and a politics based on personal ethics and ecological awareness. As well as having an ancient and multicultural heritage, vegetarianism can now be seen to represent one of the key moral, political and ecological issues of the late modern period.

SUMMARY OF MAIN POINTS

- Vegetarianism is not just a contemporary social movement, but is one with an ancient history encompassing many different cultures.
- Definitions of what constitutes a vegetarian vary widely.
- Sociology has provided many useful theories and concepts that contribute to an understanding of vegetarianism. Of particular note are: theories of oppression and liberation and the concept of speciesism; sociology of denial; the civilising process; and life politics.
- There is evidence indicating that the numbers of voluntary vegetarians is increasing worldwide at the same time as the amount of meat being consumed is increasing.

SOCIOLOGICAL REFLECTION

- What are your reasons for being or not being vegetarian?
- Do you agree with Singer's idea of animal rights and the notion of speciesism?
- Does Cohen's notion of the sociology of denial help to explain why more people are not vegetarian?

DISCUSSION QUESTIONS

1. What variations of vegetarianism exist?
2. What might be some reasons for the long period of neglect of meat-eating and vegetarianism within sociology?
3. What has aesthetics to do with diet in general, and with the rejection of meat in particular?
4. Discuss some of the social processes involved in cultural denial. How does this process work to reinforce meat-eating in Western societies?
5. Discuss some of the health and/or environmental reasons put forward to support a vegetarian diet.

Deidre Wicks

6.   Relate the ideas of Giddens concerning life politics and emancipatory politics to the issue of meat rejection.

Further investigation

1.   Turning animals into meat has become hazardous for human and non-human life forms. Discuss this statement in relation to the impact of meat production on the environment.
2.   How does the theoretical approach of Norbert Elias contribute to an understanding of the growth of vegetarianism in modern Western countries?

FURTHER READING AND WEB RESOURCES

Books

Beardsworth, A. & Keil, T. 1997, *Sociology on the Menu*, Routledge, New York.

Patterson, C. 2002, *Eternal Treblinka: Our Treatment of Animals and the Holocaust*, Lantern Books, New York.

Pollan, M. 2006, *The Omnivore's Dilemma*, Bloomsbury, London.

Singer, P. 1975, *Animal Liberation: A New Ethics for Our Treatment of Animals*, Avon, New York.

—— & Mason, J. 2006, *The Ethics of What We Eat*, Text, Melbourne.

Spencer, C. 1995, *The Heretic's Feast*, University of New England, Hanover, NH.

Websites

Animals Australia: www.animalsaustralia.org/

Compassion in world farming: www.ciwf.org.uk/

Ethical consumer: www.ethicalconsumer.org/

International Vegetarian Union (IVU): www.ivu.org/

Vegan.com: www.vegan.com

Vegetarian.com: www.vegetarian.com

Vegetarian Nutrition Dietetic Practice Group: www.vegetariannutrition.net

REFERENCES

Adams, C. 2002, *The Sexual Politics of Meat. A Feminist-Vegetarian Critical Theory*, Continuum, New York.

BBC News 2006, 'New Way to Stop Food Poison Bugs', http://news.bbc.co.uk/1/hi/health/4609022.stm [accessed 2 October 2007].

Beardsworth, A. & Keil, T. 1992, 'The Vegetarian Option: Varieties, Conversions, Motives and Careers', *The Sociological Review*, vol. 40, pp. 253–93.

—— 1997, *Sociology on the Menu*, Routledge, New York.

Berriman, M. 1996, 'Mad Cow Disease, the Watergate of the Meat Industry', *New Vegetarian and Natural Health*, winter edition, pp. 47–8.

Cho, E., Chen, W.Y., Hunter, D.J., Stampfer, M.J., Colditz, G.A., Hankinson, S.E. & Willett, W.C. 2006, 'Red Meat Intake and Risk of Breast Cancer Among Premenopausal Women', *Archives of Internal Medicine*, vol. 166, pp. 2253–9.

Coetzee, J.M. 2001, *The Lives of Animals*, Princeton University Press, Princeton.

Cohen, S. 2001, *States of Denial. Knowing About Atrocities and Suffering*, Polity Press, Cambridge.

Cartmill, M. 1993, *A View to a Death in the Morning: Hunting and Nature Through History*, Harvard University Press, Mass.

Department of Agriculture, Fisheries & Food (Ireland) 2007, 'Report prepared on foot of reading of BSE results from 01/01/07 to 03/06/07' http://www.agriculture.gov.ie/index.jsp?file=areasofi/bse/bse_confirmations.xml, date accessed: 30.11.07.

Elias, N. 2000, *The Civilizing Process*, Blackwell Publishing, Oxford.

Fieldhouse, P. 1995, *Food and Nutrition: Customs and Culture*, Croom Helm, Kent.

Gaita, R. 2002, *The Philosopher's Dog*, Text, Melbourne.

Garces, L. 2002, *The Detrimental Impacts of Industrial Animal Agriculture—A Case For Humane And Sustainable Agriculture*, Compassion in World Farming Trust, Hampshire.

Giddens, A. 1991, *Modernity and Self-Identity: Self and Society in the Late Modern Age*, Polity Press, Cambridge.

Gold, M. 2004, *The Global Benefits of Eating Less Meat*, Compassion in World Farming Trust, Hampshire.

Jeffries, S. 2001, 'Have the French Lost their Appetite?', *Observer* 'Food Monthly', June 10, http://observer.guardian.co.uk/foodmonthly/story/0,,502824,00.html [accessed 4 October 2007].

Institute of Marine Research 2005, 'Salmon Lice Spread by Currents—But Where do They Go?', www.imr.no/english/news/news_2005/salmon_lice_spread_by_currents__but_where_do_they_go [accessed 4 October 2007].

Lawrence, G., Vanclay, F. & Furze, B. (eds) 1992, *Agriculture, Environment and Society: Contemporary Issues for Australians*, Macmillan, Melbourne.

Lee, J. 2007, 'Pigs Sentenced to 10 More Cramped Years', *Sydney Morning Herald*, 23 April 2007, www.smh.com.au/news/environment/pigs-sentenced-to-10-more-cramped-years/2007/04/22/1177180487707.html

Leemann, P. 2000, *Joia. Colours, Flavours and Consistency in Natural Haute Cuisine*, Editrice Abitare Segesta, Milan.

Lukes, S. 1974, *Power. A Radical View*, Macmillan, London & Basingstoke.

Marcus, E. 2001, *Vegan. The New Ethics of Eating*, McBooks Press, New York.

Maurer, D. 1995, 'Meat as a Social Problem: Rhetorical Strategies in the Contemporary Vegetarian Literature', in D. Maurer & J. Sobal (eds), *Eating Agendas: Food and Nutrition as Social Problems*, Aldine de Gruyter, New York.

McLennan, W. & Podger, A. 1997, *National Nutrition Survey Selected Highlights Australia 1995*, Australian Bureau of Statistics, Department of Health and Family Services, Canberra.

Merchant, C. 1980, *The Death of Nature*, Wildwood House, London.

—— 1983, *Animals and Why They Matter*, Penguin Books, Melbourne.

Murcott, A. (ed.) 1983, *The Sociology of Food and Eating*, Gower, Aldershot.

Noske, B. 1997, *Beyond Boundaries. Humans and Animals*, Black Rose Books, Montreal.

Patterson, C. 2002, *Eternal Treblinka. Our Treatment of Animals and the Holocaust*, Lantern books, New York.

Phillips, P. 2003, *Humanity Dick. The Eccentric Member for Galway*, Parapress Ltd, Kent.

Pollan, M. 2006, *The Omnivore's Dilemma. The Search for a Perfect Meal in a Fast-Food World*, Bloomsbury, London.

Purvis, A. 2003, 'Farmed fish', *Observer* 'Food Monthly', 11 May, http://observer. guardian.co.uk/foodmonthly/story/0,,951686,00.html [accessed 04 October 2007].

Rifkin J. 1993, *Beyond Beef: The Rise and Fall of the Cattle Culture*, Plume, New York.

Schlosser, E. 2001, *Fast Food Nation*, Penguin, London.

Singer, P. 1975, *Animal Liberation: A New Ethics for Our Treatment of Animals*, Avon, New York.

—— 2000, *Ethics into Action*. Henry Spira and the Animal Rights Movement, Rowman & Littlefield Publishers, Inc. Maryland.

—— & Mason, J. 2006, *The Ethics of What We Eat*, Text, Melbourne.

Smith, J. 1997, *Hungry For You*, Vintage, London.

Spencer, C. 1995, *The Heretic's Feast*, University Press of New England, Hanover.

Swan, S.H., Liu, F., Overstreet, J.W., Brazil, C. & Skakkebaek, N.E. 2007, 'Semen Quality of Fertile U.S. Males in Relation to Their Mothers' Beef Consumption During Pregnancy', *Human Reproduction*, vol. 22, no. 6, pp. 1497–502.

Taylor, E.F., Burley, V.J., Greenwood, D.C. & Cade, J.E. 2007, 'Meat Consumption and Risk of Breast Cancer in the UK Women's Cohort Study', *British Journal of Cancer*, vol. 96, pp. 1139–46.

WHO—*see* World Health Organization.

Willetts, A. 1997, '"Bacon Sandwiches Got the Better of Me": Meat-eating and Vegetarianism in South-east London', in P. Caplan (ed.), *Food, Health and Identity*, Routledge, London.

World Health Organization 2007, 'Bovine spongiform encephalopathy (BSE)', WHO website, www.who.int/zoonoses/diseases/bse/en/ [accessed 4 October 2007].

CHAPTER 14

Food and Ageing

Wm. Alex McIntosh and Karen S. Kubena

OVERVIEW

- Why are older people at risk of hunger and poor nutrition?
- How do social isolation and stress affect older people's nutrition?
- How do social relationships reduce the risk of hunger and poor nutrition among older people?

Older people are a group at high risk of food insecurity, hunger and poor nutrition. They are particularly vulnerable because they generally have fewer socioeconomic resources than younger people and are more prone to isolation, disability, and stress. These problems tend to be even more prevalent among older people who are members of ethnic minorities. In addition, many countries, including the United States of America, have recently reduced funding for food-assistance programs such as food stamps and congregate meals. Private charities have been unable to compensate for these cutbacks. Many older people, however, are able to compensate for their lack of resources and physical isolation through their social networks. Older people who live alone may find mealtime companionship among their friends and neighbours. In addition, relatives and neighbours provide many disabled older people with shopping and cooking assistance.

Key terms

activities of daily living	nutritional risk	social network
ageism	postmodern society	social support
disabilities	role	socioeconomic status (SES)
food insecurity	social control	status
life chances	social isolation	stigma

Introduction

Older people are an important group for sociological study for a number of reasons. First, older people represent one of the fastest-growing segments of the population of most developed countries. The populations of most developed countries are growing older. In the USA, the number of people aged 65 or older constituted 13 per cent of the population in 2000; it has been predicted that, by 2050, over 20 per cent of the population will be in this age group, thanks to better diets as well as better health and health care (FIFARS 2000). The proportion of people aged 85 or above is expected to increase at an even faster rate during this same period. The growth of the older population and their increasing needs will have an impact on every aspect of society.

Second, because of filial obligations supported by laws, traditions and social norms, older people are a group whose needs continue to be the responsibility of both families and the state. However, as older people live longer, and as financial and time constraints place a greater burden on families and government programs, it will become more and more difficult to meet these obligations.

Third, age is a social category and is related to **status** and **role**, two of sociology's most fundamental concepts. Typical roles include patient, physician, grandmother and daughter. Age determines a role, 'independent of capacities and preferences' of the incumbent (Moen 1996, p. 171). Status represents the prestige or respect accorded to individuals occupying these social positions. The respect that an individual receives for performing a role is somewhat independent of actual performance; simply occupying the position itself accords a certain amount of prestige. 'Age', 'ageing' and 'elderly' are all words with supposed biological meanings, yet each represents a socially defined category. In fact, much of what passes as biological wisdom in defining 'older people' has more to do with socially generated beliefs and norms. In addition, because age is a social category, it contains an evaluative component. The terms 'age', 'ageing', and 'elderly' are all associated with negative expectations about abilities and quality of life, among other things (Palmore 1990). Ageing is also viewed as a process of declining status; it is seen as biologically driven downward mobility. This is, in part, true. Many older people experience a decline in their health as they age, and many face declining incomes in the form of retirement reimbursements. But ageing also has a negative status because of its relationship to what is currently one of the most desirable statuses in Western society: youth. There is considerable evidence that older people encounter **ageism**, or prejudice and discrimination based on age.

Because of the increasing size of the elderly population and the difficult economic circumstances that many older people face, sociologists and nutritionists have turned their attention to older people's food habits, nutritional status and health. Several important themes have emerged from their studies. The first is that of **socioeconomic status (SES)**. It is widely believed that inadequate resources are the reason for **food**

insecurity and risk of malnutrition (McIntosh 1996; Weddle et al. 1996). A second theme is **social isolation**. Isolation from others is thought to deprive an individual of help, companionship and motivation for self-care. The third theme represents the opposite of isolation: social integration and **social support**. A multiplicity of ties to others not only increases contact with other human beings, but also ensures companionship and access to resources such as transportation and help with cooking. Some believe that the nature of an older person's **social network** has greater consequence for them than the help that network provides; others have argued that the greatest impact of help from others lies in how it is perceived by its recipients.

The fourth, and most recent, theme to emerge in the sociology of nutrition is that of stressful life events. All human beings experience change, and some of these changes are upsetting and disrupting (Thoits 1995). Older people are not immune to such events, and they are most likely to experience events such as the death of a loved one. Such stressors have a negative impact on health, including nutritional status. The debate here centres on whether some stressors have a more deleterious effect than others have, and whether some individuals are better equipped than others to deal with negative life changes. Some old people are able to cope with the help of their social support network. Such aid comes into play for another kind of crisis that confronts many older people: reduced functional capacity.

Disability, its effects, and the social responses to it represent a fifth theme in the literature. As people age, the probability of contracting one or more chronic illnesses increases (Verbrugge 1990). A number of such illnesses have symptoms that limit mobility or some other aspect of body functioning (Manton 1989). Some older people are able to cope with these threats to independence through their own efforts. 'Self-care' involves those changes that individuals choose to make as a means of improving health and dealing with symptoms of illness—for example, dietary and exercise modifications. Certain limitations, however, may make it more difficult for some individuals to engage in self-care. In such cases, the social network's services become vitally important.

Sixth, sociologists have renewed their interest in the body as a reflection of various socially defined attributes of worth. These values play a major role in determining individuals' perceptions of themselves. Sociologists refer to this self-perception as 'the self'. Body image, or body self, has increased in importance in the formation of the self. Anthony Giddens (1991) and others have argued that individuals have found it increasingly difficult to affect their political and economic environments and so have turned to the self and the body as things upon which they can have an impact. Much of this concern is directed at manipulating body weight in an attempt to achieve physiologically improbable goals.

Finally, it should be noted that sociological approaches to food and nutrition tend to take a 'social problems' orientation. Concern centres on the social causes and consequences of food insecurity, hunger, malnutrition, overnutrition and so on.

Wm. Alex McIntosh and Karen S. Kubena

This chapter reviews the literature that has developed around the themes mentioned above, beginning with the notion that food and nutrition problems may be conceived of as social problems.

Ageing and associated food and nutrition problems

A number of nutritional problems confront older people, and they are usually presented in biological terms. Without doubt, these nutritional problems have clear biological causes and consequences; however, unless social and economic factors are also considered, our understanding of older people's nutrition is incomplete.

People's nutritional needs change as they age (Fiatarone & Evans 1993). Older people have decreased energy requirements but greater protein requirements. General concerns in this area have focused on the inability of some older people to meet their nutrient needs and on the effects of nutrient deficiency on, for example, immune function (Kubena & McMurray 1996). Mobility of elderly individuals is dependent on their having adequate bone mass and normal muscle function. Bone loss and impaired muscle function can be caused by inadequate dietary intake of vitamin D (Jassen et al. 2002) and calcium (Dawson-Hughes & Harris 2002). Increasingly, research is suggesting a role for adequate nutrition in maintaining cognitive functioning (Smith 2002). The lower intake of nutrients among the elderly is partly a result of the decreased income that some receive as they age, but it is also a consequence of misconceptions within this age group regarding their nutrient needs. One source of these misconceptions is the marketing messages of our consumer society. Products and advertisements both provide a contradictory array of information regarding the way that nutrition, health and ageing are related.

Loosely associated with the declining ability of some older people to meet their nutritional needs are the problems of *hunger* and *food insecurity*. In the USA, the definitions of these terms are less rooted in biology than in norms. 'Hunger' is defined and measured in terms of the inability to buy all the food one would like or of sending one's children to bed hungry. For some, hunger is an acute, emergency situation, the result of a temporary shortfall in resources. For others, hunger is chronic. Some older people, for example, have reported that they commonly run short of money to purchase food during the last week of every month. While there is no evidence that such food insufficiency increases the likelihood of chronic disease, there is evidence that it increases the likelihood of infections such as pneumonia.

Food insecurity is a broader concern, affecting all those who believe that hunger is just around the corner. The food-insecure are those who anticipate deprivation, or the inability to achieve a diet that they consider adequate. Currently, 6 per cent of elderly households are considered to be food-insecure (Nord 2002). Once again, inadequate resources appear to be the driving force behind food insecurity.

Low income, costly medical bills, lack of transportation, and the absence of nearby grocery stores have been associated with food insecurity in the elderly (Rowley 2000). Furthermore, several studies of food-insecure elderly people indicate that such people are more likely to experience poorer quality diets, be underweight and be anaemic (Rose & Oliveria 1997; Klesges et al. 2001; Lee & Frongillo 2001; American Dietetic Association 2002). We suggest that, while those who concern themselves with hunger and food insecurity probably have negative biological consequences in mind, it is, once again, a normative interpretation that has led people to define these conditions as problems. Hunger and food insecurity are thought to be the result of the inequitable distribution of resources and the denial of inalienable rights. According to this position, all people, including older people, have a 'right to food', which is said to incorporate 'the right of everyone to an adequate standard of living' and 'the right to be free from hunger' (Alston 1994, p. 209).

Declining ability may also result from changes in body size. Both being over-weight and being underweight, and the associated health problems, can make it more difficult for older people to perform their various roles. In addition, there is strong evidence that body weight affects the probability of death. Older people who are greatly over or under the weight standard for their age, height and gender have a greater risk of dying than older people closer to standard (Flegal 1996).

Weight is also a highly salient social marker, partly because of the association of slimness with youth but also because what is defined socially as excessive body weight connotes a negative social status. To begin with, the weight itself is considered unattractive. In addition, overweight is perceived to be a marker of more deep-seated undesirable traits, such as greed, dishonesty, and lack of ambition and self-control (see Chapter 17).

Both chronic illnesses and medications affect appetite, the sense of taste, the absorption of nutrients and the need for nutrients. There are social issues here as well, regarding the decline in social relationships that occurs when an individual becomes disabled and the effect that this decline and the disability has on the individual's ability to shop, prepare meals and eat. Furthermore, there is some evidence that older people are overmedicated because they are too passive when confronting medical authority.

Access to resources

Socioeconomic status

A person's SES depends on their wealth, prestige and power; differential access to these things leads to differences in lifestyle and **life chances** (Gerth & Mills 1946). Those with greater wealth and status enjoy better life chances than those with less of these, simply because they can afford better health practices and health care. Greater resources also permit expanded lifestyle choice in such areas as dwellings,

Wm. Alex McIntosh and Karen S. Kubena

food purchases, clothing and vacations. An individual's SES is usually conceptualised and measured by that individual's education, occupation, and income. Education and occupation are primary determinants of income, and they are also sources of prestige. Gender, ethnicity and age also influence a person's status. Each of these characteristics affects access to wealth, prestige and power, and each is associated with distinctive aspects of lifestyle and life chances.

In the USA, old age was commonly associated, until recently, with poverty—as many as 25 per cent of older people were classified as poor (Crystal 1996, p. 394). Increases in social security benefits and other changes have halved this proportion. But great inequities remain among retired people in the USA, with former white-collar workers generally in a better financial position than former blue-collar workers. Furthermore, many of those in the lowest 20 per cent of incomes are still considered to be above the poverty line (Crystal 1996, p. 397). Those in this group tend to lack health insurance, but are not considered poor enough to qualify for means-tested programs like Medicaid or food stamps. Janet Poppendieck (1998) found that while only 10 per cent of the poor are older people, this group constitutes 22 per cent of soup-kitchen clientele.

As previously mentioned, malnutrition exists among poor older people (Weddle et al. 1996). In fact, low SES is related to low levels of nutrition knowledge, poorer eating habits, inadequate diets and poorer nutritional status (Wolinsky et al. 1990; Quinn et al. 1997; Howard et al. 1998; Guthrie & Lin 2002). Finally, food-insecure elderly people are more likely to be poor and in need of food assistance (Lee & Frongillo 2001).

Ethnicity and class

Ethnicity is a social status that has implications for the distribution of resources. Social scientists argue that the combination of low income and ethnicity constitutes 'double jeopardy'. Others have used this same argument to claim that older people who are members of minorities experience double jeopardy, and it is a relatively short logical leap to argue that poor older people from minority groups are subject to triple jeopardy. In the USA, poverty rates have remained highest among older black and Hispanic people, with 26 per cent and 21 per cent living in poverty respectively (FIFARS 2000). The effects of double and triple jeopardy are reflected in older people's nutritional status. Nancy Schoenberg and her colleagues (1997), for example, found rural black people to be at greater **nutritional risk** than urban black people or white people in general.

Class conflict

Social class is no mere marker of the distribution of resources. Because resources are scarce, struggles ensue over their distribution, usually along class lines. Food and medical care are two such resources that politicians frequently consider redistributing according to social categories, such as those of children, older people, women and war veterans. In an era of declining social-welfare funding, struggles over food-stamp eligibility and access to subsidised medical care once again reflect class, generational and ethnic group interests, among other interests.

In the past, after a great deal of political struggle, a number of programs to benefit older people were established in the USA. Meals on Wheels and Congregate Meals were designed to provide one meal per day containing at least one-third of the recommended daily allowances of most nutrients. Critics have sparked considerable debate over the efficacy of these programs, and some have even questioned their fairness.

Debates aside, budget cuts and decentralisation have left many US states unable to fund feeding programs to meet current needs. Forty-one per cent of Meals on Wheels programs report, for example, that they now maintain lengthy waiting lists (Ponza et al. 1997). Many food-pantry and soup-kitchen participants report that they use such food charities because they are unable to access government programs such as food stamps.

Ageism and stigma

Social statuses contain evaluative as well as cognitive components: not only do we hold certain beliefs about people with particular statuses, but we also make judgments regarding the worth of people holding those statuses. Age is a social status, and various age groups reflect differentially valued statuses. Groups accorded negative status and negative evaluations frequently encounter prejudice and discrimination. When it comes to race and gender, these are referred to as 'racism' and 'sexism' respectively. 'Ageism' is their counterpart when it comes to negative evaluations of old age. At present, youth is generally regarded as more valuable in Western societies, and so young people are accorded more status than older people. Perhaps one of the most undesirable statuses to inhabit is that of old age. Numerous negative evaluations are attached to this status. As with many negatively evaluated statuses, the basis of the negative evaluations is socially determined.

The stereotypes associated with ageism are similar to those associated with racism and sexism in that they question the abilities of the status-holder relative to the abilities of others. Those holding negatively evaluated statuses are usually judged, in a biological sense, as having lesser physical and mental abilities, and this negative evaluation is thus considered to be both natural and immutable. Many believe that because some older people have physical or mental limitations, all older people are so limited. These assumptions lead to a denigration of older people's capabilities and worth. It is assumed that older people are unable to care for themselves. Such negative evaluations hinder older people's ability to obtain employment and result in

Wm. Alex McIntosh and Karen S. Kubena

intergenerational struggles over the allocation of resources. Much of the debate over the extent to which current and future resources should be devoted to retirement benefits and to subsidised access to food and medical care has reflected a continuing debate over the worth of older persons. This debate is cast in either equality or equity terms. Equality arguments have endorsed the sharing of resources based on need (Poppendieck 1998). Equity arguments, by contrast, have advocated the sharing of resources based on the size of the contribution each individual makes to society or has made at some time in the past (Gokhale & Kotlikoff 1998).

The unequal distribution of resources is brought about by social as well as economic and political factors. Those persons eligible for aid, including older people, often refuse it because of the **stigma** associated with poverty and welfare. Simply put, those who are less well-to-do are less admired than those who are better off. In the USA, where poverty is viewed as being the result of irresponsible behaviour rather than unequal resource distribution, the working poor are accorded more respect than the non-working poor. The poor who get by on charity and/or welfare receive the least respect. The public associates a wide range of negative characteristics with welfare recipients, culminating in the pejorative label 'the undeserving poor'. Those who provide benefits such as food stamps hold many of these stereotypes, as do a number of those who work for private charities such as food pantries and soup kitchens (Poppendieck 1998).

Social resources

Social networks

A person's social network consists of his or her friends, relatives, spouses, children, co-workers, neighbours, fellow members of voluntary organisations, fellow church members and so on. These tend to be the individuals with whom a person has the most contact or from whom the person receives the most support or help (Berkman & Glass 2000; Brissette et al. 2000). 'Social support' refers to both instrumental aid (goods and services) and expressive aid (emotional support and companionship). Social support also includes efficacious **social control**: network members may attempt to persuade or cajole an individual to engage in desirable behaviour, such as reducing dietary fat (Brissette et al. 2000).

People who receive social support become ill less frequently and recover more quickly and successfully when they do become ill. The most striking effect of social support appears to be the lessening of the risk of death. Numerous studies have found that those with social support are likely to live longer than those who lack it (Schoenbach et al. 1986; Seeman et al. 1993; Yasuda et al. 1997). More recently, we and our colleagues have found a connection between social support and nutritional health (McIntosh, Kubena & Landmann 1989; McIntosh, Shifflett & Picou 1989; McIntosh et al. 1995).

Social support results in part from the very structure of the social network. There is considerable debate between social-support researchers, however, about the degree to which network characteristics are more important than the aid received or the recipients' subjective evaluations of that aid. Network structure characteristics include the network's size (the number of people in it) and its density (the degree to which network members know and interact with one another). Networks that contain a small number of people who are well acquainted with one another provide greater intimacy and emotional support. At the same time, some studies suggest that larger networks generate more support (Faber & Wasserman 2002). In our study of 424 free-living Houston elderly, we found that those older people with large social networks tended to receive more social support, although men received greater benefits from greater network size than did women. Older men with large networks got more advice about food and cooking, more help with grocery shopping and cooking, and more mealtime companionship than men with smaller networks, and their iron status was better than that of men with smaller networks. Older women with denser networks tended to have more company during meals. Other researchers have found that larger, denser networks are not necessarily beneficial for the elderly when it comes to making healthy changes in their diets. Such networks may block these efforts through social control (Silverman et al. 2002).

Social support and nutrition

Certain kinds of social support appear to be associated with nutritional health, particularly that of older people. Instrumental aid, such as transportation for grocery shopping, help with meal preparation, companionship during meals, loans of food, and advice about cooking, diets and food, has the potential to maintain or improve the nutritional health of individuals. It is precisely this sort of help that older people frequently need. In Houston, older people with a greater number of companions in their networks had better appetites and more muscle mass (McIntosh, Kubena & Landmann 1989). Those who received help with shopping, cooking and housekeeping were at lower nutritional risk (fewer impediments to eating a healthy diet) than those who received little or no such help. And those who had more people in their social network giving them advice about food and nutrition tended to have higher vitamin B-6 status. Elderly people who had a greater number of companions had lower nutritional risk (Hendy et al. 1998).

Social isolation and loneliness

Living alone (social isolation) represents a clear trend among older people. In 1960, about 20 per cent of older people in the USA lived alone, but by 1998 the proportion had increased to 37 per cent (FIFARS 2000). Forty-one per cent of elderly women lived alone; this is partly the result of the mortality differential between males and females—women, on average, live longer than men. Our own data on older people in Houston indicate that 12 per cent of the men and 50 per cent of the women lived alone, and that the propensity to live alone increased with age, especially for women. Others note, however, that many older people live close to one of their children, and approximately 40 per cent keep in daily phone contact with one of their offspring (Moody 1994). Because many older people live alone, they are frequently thought to be at risk of loneliness and poor nutrition. There are documented health consequences of living alone. Those older people who live alone because of the recent death of their spouse, for example, have an increased risk of mortality (Rogers 1996).

Nutrition researchers have argued that without the social contact that typically comes with shared living arrangements, the motivation to cook food or to eat regular meals may be reduced. Maradee Davis and her colleagues (1985) found that older people who lived alone were more likely to eat an inadequate diet than those living with a spouse. Similarly, Susan Murphy and others (1990) observed that older women had a higher energy intake if they lived with a spouse. Dellmar Walker and Roy Beauchene (1991) found among older people in Georgia that the greater the loneliness experienced, the poorer the diet in terms of iron, protein, phosphorous, riboflavin, niacin and ascorbic acid (vitamin C). In New York, older men skipped more meals if they lived alone (Frongillo et al. 1992). In Houston, we measured dietary adequacy by determining the degree to which the dietary intake of older people over a three-day period met 67 per cent of the recommended dietary allowances (RDAs) for this age group. We found that both older women and older men were likely to fall below 67 per cent of the RDA for a number of nutrients if they lived by themselves. Elderly people who ate a greater number of meals with others each day were less likely to experience nutritional risk (Hendy et al. 1998). In addition, Green and Wang (1995) found that elderly people who skip meals have less adequate diets than those who miss no meals. Meal skipping is more common among those elderly people who live alone. Finally, old people who report being lonely also report forgetting to eat and experiencing loss of appetite (Wylie 2000).

Disability and functioning

All human beings are susceptible to impairments caused by chronic illness, injury or accident; impairments involve bodily abnormalities that may limit movement of limbs or cause generalised muscular weakness (Jette 1996). They can limit the ability of a person to perform social roles and are often referred to as '**disabilities**'. Older people are more prone to chronic illnesses than people in other age groups, and thus their rates of impairment are higher. Furthermore, as they grow older, greater percentages of older people experience these limitations. Some impairments result in functional limitations or restrictions in performing what are considered to be everyday activities. In the USA, 39 per cent of people aged 70 or older have one or more disabilities that limit **activities of daily living**. Eleven per cent of older people experience difficulties shopping for groceries; 4 per cent have trouble preparing meals; 2 per cent experience problems with eating food (Jette 1996, p. 100). Some elderly people report having to sit down while cooking, while others have trouble manipulating cooking utensils (Wylie 2000).

Disabilities are directly associated with risk of poor nutritional status, and thus some of the tools devised to measure nutritional risk include measures of disability, such as difficulty chewing or swallowing. Certain foods may be avoided as a result of such difficulties, as a study by Mary-Ellen Quinn and others (1997) demonstrated. Other studies have found a relationship between inadequate diet and level of disability (Walker & Beauchene 1991). The Houston study found that older people who had difficulties in using their upper bodies or difficulties in walking tended to have more body fat and less muscle mass. Such people also tended to be less physically active and have less adequate diets. Elderly people with dentures tend to eat more fats, sweets and snacks (Vitolins et al. 2002).

There is considerable debate over whether disability leads to an increase or decrease in social support. Some studies provide evidence of a shrinking social network and increased social isolation, with the only help with daily activities being supplied by remaining kin. Furthermore, as the burden of such help grows, the caregiver is in danger of experiencing resentment and burnout. Others argue that disabilities actually mobilise social networks into action, increasing the level of support supplied (Kivett et al. 2000). Our own Houston data confirm the latter hypothesis. The greater the level of disability, the more help with grocery shopping, cooking and other activities of daily living the older person received, regardless of gender (McIntosh et al. 1988). In addition, people with disabilities were less likely to experience the nutritional problems mentioned above when they had social support from others. For example, although those with limited mobility were less likely to eat breakfast and more likely to have lower muscle mass but more body fat, these negative effects were offset, to a degree, by their having more friends in their social network and receiving help with activities of daily living. Finally, the elderly tend to experience fewer obesity-related physical disabilities if they had adequate confidant support (Surtees et al. 2004).

Stress, strain and health

Human beings experience a great number of changes in their lives—marriage, having children, getting and losing jobs, retirement, illness and so on (Thoits 1995). A number of these changes are welcomed; others are not. The unwelcome changes are thought to be 'stressors'. Stressors are threats, demands or constraints on individuals that 'tax or exceed their resources for managing them' (Burke 1996, p. 146). One kind of stressor is a 'life event', a discrete, observable event that leads to a major change in life. Divorce, job loss and the death of a spouse are examples of such potentially life-shattering changes.

Wm. Alex McIntosh and Karen S. Kubena

There is a well-established link between poor health and stressors (House et al. 1988). Various forms of illness—such as coronary heart disease, hypertension, cancer and depression—have been found to be associated with various stressful events, such as job loss, marital conflict and the death of a spouse or close friend (Marmot & Theorell 1988; Umberson et al. 1992). Definitions of 'stress' often emphasise disequilibrium in the organism, which results from exposure to stressors. William Krehl (1964, p. 4) has described nutrition as 'the sum of all the processes by which an organism ingests, digests, absorbs, transports, and utilizes food substances'. Therefore, anything that disrupts nutrient ingestion, digestion, absorption, transportation or utilisation by the body is a potential stressor.

Research suggests that stressful life events do indeed interfere with nutrition. In our study of older Virginians (McIntosh, Shifflett & Picou 1989), we found that financial worries led to depressed appetite, which in turn was associated with lower intake of energy and protein. More recently, Payette and others (1995) observed a relationship between a high level of self-assessed stress and a lower intake of protein. We found, in Houston, that the two kinds of events that seemed to have the greatest negative effect on older people's nutrition were financial difficulties and general, unspecified problems in relations with various family members. Financial problems had a negative effect on body fat, muscle mass, iron status, and the frequency of eating breakfast among older women, and older men had higher body fat and snacked more if they had recently experienced family troubles.

Social identity and age

All human beings develop a sense of identity, persona or self. Much of this sense of self derives from social interactions with others. Individuals, however, have some control over the perceptions of others and actively attempt to influence those perceptions. While there is disagreement over the degree to which an individual can 'manage the impressions of others', it is clear that, within limits, this management is achievable.

Western societies, particularly the USA, place a high value on youthfulness. Mass-media programming and advertising have perhaps exacerbated this emphasis, by mostly featuring young actors, presenters and models (Turrow 1997). But as the older population has grown and its economic fortunes have improved, producers and advertisers have discovered a vast, insufficiently tapped market in older people, especially the so-called 'young-old' (those under 70 years of age). Their approach to older people has been to stress that older people are still as capable, in many ways, as the young. According to Mike Featherstone and Mike Hepworth (1995), this has had a positive effect in that it has helped reduce the perception of older people as less capable human beings. However, it must be pointed out that producers have attempted to market their products in terms of identity manipulation—that is, they have developed products to help older people disguise their age.

Sociologists have increasingly been taking the body's social dimensions seriously. Chris Shilling (1994), for example, has put forward the notion that bodies are judged unequally; thus differentials in body size and shape constitute a form of inequality. Linda Jackson's (1992) review of extant research indicates that body appearance has a significant impact on how others judge an individual. Pierre Bourdieu (1979/1984) has hypothesised that bodies reflect social class in that they represent the owner's relationship to the worlds of necessities and taste. Among the lower classes, a heavy body represents a diet high in fat but low in cost. Bourdieu refers to this as the diet of necessity. Taste makes necessity a virtue. Bodies also reflect 'bodily orientation'. Members of the working class take a more instrumental approach to their body in that they make direct use of their body's capacities in making their living. The implication for eating is that heavy foods in large quantities are desirable because of their perceived contribution to strength. The dominant classes, according to Bourdieu (1979/1984), prefer slender bodies and are willing to defer gratification to achieve them.

In old age, working-class individuals may experience a decline in both income and bodily function. A middle-class individual may worry about being replaced by a person with a younger body. Upper-class individuals may view middle and old age as a time to enjoy the fruits of their labour and may expect to have not only the money but also the physical capacity to do so.

The body in **postmodern society** is said to have become more malleable, in the sense that it can be manipulated in a person's quest for a new or altered identity. Surgery, diets, exercise and drugs have all been called upon in attempts to make the body appear more youthful (see Chapter 15). Older people are equally inclined to make such attempts (Biggs 1997). Older people are slightly less likely to participate in exercise programs, but after differences in disability levels are accounted for their participation levels are higher than those of many other age groups. Older women have been found to worry about weight gain for appearance as well as health reasons. But for these women, 'health tends to be a valid justification for being concerned with one's weight, while an appearance orientation is deemed to be indicative of vanity' (Clarke 2002). Featherstone and Hepworth (1995) argue that with increasing age, the physical constraints on the ability to alter appearance grow. As they put it, the body becomes an unchanging mask that its occupant can no longer escape.

Conclusion

While much is known about the effects of SES on nutrition, research is just beginning on how social networks help older people maintain a healthy diet and avoid nutritional risk. Similarly, the negative effects of both stressors and disabilities on older people's nutrition are not fully understood. Finally, older people's efforts to manage their identities through diet and exercise remain an important, but relatively unexplored, area of sociological research.

Wm. Alex McIntosh and Karen S. Kubena

SUMMARY OF MAIN POINTS

- While older people's energy needs tend to be lower than those of people from other age groups, their need for nutrients is as high or higher.
- Older people's nutrition can be compromised by chronic illness, disabilities, and interactions between drugs and nutrients.
- Older people are at greater risk of serious consequences from food-borne illnesses than younger people.
- Older people's nutrition is also negatively affected by poverty, stressful life events and social isolation.
- Social networks supply aid of various kinds, such as transportation to buy groceries, help with meal preparation and companionship during meals. Both network structure and the help that networks provide have a positive impact on older people's nutrition. Social support helps people overcome the constraints imposed by living alone, functional limitations and stressful events.
- Older people perceive their weight, as do others in modern society, as a means through which they can re-create their selves. Consumer culture has some influence on the choices that older people and others make when selecting 'selves' to pursue. As they age, however, their ability to control their appearance declines.

SOCIOLOGICAL REFLECTION

- If you have grandparents, have you thought about the quality of their diets and their nutritional health?
- Do your grandparents frequently eat alone or skip meals?
- What kind of social support do your grandparents receive, if any? Are there key aspects of support missing from your grandparents' lives? Could your immediate family and/or you do something to fill this gap?
- Have your grandparents recently experienced stressful life events such as a decline in their economic circumstances? Do you think these experiences might have had an effect on their eating habits?

DISCUSSION QUESTIONS

1. What are the main nutritional problems faced by older people?
2. What are the sources of low socioeconomic status and isolation among older people?
3. How do stress and disabilities affect older people's nutrition?
4. How does social support help older people overcome such problems as lack of resources, isolation, disability and stress?

5. Why are older people concerned with their physical appearance, and what do they do to maintain that appearance?

Further investigation

1. Compare and contrast the effects of social and economic resources on the nutritional health of the elderly. How might the absence of both social and economic resources interact to make an elderly person's situation worse?
2. Discuss the normative/moral issues connected to the status of elderly people in society and how the normative order contributes to the nutritional health of the elderly.

FURTHER READING AND WEB RESOURCES

Books

Blaxter, M. 1990, *Health and Lifestyles*, Routledge, New York.

Kosberg, J.I. & Kayne, L. 1997, *Elderly Men: Special Problems and Professional Challenges*, Springer, New York.

Litwak, E. 1985, *Helping the Elderly: The Complementary Roles of Informal Networks and Formal Systems*, Guilford Press, New York.

Sokolovsky, J. 1997, *The Cultural Context of Aging: Worldwide Perspectives*, Bergin & Garvey, Westport.

Articles

Peters, G.R. & Rappaport, L.R. 1988, 'Food, Nutrition, and Aging: Behavioral Perspectives', *American Behavioral Scientist*, vol. 32, no. 1, special issue, pp. 1–88.

Journals

Ageing and Society: www.journals.cambridge.org/jid_ASO

Agriculture, Food, and Human Values: www.afhvs.org/journal.html

Appetite: www.elsevier.com/wps/find/journaldescription.cws_home/622785/description #description

Food, Culture and Society: www.bergpublishers.com/us/food/food_about.htm

The Gerontologist: http://gerontologist.gerontologyjournals.org/

Journal of Aging and Health: http://jah.sagepub.com/

Journal of the American Dietetic Association: www.adajournal.org/

Journal of Gerontology: www.geron.org/journals/medical.html

Journal of Health and Social Behavior: www.asanet.org/cs/root/leftnav/publications/ journals/journal_of_health_and_social_behavior/homepage

Journal of Nutrition Education and Behavior: http://www.jneb.org/

Journal of Nutrition for the Elderly: www.haworthpress.com/store/product.asp?sku=J052

Wm. Alex McIntosh and Karen S. Kubena

Websites

Association for the Study of Food and Society: http://food-culture.org/

New England Research Institute: www.neri.org

REFERENCES

Alston, P. 1994, 'International Law and the Right to Food', in B. Harriss-White & R. Hoffenberg (eds), *Food: Multidisciplinary Perspectives*, Blackwell, New York.

American Dietetic Association 2002, 'Position of the American Dietetic Association: Domestic Food and Nutrition Security', *Journal of the American Dietetic Association*, vol. 102, no. 12, pp. 1840–7.

Berkman, L.F. & Glass, T. 2000, 'Social Integration, Social Networks, Social Support, and Health', in L.F. Berkman & I. Kawachi (eds), *Social Epidemiology*, Oxford University Press, New York.

Biggs, S. 1997, 'Choosing Not to Be Old? Masks, Bodies, and Identity Management in Later Life', *Ageing and Society*, vol. 17, September, pp. 553–70.

Bourdieu, P. 1979/1984, *Distinction: A Social Critique of the Judgement of Taste*, Harvard University, Cambridge, Massachusetts.

Brissette, I., Cohen, S. & Seeman, T. 2000, 'Measuring Social Integration and Social Networks', in S. Cohen, L.G. Underwood & B.H. Gottlieb (eds), *Social Support Measurement and Intervention: A Guide for Health and Social Scientists*, Oxford University Press, New York.

Burke, P. 1996, 'Social Identities and Psychosocial Stress', in H.B. Kaplan (ed.), *Psychosocial Stress: Perspectives on Structure, Theory, Life-Course, and Methods*, Academic Press, San Diego.

Clarke, L.H. 2002. 'Older Women's Perceptions of Ideal Body Weights: The Tensions between Health and Appearance Motivations for Weight Loss', *Ageing and Society*, vol. 22, no. 6, pp. 751–73.

Crystal, S. 1996, 'Economic Status of the Elderly', in R.H. Binstock & L.K. George (eds), *Handbook of Aging and the Social Sciences*, 4th edition, Academic Press, San Diego.

Davis, M.A., Randall, E., Forthofer, R.N., Lee, E.S. & Margen, S. 1985, 'Living Arrangements and Dietary Patterns of Older Adults in the United States', *Journal of Gerontology*, vol. 40, no. 4, pp. 434–9.

Dawson-Hughes, B. & Harris, S.S. 2002, 'Calcium Intake Influences the Association of Protein Intake with Rates of Bone Loss in Elderly Men and Women', *American Journal of Clinical Nutrition*, vol. 75, no. 6, pp. 773–9.

Faber, A.D. & Wasserman, S. 2002, 'Social Support and Social Networks: Synthesis and Review', *Social Networks and Health*, vol. 8, pp. 29–72.

Featherstone, M. & Hepworth, M. 1995, 'Images of Positive Ageing: A Case Study of Retirement Magazine', in M. Featherstone & M. Hepworth (eds), *Images of Ageing: Representations of Later Life*, Routledge, New York.

Federal Interagency Forum on Aging Related Statistics 2000, *Older Americans 2000: Key Indicators of Well-being*, Washington, DC.

Fiatarone, M. & Evans, W. 1993, 'The Etiology and Reversibility of Muscle Dysfunction in the Aged', *Journal of Gerontology*, vol. 47, September, pp. 77–83.

FIFARS—*see* Federal Interagency Forum on Aging Related Statistics.

Flegal, K.M. 1996, 'Trends in Body Weight and Overweight in the US Population', *Nutrition Reviews*, vol. 54, no. 4 (supp.), pp. 97–100.

Frongillo, E.A., Jr, Rauschenbach, B.S., Roe, D.R. & Williamson, D.F. 1992, 'Characteristics Related to Elderly Persons' Not Eating for 1 or More Days: Implications for Meal Programs', *American Journal of Public Health*, vol. 82, no. 4, pp. 600–2.

Gerth, H. & Mills, C.W. 1946, *From Max Weber: Essays in Sociology*, Oxford University Press, New York.

Giddens, A. 1991, *Modernity and Self-identity: Self and Society in the Late Modern Age*, Stanford University Press, Stanford, California.

Gokhale, J. & Kotlikoff, L.J. 1998, 'Medicare from the Perspective of Generational Accounting', paper presented at the Medicare Reform: Issues and Answers conference, Bush School of Government and Public Service, Texas A&M University, College Station, 3 April.

Green, B.L. & Wang, M.Q. 1995, 'The Effects of Missing Meals on the Dietary Adequacy of the Elderly: The 1987–1988 National Food Consumption Survey', *Wellness Perspectives*, vol. 11, no. 4, pp. 64–8.

Guthrie, J.F. & Lin, B.-H. 2002, 'Overview of the Diets of Lower- and Higher-Income Elderly and Their Food Assistance Options', *Journal of Nutrition Education and Behavior*, vol. 34, supp. 1, pp. S31–S41.

Hendy, H.M., Nelson, G.K. & Greco, M.D. 1998, 'Social Cognitive Predictors of Nutritional Risk in Rural Elderly Adults', *International Journal of Aging and Human Development*, vol. 47, no. 4, pp. 299–327.

House, J.S., Umberson, D. & Landis, K. 1988, 'Structures and Processes of Social Support', *Annual Review of Sociology*, vol. 14, pp. 293–318.

Howard, J.H., Gates, G.E., Ellersieck, M.R. & Dowdy, R.P. 1998, 'Investigating Relationships between Nutritional Knowledge, Attitudes and Beliefs, and Dietary Adequacy of the Elderly', *Journal of Nutrition for the Elderly*, vol. 17, no. 4, pp. 35–52.

Jackson, L.A. 1992, *Physical Appearance and Gender: Sociological and Sociocultural Perspectives*, State University of New York, Albany.

Jassen, H.C., Samson, M.M. & Verhaar, H.J.J. 2002, 'Vitamin D Deficiency, Muscle Function, and Falls in Elderly People', *American Journal of Clinical Nutrition*, vol. 75, no. 4, pp. 611–15.

Jette, A. 1996, 'Disability Trends and Transitions', in R.H. Binstock & L.K. George (eds), *Handbook of Aging and the Social Sciences*, 4th edition, Academic Press, San Diego.

Kivett, V.R., Stevenson, M.L. & Zwane, C.H. 2000, 'Very-old Rural Adults: Functional Status and Social Support', *Journal of Applied Gerontology*, vol. 19, no. 1, pp. 58–77.

Klesges, L.M., Pahor, M., Shorr, R.J., Wan, J.Y. & Williamson, J.D. 2001, 'Financial Difficulty in Acquiring Food among Elderly Disabled Women: Results from the Women's Health and Aging Study', *American Journal of Public Health*, vol. 91, no. 1, pp. 68–75.

Krehl, W.A. 1964, 'Nutrition in Medicine', *American Journal of Clinical Nutrition*, vol. 15, no. 2, pp. 191–4.

Kubena, K. & McMurray, D. 1996, 'Nutrition and the Immune System: A Review of Nutrient–Nutrient Interactions', *Journal of the American Dietetic Association*, vol. 96, no. 11, pp. 1156–64.

Lee, J.S. & Frongillo, E.A., Jr. 2001, 'Nutritional and Health Consequences are Associated with Food Insecurity among U.S. Elderly Persons', *Journal of the American Dietetic Association*, vol. 131, no. 5, 1503–9.

Manton, K. 1989, 'Epidemiological, Demographic, and Social Correlates of Disability among the Elderly', *Milbank Memorial Quarterly*, vol. 67, supp. 2, part 1, pp. 13–58.

Marmot, M. & Theorell, T. 1988, 'Social Class and Cardiovascular Disease', *International Journal of Health Service*, vol. 8, no. 4, pp. 1–13.

McIntosh, W.A. 1996, *Sociologies of Food and Nutrition*, Plenum, New York.

——, Kaplan, H.B., Kubena, K.S. & Landmann, W.A. 1995, 'Life Events, Social Support, and Immune Response in Elderly Individuals', in J. Hendricks (ed.), *Health and Health Care Utilization in Later Life*, Baywood, Amityville, New York State.

——, Kubena, K.S. & Landmann, W.A. 1989, *Social Support, Stress, and the Diet and Nutrition of the Aged: Final Report to the National Institute on Aging*, Department of Rural Sociology, Texas A&M University, College Station.

——, Kubena, K.S., Landmann, W.A. & Dvorak, S. 1988, *A Comparative Assessment of the Social Networks of Elderly Disabled and Non-disabled*, paper presented at the annual meeting of the American Sociological Association, Atlanta, August.

——, Shifflett, P.A. & Picou, J.S. 1989, 'Social Support, Stress, Strain, and the Dietary Intake of the Elderly', *Medical Care*, vol. 21, no. 2, pp. 140–53.

Moen, P. 1996, 'Gender, Age, and the Life Course', in R.H. Binstock & L.K. George (eds), *Handbook of Aging and the Social Sciences*, 4th edition, Academic Press, San Diego.

Moody, H.R. 1994, *Aging: Concepts and Controversies*, Pine Forge Press, Thousand Oaks, California.

Murphy, S.P., Davis, M.A., Neuhouse, J.M. & Lein, D. 1990, 'Factors Influencing the Dietary Adequacy and Energy Intake of Older Americans', *Journal of Nutrition Education*, vol. 22, no. 6, pp. 284–91.

Nord, M. 2002, 'Food Security Rates are High for Elderly Households', *Food Review*, vol. 25, no. 2, pp. 19–24.

Palmore, E. 1990, *Ageism: Negative and Positive*, Springer, New York.

Payette, H., Gray-Donaldson, K., Cyr, R. & Boutier, V. 1995, 'Predictors of Dietary Intake in a Functionally Dependent Elderly Population in the Community', *American Journal of Public Health*, vol. 85, no. 5, pp. 667–83.

Pierce, M.B., Sheehan, N.W. & Ferris, A.M. 2002, 'Nutrition Concerns of Low-Income Elderly Women and Related Social Support', *Journal of Nutrition for the Elderly*, vol. 21, no. 3, pp. 37–53.

Ponza, M., Ohls, J.C. & Millen, B.E. 1997, *Serving the Elderly at Risk, The Older Americans Act Nutrition Programs, National Evaluation of the Elderly Nutrition Program, 1993–1995*, Agency on Aging, National Aging Information Center, Washington, DC.

Poppendieck, J. 1998, *Sweet Charity? Emergency Food and the End of Entitlement*, Viking Penguin, New York.

Quinn, M.E., Johnson, M.A., Poon, L.W., Martin, P. & Nickols-Richardson, S.M. 1997, 'Factors of Nutritional Health-seeking Behaviors: Findings from the Georgia Centenarian Study', *Journal of Aging and Health*, vol. 9, no. 1, pp. 90–104.

Rogers, R. 1996, 'The Effects of Family Composition, Health, and Social Support Linkages on Mortality', *Journal of Health and Social Behavior*, vol. 37, no. 4, pp. 326–38.

Rose, D. & Oliveria, V. 1997, 'Nutrient Intakes of Individuals from Food Insufficient Households in the United States', *American Journal of Public Health*, vol. 87, no. 12, pp. 1956–61.

Rowley, T.D. 2000, *Food Assistance Needs of the South's Vulnerable Populations*, Southern Rural Development Center, Mississippi State University, Starkville, Mississippi.

Schoenbach, V.J., Kaplan, B.H. & Kleinbaum, D.G. 1986, 'Social Ties and Mortality in Evans County, Georgia', *American Journal of Epidemiology*, vol. 123, no. 4, pp. 577–91.

Schoenberg, N.E., Coward, R.T., Gilbert, G.H. & Mullens, R.A. 1997, 'Screening Community-dwelling Elders for Nutritional Risk: Determining the Influence of Race and Residence', *Journal of Applied Gerontology*, vol. 16, no. 2, pp. 172–89.

Seeman, T.E., Berkman, L.F., Kohout F., LaCroix, A. & Blazer, D. 1993, 'Intercommunity Variations in the Association between Social Ties and Mortality in the Elderly: A Comparative Analysis of Three Communities', *Annual Review of Epidemiology*, vol. 3, pp. 325–35.

Shilling, C. 1994, *The Body and Social Theory*, Sage, Newbury Park, New York State.

Silverman, P., Hecht, L. & McMillin, J.D. 2002, 'Social Support and Dietary Change among Older Adults', *Ageing and Society*, vol. 22, no. 1, pp. 29–59.

Smith, A.D. 2002, 'Homocystine, B vitamins, and Cognitive Deficit in the Elderly', *American Journal of Clinical Nutrition*, vol. 75, no. 6, pp. 785–6.

Surtees, P.G., Wainwright, N.W.J., Kaw, K.-T. 2004, 'Obesity, Confidant Support, and Functional Health: Cross-Sectional Evidence from the EPIC-Norfolk Cohort', *International Journal of Obesity*, vol. 28, March, pp. 748–58.

Thoits, P.A. 1995, 'Stress, Coping, and Social Support Processes: Where are We? What Next?', *Journal of Health and Social Behavior*, vol. 36 (supp.), pp. 53–79.

Turrow, J. 1997, *Breaking up America: Advertisers and the New Media World*, University of Chicago Press, Chicago.

Umberson, D., Wortman, C. & Kessler, R. 1992, 'Widowhood and Depression: Explaining Low-term Gender Differences in Vulnerability', *Journal of Health and Social Behavior*, vol. 33, no. 1, pp. 10–24.

Verbrugge, L.M. 1990, 'The Iceberg of Disability', in S.M. Stahl (ed.), *The Legacy of Longevity: Health and Health Care in Later Life*, Sage, Newbury Park, New York State.

Vitolins, M.Z., Quandt, S.A., Bell, R.A., Arcury, T.A. & Case, L.D. 2002, 'Quality of Diets Consumed by Older Rural Adults', *Journal of Rural Health*, vol. 18, no. 1, pp. 49–56.

Walker, D. & Beauchene, R. 1991, 'The Relationship of Loneliness, Social Isolation, and Physical Health of Independently Living Elderly', *Journal of the American Dietetic Association*, vol. 90, no. 12, pp. 1667–72.

Weddle, D., Wellman, N. & Shoaf, L. 1996, 'Position of the American Dietetic Association: Nutrition, Aging, and the Continuum of Care', *Journal of the American Dietetic Association*, vol. 96, no. 10, pp. 1048–52.

Wolinsky, F., Coe, R.M., McIntosh, W.A., Kubena, K.S., Prendergast, J.M., Chavez, M.N., Miller, D.K., Romeis, J.C. & Landmann, W.A. 1990, 'Progress in the Development of a Nutritional Risk Index', *Journal of Nutrition*, vol. 120, pp. 1549–53.

Wylie C. 2000, 'Health and Social Factors Affecting the Food Choices and Nutritional Intake of Elderly People with Restricted Mobility', *Journal of Human Nutrition and Dietetics*, vol. 13, no. 5, pp. 363–71.

Yasuda, N., Zimmerman, S.I., Hawkes, D., Fredman, L., Hebel, J.R. & Magaziner, J. 1997, 'Relation of Social Network Characteristics to 5-Year Mortality among Young-Old versus Old-Old White Women in an Urban Community', *American Journal of Epidemiology*, vol. 145, no. 6, pp. 516–23.

PART 5
Food and the Body: Civilising Processes and Social Embodiment

When you don't have any money, the problem is food. When you do have money, it's sex. When you have both, it's health.

J. P. Donleavy, *The Ginger Man* (1955)

Certainly these days, when I hear people talking about temptation and sin, guilt and shame, I know they're referring to food rather than sex.

Carol Sternhell, quoted in Rothblum (1994, p. 53)

Food is abundant in developed countries, and food manufacturers use the media to continuously and persuasively encourage people to enjoy the full pleasures of food consumption. Consumers have embraced this trend, and the last decade has seen the rise of the celebrity chef and recipe books featuring strongly on bestselling book lists. Counter to the food hedonism trend, the disciplining of the body emerged in the late twentieth century. The increasing focus on the body has contributed to healthism, an ideology that views health as the primary human goal. The sins of gluttony and sloth have had renewed attention and can be seen in secular attitudes of lipophobia (fear of fat). For some people, particularly women, these attitudes have translated into a lifelong quest for the holy grail of the 'thin ideal', which at its most extreme can be seen in sufferers of eating disorders. Others face the daily stigma of obesity, where fatism—open prejudice against overweight people—remains widespread. These attitudes are reflected in the health messages espoused by various health authorities, health 'experts' and diet-related industries. Regimes of body control, particularly through the regulation of food intake, are common features of Western culture. The connections between food and the body, in terms of food culture and the social construction of body ideals (and body taboos), are the focus of this final part of the book. Specifically, this section consists of three chapters:

- Chapter 15 explores the social construction of the thin ideal in Western societies and how women adopt, modify or resist the social pressure of rigid regimes of body management and dieting. In particular, body acceptance is considered as an alternative discourse through which women resist the thin ideal. This chapter provides the foundation for the next two chapters that examine more extreme issues around the body.
- Chapter 16 examines eating disorders, highlighting the limitations of the medical model, and discusses the contributions of feminist and social constructionist approaches.
- Chapter 17 provides a sociological analysis of the stigmatisation of obesity and discusses how individuals cope with a 'fat identity'.

CHAPTER 15

Constructing the Female Body: Dieting, the Thin Ideal and Body Acceptance

Lauren Williams and John Germov

OVERVIEW

- What are the social origins of the thin ideal for women and how is it perpetuated?
- How do women respond to the thin ideal?
- Is body acceptance an effective response to the thin ideal?

Gender differences in food consumption remain one of the clearest examples of the social appetite—in short, women often eat differently to men. The social norms governing women's appearance and behaviour result in concern about the implications of food consumption for the look of the female body. The thin ideal is the desired aesthetic look for women's bodies in contemporary Western societies and its pursuit—primarily through dieting—significantly influences women's food choices. This chapter examines why dieting is predominantly a female behaviour by exploring the historical, structural, cultural and critical factors that have contributed to the development of, and resistance to, the thin ideal. The ability of some women to achieve body acceptance is conceptualised using Anthony Giddens' theory of self-identity to explain how certain social processes enable women to exercise their agency.

Key terms

agency
body acceptance
body image
body mass index (BMI)
eating disorders
emancipatory politics
epidemiology
fatism

feminist
gender socialisation
life politics
maternal ideal
muscular ideal
obesity
patriarchy
post-structuralist

reflexive modernity
social construction
social control
social embodiment
stigma
structuralist
thin ideal

Introduction: The thin ideal and the sexual division of dieting

The term '**thin ideal**' refers to the social desirability of a slender body shape in Western societies. A thin body is considered the epitome of beauty and sexual attractiveness, and has been linked to social status, health and even moral worth. In today's advanced capitalist societies, food is readily available and social worth is increasingly measured by a person's ability to resist excess. The moralistic censure of sloth and gluttony is a remnant of earlier Christian values that focused on purifying the soul and disciplining the body through abstinence and penance, and on purging oneself of excess (Schwartz 1986; Turner 1992).

As the overriding aesthetic ideal of female beauty, the thin ideal has significant implications for women's eating patterns. Dieting, or the conscious manipulation of food choice and eating patterns to reduce or maintain weight, is a common response to the thin ideal. Since the thin ideal is directed at women, it is unsurprising that dieting is primarily a female act. Women often assess food in terms of its dieting value, dividing foods into 'dieting' (good) and 'fattening' (bad) foods (Sobal & Cassidy 1987; McKie et al. 1993; Germov & Williams 1996a). Several authors have described the gendered nature of eating, particularly women's ambivalent relationship with food, their bodies, and the provision of food for significant others (Burgoyne & Clarke 1983; Murcott 1983; Charles & Kerr 1988; DeVault 1991). At its most extreme, gendered eating and body discipline presents as **eating disorders** (see Chapter 16; Hepworth 1999). Dieting requires a considerable investment of time and money, as well as emotional and physical resources. Kelly Brownell and Judith Rodin (1994) note that the unsuccessful nature of diets can lead to a cycle of 'yo-yo' dieting or 'weight cycling', with detrimental physiological and psychological consequences. For many women, dieting results in a lifelong 'tug of war' with food, to the extent that the act of eating is imbued with feelings of guilt, anxiety and deprivation.

The number of people seeking weight control has been measured in Western nations. Table 15.1 shows the evidence from population studies of the proportion of women and men who reported seeking to lose or maintain weight, and their methods of doing so, in the United States of America, Europe, the United Kingdom and Australia.

In a substudy of the Australian Longitudinal Study on Women's Health (ALSWH), Lauren Williams and colleagues found that 74 per cent of more than 11 000 women in the mid-age cohort (47–52 years) reported trying to control their weight, and that only one in five of these women was happy with her weight (Williams et al. 2007). Forty-three per cent wanted to lose more than 6 kilograms in weight. Dietary restriction was used more frequently than exercise, and two-thirds of those seeking weight control used a combination of two or more weight control practices. (Further detail on the combinations of weight control practices used are included in Table

Table 15.1   Population studies of women and men engaged in weight control in Europe, the UK, the USA and Australia

Research group and study purpose	Sample and method	Findings
United Kingdom		
Wardle. et al. 2000 : Examined whether respondents were trying to control their weight, and whether they performed any of a list of 11 dietary practices.	N=1894 (938 male; 956 female) Mean age 46.8y Data collected by interview as part of Omnibus Survey by Office of National Statistics UK in 1999. Stratified probability sample, women and men selected by random sampling of private households. 70% response rate	36% of people were 'watching their weight to avoid weight gain' (36% of women, 36% of men) 28% were trying to lose weight (36% of women, 21% of men) The five most common dietary practices reported by women trying to lose weight: • 76% plenty fruit and vegetables • 73% limit fried food • 72% limit fats • 69% eat breakfast • 67% avoid sweets The five most common dietary practices reported by men trying to lose weight: • 65% plenty fruit and vegetables • 65% eat breakfast • 62% avoid sweets • 57% limit fried food • 56% limit fats
Europe		
McElhone et al. 1999: Assessed body satisfaction (against silhouettes) and five weight loss strategies	N=15 239 (7098 male; 7907 female) Aged over 15 years The survey was conducted in the 15 member states of the EU between March and April 1997 with approximately 1000 participants per country. Interview-assisted Omnibus survey.	44% of respondents wanted to be 'lighter' (51% of women; 36% of men) and a further 10% 'considerably lighter' (13% of women; 8% of men) Weight loss methods used by women wanting to be lighter or considerably lighter: • Diet: 17% (lighter) and 27% (considerably lighter) • Exercise: 10% and 8% • Diet and exercise: 10% and 12% • Medication: 1% and 1% • Other methods: 7% and 7% Weight loss methods used by men wanting to be lighter or considerably lighter: • Diet: 11% (lighter) and 16% (considerably lighter) • Exercise: 11% and 12% • Diet and exercise: 8% and 9% • Medication: 0 and 0 • Other methods: 4% and 5%

Table 15.1 Population studies of women and men engaged in weight control in Europe, the UK, the USA and Australia (continued)

Research group and study purpose	Sample and method	Findings
USA		
Serdula et al. 1999: Examined prevalence of weight loss and maintenance, and strategies used to control weight (in terms of dietary change or exercise)	N=107 804 (46220 male; 61584 male) Adults over 18 years Part of the Behavioural Risk Factor Surveillance System that uses telephone to survey a representative random sample from across USA. 77.9% response rate.	36.43% trying to lose weight (28.8% of men; 43.6% of women) 33.7% trying to maintain (keep from gaining) weight (35.1% of men; 34.4% of women) Strategies used by those trying to lose weight: • Modified diet: 86.6% of men and 92.2% of women • Ate less fat only: 34.9% of men and 40.0% of women • Physical activity: 66.9% of men and 65.7% of women • Exercise for 150 mins/wk and eat fewer calories: 21.5% men and 19.4% women Strategies used by those trying to maintain weight: • Modified diet: 59.5% of men and 70.8% of women • Ate less fat only: 31.7% of men and 42.6% of women • Physical activity: 52.0% of men and 48.1% of women • Exercise for 150 mins/wk and eat fewer calories: 13.0% men and 10.0% women
Australia		
Williams et al. 2007: Assessed prevalence and effectiveness of 12 weight control practices	N=11 589 women aged 47–52 Part of the Australian Longitudinal Study on Women's Health. Representative national sample, completing a written survey every three years.	74% of the cohort (8556 women) reported trying to control their weight (weight loss or maintenance), 81% of those were seeking weight loss The five most common combinations of practices used by women trying to lose weight: • Exercise + cut size of meals and snacks+ cut down on fats and sugars (41%) • Cut size of meals and snacks + cut down on fats and sugars (20.0%) • Exercise + cut size of meals and snacks + cut down on fats and sugars + commercial weight loss program (9.3%) • Cut down on fats and sugars (7.4%) • Exercise (5.0%) The five most common combinations of practices used by women trying to maintain weight: • Exercise + cut size of meals and snacks+ cut down on fats and sugars (33.5%) • Cut size of meals and snacks + cut down on fats and sugars (15.3%) • Exercise (14.0%) • Cut down on fats and sugars (12.5%) • Exercise + cut down on fats and sugars (9.0%)

15.1.) The majority of the cohort, using a variety of weight control combinations, gained more weight on average over a two-year period than the 26 per cent of women who reported doing nothing to control their weight. This provides some **epidemiological** evidence to the thesis that dietary restraint results in ultimate weight gain (Tiggemann 2004).

Many women who diet are actually within the medically defined 'healthy weight range' for their height according to the **body mass index** (see Box 15.1). Surveys

BOX 15.1

Body Mass Index (BMI) and definitions of overweight

In the health sciences, 'overweight' and 'obese' are generally defined in terms of BMI. A person's BMI is calculated by dividing their weight in kilograms by their height in metres squared:

$$BMI = \frac{weight (kg)}{height (m2)}$$

For example, if a person weighed 67 kilograms and was 1.6 metres tall, their BMI would be 26.17 (67 divided by 2.56). The World Health Organization (WHO), using BMI, has defined the following weight ranges for both women and men:

BMI range	WHO category
<18.50	Underweight
18.50–24.99	Normal
25.00–29.99	Grade I overweight
30.00–34.99	Grade IIa* overweight
35.00–39.99	Grade IIb* overweight
40+	Grade III* overweight

* BMI greater than 30 is often referred to as 'obese'

Source: WHO (2000)

A 'normal' or 'healthy' weight range is generally considered to be a BMI of between 18.5 and 24.9, 'underweight' is below 18.5, 'overweight' is equal to or above 25 and 'obese' is equal to or above 30. These international standards are relatively new and different cut-offs for each category have been used by researchers in different parts of the world. While BMI can be useful for population-wide epidemiological studies, concerns have been raised about the appropriateness of a standard BMI measure for individuals because of the physiological differences between women and men and between some ethnic groups.

Lauren Williams and John Germov

in Australia throughout the 1980s and 1990s showed that more men than women were above their healthy weight range, even though more women attempted to diet (National Heart Foundation 1990; Australian Bureau of Statistics 1997). Australian figures based on objectively measured height and weight show that 67 per cent of men and 52 per cent of women aged 25 or over were overweight or **obese** (Dunstan et al. 2000). More recent data show that this relationship persists, with more men than women overweight or obese (AIHW 2006).

Why is the thin ideal so pervasive?

Why is seeking to conform to the thin ideal a female project? **Feminist** writers have generally approached this vexed question either from the opposing philosophical perspectives of **structuralist** feminism (liberal, Marxist and radical feminism) or **post-structuralist** feminism. Structuralist theories assume that the lives of individuals are primarily determined by the society in which they live. The focus is on the large-scale features of society—such as the economy, political system and dominant culture—and on how these structures shape individual and group behaviour. Post-structuralist theories developed as a critique of these structuralist approaches on the premise that they fail to adequately theorise how individuals shape society. Post-structuralist approaches generally abandon the search for universal causes (Annandale & Clarke 1996). Post-structuralist theorists focus on human **agency** and **social construction**. Women are not conceived of as passive adherents to the thin ideal, but rather, 'It is women themselves who practise this discipline on and against their own bodies … This self-surveillance is a form of obedience to patriarchy … [a woman becomes] a body designed to please or excite' (Wearing 1996, p. 88).

The pressure to conform to the thin ideal cannot be explained by either perspective in isolation. The thin ideal clearly has structural elements, perpetuated by various social institutions and commercial interests, such as the media, fashion and cosmetics industries. The health sector has also participated in the development and perpetuation of the thin ideal, with anti-fat messages that equate health with thinness. These structural factors have clear antecedents in the historical development of **patriarchy**, particularly in terms of the social regulation of the female body (Schwartz 1986; Turner 1992). However, post-structural factors, which represent women's subjectivity and agency—that is, the way women respond to the social pressure of the thin ideal on a daily basis—also play an important role.

This chapter aims to bridge these two perspectives by discussing the interplay between the patriarchal social structure and female agency; how the thin ideal shapes women's attitudes to food and eating, and how women adopt, modify or reject these social ideals. Before exploring these issues further, the next section considers the historical antecedents and cultural determinants of the thin ideal.

Thin ideal antecedents: A brief historical overview

How and why did the thin ideal emerge, and why were women singled out as its subjects? While the thin ideal is a relatively recent phenomenon, the historical antecedents of the **social control** of women's bodies are well documented (Rubin 1975; Ehrenreich & English 1979; Turner 1992; Corrigan & Meredyth 1994; Hesse-Biber 1996). The socially desired body ideal may change over time, in terms of size and shape, but the existence of an ideal for women to aspire to has remained constant.

The female ideal of the nineteenth century was a large, curved body, which connoted fertility, wealth and high status (Bordo 1993; Seid 1994). While poor women were occupied with physical work, the voluptuous women of the middle and upper classes were often viewed as objects of art, luxury, status, virtue and beauty. Fatness was linked to emotional stability, strength (stored energy), good health and refinement; to leisure rather than labour. The undergarment industry came to the rescue of the naturally thin woman with products such as inflatable rubber attachments (complete with dimples) to give that rounded, full-figured look (Seid 1994). These appearance norms for women reinforced patriarchal beliefs about female sexuality (Rothblum 1994).

The first break with the voluptuous tradition of the nineteenth century came in the 1920s with the 'flappers'. These thin women were financially and sexually independent, partly as a result of World War I, which left many women in charge of their dead husbands' estates. The term 'flapper' was used to trivialise the 'new independent woman', as Banner (1983, p. 279) states:

> On the one hand, she indicated a new freedom in sensual expression by shortening her skirts and discarding her corsets. On the other hand, she bound her breasts … and expressed her sensuality not through eroticism, but through constant, vibrant movement … The name 'flapper' itself [was drawn] from a style of flapping galoshes popular among young women before the war; it connoted irrelevant movement and raised the spectre of a seal with black flapping paws.

Thus, these women rejected the dominant patriarchal ideal of feminine appearance—and the passivity that went with it—and assumed a more masculine ideal; the new liberated woman was to dress, act and look more like a man (thin and without curves) (Hesse-Biber 1991; 1996). However, when women lose their curves they tend to become smaller and can appear physically weak. This phase in the redefinition of women's bodies occurred during a time of female political activism in the USA and the UK, as the suffragette movement pressed for women's right to vote. While women entered the public sphere and increased their profile and power, the ideal female body inversely decreased in size.

Other factors contributed to the emergence of the thin female ideal. The food shortages caused by the Great Depression in 1929, followed by World War II, led to austerity measures and a subsequent concern with the link between food and health. These decades marked the start of calorie-counting and use of food for its energy value (Schwartz 1986). Such measures imposed a dieting mentality on the population, especially women, as the primary gatekeepers of food in the family. The prosperity that followed the end of World War II, together with the rise of the food manufacturing industry, saw the balance shift back to food abundance during the 1950s in Western societies. As a number of authors have noted (Beller 1977; Mennell 1985), when food is scarce, cultural ideals favour a large body, whose 'abundance' symbolises wealth and status. Conversely, in times of plenty, social values shift towards disciplining food intake, and the thin body becomes the ideal.

The contemporary thin ideal

The contemporary thin ideal was born in the 1960s and was epitomised by the model Twiggy (whose name alluded to her slight frame) as well as by actresses such as Audrey Hepburn and Grace Kelly. By the 1970s, a rare coalescence of factors emerged to reinforce the thin ideal: medical science, government authorities and the fashion industry all adopted an anti-fat stance. At the same time, medical and epidemiological studies began to find links between obesity and premature mortality. In Chapter 17, Jeffery Sobal discusses the changing social attitudes towards 'fat' and the rise of obesity **stigmatisation**. While dieting and the cultural aversion to 'fat' have historical underpinnings that predate contemporary health warnings (see Schwartz 1986), the well-intentioned anti-fat messages of health professionals and government agencies may have reinforced and legitimised the thin ideal (Germov & Williams 1996a).

Roberta Seid (1994) argues that the second wave of feminism in the 1970s initially embraced a super-fit, thin ideal as a celebration of women's strength and control. Such body control was regarded as a positive symbol of femininity, in contrast to the aesthetics of previous centuries, which conceptualised women as invalids (the 'weaker sex') or as maternal icons (useful for their reproductive capacity). Both of these stereotypes were used to support orthodox views that women should be 'protected' from physical and intellectual labour, and that they were dependent on men. Actress Jane Fonda was a vocal feminist in the 1970s and 1980s, and promoted health and beauty through physical fitness by positing the thin ideal as a break from the **maternal ideal**. Marjorie Ferguson's content analysis of women's magazines at that time (1983, p. 113) notes the influence of the self-help movement on contemporary femininity, bringing about a shift in editorial emphasis 'towards greater self-realisation, self-determination, and the presentation of a more independent and assertive femininity'. This development, which paralleled the growth of consumerism and individualism in advanced capitalist societies, reflected the magazines' profitable marketing strategy of teaming the thin ideal with women's sexual and economic liberation. As Fonda and various imitators discovered, the focus on female self-help and independence through body discipline tapped into a new market of potential consumers. Fonda, who has admitted suffering from an eating disorder and having had cosmetic surgery, presents an interesting case study of a celebrity, well known for advocating women's emancipation from patriarchy (in terms of economic and sexual liberation) while at the same time playing a significant part in reinforcing their subjugation to the patriarchal thin ideal—liberation from the beauty myth was seemingly not part of her agenda.

Body backlash: The continued social control of women's bodies

Susan Faludi (1991) and Naomi Wolf (1990) argue that it is no accident that the current thin ideal emerged during the second wave of feminism, a period of increased female sexual and socioeconomic liberation. As Sharlene Hesse-Biber states, 'when women are "demanding more space" in terms of equality of opportunity, there is a cultural demand that they "should shrink"… Thinness may be considered a sign of conforming to a constricting feminine image, whereas weight may convey a strong, powerful image' (1991, p. 178). This echoes the era of the flappers where the rise of women's political and social status resulted in a female body ideal that was diminutive and weak. However, as we shall see later, this time around the social control over women's bodies has not only been exercised through the external industries of fashion, cosmetics, fitness and the media, but through the internalisation of the thin ideal by women.

Popular portrayal of the thin ideal

Models and celebrities have been the overt public face of changes in beauty standards over recent decades. Compare, for example, the figure of Marilyn Monroe in the 1950s with that of Elle Macpherson in the 1980s, and contemporary figures such as Kate Moss, Eva Herzigova, Heidi Klum and Paris Hilton. Content-analysis studies of magazines, beauty pageants, Hollywood movies and television programs have consistently found that the female beauty ideal has become thinner with time (Silverstein et al. 1986; Morris et al. 1989). Moreover, experimental studies have found that exposure to media images of thin bodies increases female body dissatisfaction (Groesz et al. 2002).

Figures 15.1, 15.2 and 15.3 show three cover designs of Australia's popular women's magazine *Cleo* to trace the presentation of women by the structural interests of the media, advertising and fashion industries over the past 30 years, from the 'self-help days' of the early 1970s to the engineered 'insecurity' of the early 1990s and the new millennium.

Figure 15.1   *Cleo* magazine cover, January 1973

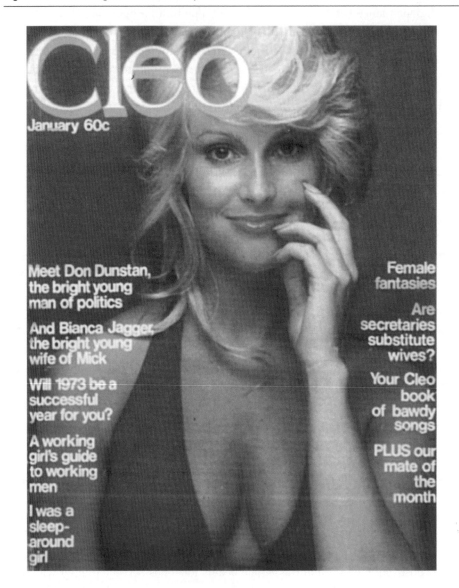

- Meet Don Dunstan, the bright young man of politics
- And Bianca Jagger, the bright young wife of Mick
- Will 1973 be a successful year for you?
- A working girl's guide to working men
- I was a sleep-around girl
- Female fantasies
- Are secretaries substitute wives?
- Your Cleo book of bawdy songs
- PLUS our mate of the month

Figure 15.2 *Cleo* magazine cover, January 1983

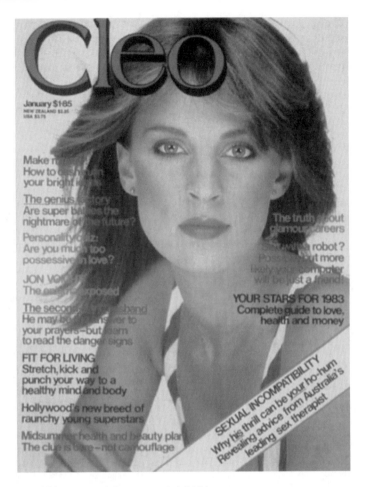

- Make money! How to cash in on your bright ideas
- The genius factory: Are super babies the nightmare of the future?
- Personality quiz: Are you too possessive in love?
- JON VOIGHT: The engima exposed
- The second-hand husband: He may be the answer to your prayers—but learn to read the danger signs
- FIT FOR LIVING: Stretch, kick and punch your way to a healthy mind and body
- Hollywood's new breed of raunchy young superstars
- Midsummer health and beauty plan: The clue is care—not camouflage
- The truth about glamour careers
- Sex with a robot? Possible, but more likely your computer will just be a friend!
- YOUR STARS FOR 1983: Complete guide to love, health and money
- SEXUAL INCOMPATIBILITY: Why <u>his</u> thrill can be <u>your</u> ho-hum. Revealing advice from Australia's leading sex therapist

Lauren Williams and John Germov

Figure 15.3   *Cleo* magazine cover, January 1993

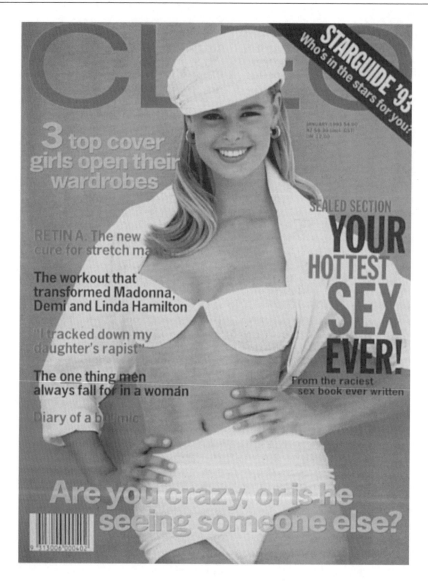

- 3 top cover girls open their wardrobes
- RETIN A: The new cure for stretch marks!
- The workout that transformed Madonna, Demi and Linda Hamilton
- 'I tracked down my daughter's rapist'
- The <u>one</u> thing men always fall for in a woman
- Diary of a bulimic
- Are you crazy, or is he seeing someone else?
- SEALED SECTION: YOUR HOTTEST SEX EVER! From the raciest sex book ever written
- STARGUIDE '93. Who's in the stars for you?

The image on the cover of the January 1973 *Cleo* is a sexual presentation of an attractive blonde model with a plunging halter-top. The picture stops just below the breasts. The woman has her hand to her face in a submissive gesture and is smiling into the camera with a 'knowing' look. This cover shot reflects the content of some of the headlines, which have an emphasis on sexual liberation. There is a notable absence of articles relating to dieting, exercise or the body.

The 1983 model is an attractive brunette in a head-and-shoulders shot, turned side-on below the shoulders so that we do not see her breasts. She has an almost vacant, expressionless look on her face. The image is one of attractive wholesomeness, rather than sexuality. By the 1980s, the stories no longer focus on sexual liberation, but on the need for a health and beauty plan. The magazine has learned that encouraging insecurity is the best strategy for ensuring a sustainable readership ('Are you much too possessive in love?'). The emphasis on money in the first-listed headline story reflects both the increased financial independence of women and the rise of the 'decade of greed'.

The January 1993 cover shows a three-quarter body shot in which the model's body is exposed but in a stance that is more athletic than sexy. The model is wearing a white bathing costume with full pants rather than revealing briefs. By the 1990s, the focus on body insecurity has intensified: readers are exposed to the wardrobes of models and the workouts of movie stars, neither of which most readers have any hope of attaining. Thus the thin ideal is glamorised and made apparently accessible (if you just read the health and beauty section!). The dangers of body insecurity are poignantly reflected in the 'Diary of a bulimic'. Encouragement of insecurity about men, sex and life-management continues—you need to read the 'stars' to know how to meet men, and if you already have a man, you need to ask 'are you crazy or is he seeing someone else?'

By 2003, little had changed, with the August issue of *Cleo* headlining stories on 'why sex is the new breakfast' and 'pick up tricks you can learn from a guy', a 'sealed section' on 'tattoos, piercings and designer waxes', and special features on shoes, hair and weddings (image not shown). The cover photo shows well-known actor Kate Hudson, who is thin, blonde and blue-eyed. The use of actors on covers, which has become increasingly common is, according to Cyndi Tebbel (2000), an attempt by magazines to move away from using supermodels towards what the industry terms 'real women'. Unfortunately, the bodies of these women are no more attainable than those of the models. Early in the twenty-first century, the ranks of thin ideal role models continue to swell, particularly among actors and pop singers—for example, Jennifer Aniston, Nicole Kidman, Kylie Minogue, Paris Hilton, Mischa Barton and Victoria Beckham. In the face of a constant barrage of glamorous images, it is little wonder that the number of cosmetic surgery procedures for breast augmentation, face lifts, collagen injections and liposuction continue to rise. The non-surgical procedure of botox—a wrinkle treatment based on injecting small amounts of the highly toxic botulinum (the product of the bacterium that causes botulism)—has proven to be a popular treatment, resulting in a generation of Hollywood actresses and TV personalities with faces unable to show expression.

Occasionally the mass media takes an opposing perspective on women's bodies. Figure 15.4 depicts a front cover of the Australian *Who Weekly* magazine. It is one of the few examples of the mass media being critical of the thin ideal. This picture was seized upon by the media in Australia as an example of how the (mid 1990s) trend towards the 'waif look', promoted by the modelling and fashion industry, had pushed

Figure 15.4   *Who Weekly* cover, 27 May 1996, issue no. 222 (reproduced courtesy of WHO WEEKLY)

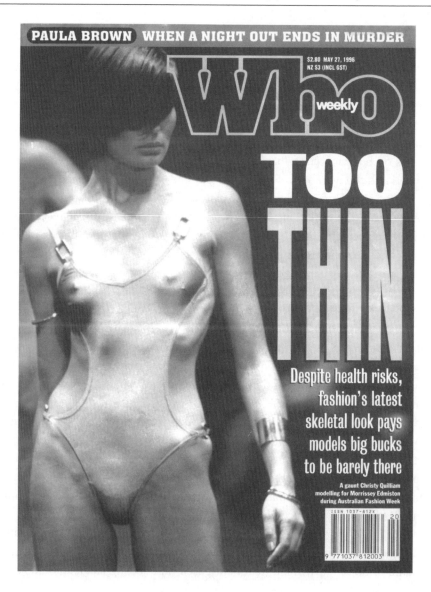

the thin ideal too far. At the time, model Sophie Dahl and actor Kate Winslet were touted as successful women who challenged the dominance of the thin ideal. In both cases this was short-lived, with both women shedding kilos to attract work. Dahl went as far as claiming she was never a role model for body diversity. Winslet has commented on her ongoing struggle to resist dieting to gain more acting work, but ultimately embraced a more conformist body shape. Clearly, examples that challenge the thin ideal remain transitory and marginal. Nonetheless, they show that the thin ideal can be undermined.

Men have also increasingly become subject to social pressure over their bodies, though their experience is quite distinct to that of women (see Box 15.2).

Men and body image: The muscular ideal

While men are also subject to social pressure regarding their bodies, particularly in the context of obesity stigmatisation, their experience is considerably different to that of women. Even though more men than women are overweight, men report less body dissatisfaction, are less concerned about their bodies, and are less likely to be on a weight loss diet (Grogan 1999). The social pressure on men is to achieve a **muscular ideal** that indicates strength and masculinity. Rather than promoting weight-loss and slenderness, the male body ideal exaggerates masculine traits to convey power and dominance. Men generally indicate a preference for a larger, more muscular body, and will sometimes undergo cosmetic surgery or take supplements detrimental to their health to achieve it (such as anabolic steroids and human growth hormone). Epitomised by Arnold Schwarzenegger in the 1980s and more recently by Dwayne Douglas Johnson ('The Rock'), the muscular ideal has become widespread, as evidenced by the ubiquitous athletic-looking male model sporting highly toned musculature, a defined chest, large biceps, and a 'six pack' of well-defined abdominal muscles.

BOX 15.2

The thin ideal for women and the muscular ideal for men are well entrenched by adolescence (Grogan 1999; Nowak et al. 2001). Women and men are exposed to these body ideals from childhood through the process of **gender socialisation**. Consider, for example, the popular Barbie doll made by Mattel. This doll, with annual sales of US$1 billion (*New York Times Magazine*, 27 May 1994; O'Brien 1997), is tall, thin, long-legged and slim-waisted and has a flat stomach, square shoulders, large eyes and curved red lips. Ken Norton and colleagues (1996) undertook a study in which they scaled the anthropometric measurements of the Barbie doll to adult size, finding that the probability of an adult woman having a Barbie-like body shape is less than one in 100 000. Interestingly, they also scaled the Ken doll (the male equivalent of

Lauren Williams and John Germov

Figure 15.5   The Body Shop's 'Ruby' Campaign (reproduced with permission of The Body Shop International PLC)

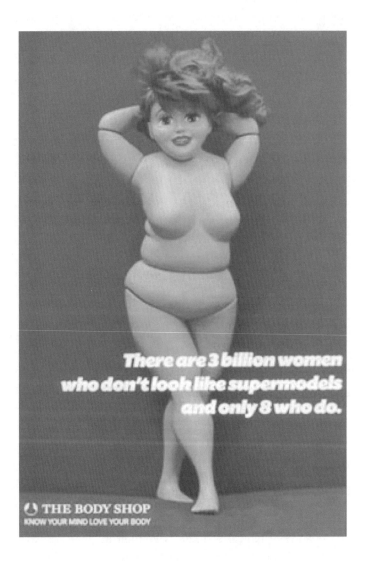

the Barbie doll, produced and marketed by the same company), and found it to have a 'more realistic' body shape, likely to be found in one in every 50 males. This makes Barbie's figure 2000 times less attainable than Ken's, reflecting the fact that women are encouraged to aspire to a more unrealistic body ideal than men. The Body Shop produced its own version of Barbie, a full-figured doll named 'Ruby', as part of its campaign for body diversity. The company was initially forced to withdraw the doll as a result of pressure from Mattel, which considered the doll's features to be too similar to those of its idealised best-seller; the Body Shop subsequently released a revised version (Smith 1998).

Factors influencing the thin ideal today

Structuralist approaches to the thin ideal

In explaining the emergence of the thin ideal, a structuralist would maintain that it is the outcome of a patriarchal society, in which powerful men and the various industries and social institutions they control (structural factors) construct the 'beauty myth' for their own material and political benefit (Wolf 1990; Bordo 1993). These structural factors clearly have an impact on cultural beliefs, particularly in terms of gender socialisation, by constructing and promoting a particular ideal of female beauty.

The rise of consumerism led the **body image** industries to develop a 'sure-fire' formula for success: promote a thin ideal of beauty that the majority of women can never attain and thereby create virtually infinite demand among consumers. With the high proportion of people worldwide trying to lose weight, and dieting being a popular strategy, the diet industry is a significant economic force. The weight-loss industry has shown an impressive ability to continually reinvent itself, as witnessed by the emergence of new 'fad diets' (the Zone diet being a recent example) and the resurgence of old fad diets such as the Atkins diet. Moreover, a plethora of 'infomercials' on late-night and daytime TV advertise exercise equipment and diet supplements that promise to give buyers model-like bodies with a minimum of effort. The pharmaceutical industry continues to release so-called 'anti-obesity' drugs, which have significant side effects and have had only modest results to date. The irony of the weight-loss industry is that its very existence depends on the failure of its products. In what other industry would customers repeatedly pay large sums of money for products and services that do not work? The weight-loss industry has been clever enough to sustain its market share by placing the blame on the consumer, with caveats that their products will only work if used in combination with 'a sensible diet and regular exercise'.

As thinness became synonymous with health and beauty, the female body became increasingly exploited by both corporate interests and government health authorities. Calls to exercise self-control over one's body for the health benefits and for the sake of social conformity expanded upon the cultural values of individualism and self-responsibility. Women's magazines thus became an important sphere of influence for perpetuating the thin ideal. An example of the extent of this influence is conveyed by the former editor of *New Woman* magazine in Australia, Cyndi Tebbel (2000), who claimed to have lost her job because the magazine featured a 'Big Issue', which supported International No Diet Day, used size-16 models, and promoted body diversity. According to Tebbel, sales of the magazine were not affected, but advertisers complained and threatened to withdraw, risking up to 50 per cent of the total revenue of the magazine (Tebbel 2000). Consequently, the magazine returned to featuring thin models and to stories promoting body insecurity. This illustrates the fact that the cosmetics, fitness and fashion industries will not tolerate a message that acts against their vested commercial interests—that is, a message challenging the dominant ideal of female beauty.

While gender is clearly a major factor in explaining the cultural preoccupation with the thin ideal, there is conflicting evidence on the role that ethnicity plays, if any. A US study by Sheila Parker and others (1995) examined the body image and dieting behaviours of African–American and white adolescent females. They found that the African–American girls exhibited significantly less body dissatisfaction, and greater appreciation of body diversity and of large female bodies, than their white counterparts, who tended to be rigid adherents to the thin ideal. While the African–American girls studied tended to have a lower prevalence of dieting and were less concerned about body weight and shape than were the white girls, this may not apply to all ethnic groups in the USA. A major US study of over 17 000 adolescent girls found that ethnicity, as opposed to skin colour, did not 'protect' against body dissatisfaction or dieting behaviour, concluding that ethnic subcultures are just as affected by the thin ideal as white mainstream culture (French et al. 1997). Similar findings have been reported in Australia, which show that ethnicity did not mediate the influence of the thin ideal within a Western society (O'Dea 1998; Ball & Kenardy 2002).

The role of female agency in perpetuating the thin ideal

In contrast to a structuralist analysis, which focuses on the external forces that exert pressure on women to conform to a thin ideal, post-structuralist feminist theorists are concerned with the role played by women themselves in reproducing and resisting the thin ideal (Bartky 1990; Blood 2005). Post-structuralists do not deny the importance of the historical and cultural factors discussed above, but, rather than viewing these factors as all-determining, they stress the importance of female subjectivity and deal with the complex and subtle facets of the social construction of women's bodies.

It is commonly stated that some women use body control to demonstrate their control over other aspects of their lives. As the January 1993 *Cleo* cover shows (Figure 15.3), the 'successful woman' is financially independent, sexually liberated and thin. However, Sandra Bartky argues that 'a tighter control of the body has gained a new kind of hold over the mind' (1990, p. 81). The thin body has become an essential symbol of modern femininity and a new form of social control of women's bodies; body regulation is self-inflicted, administered by women on themselves through dieting, starvation, excessive exercise and, at the extreme, plastic surgery. Therefore, there is a self-imposed component in the pressure to conform. Women are not simply passive sponges of coercive patriarchal structures and cultural stereotypes. In effect, the social control of women's bodies becomes internalised by the women themselves.

The desire to be seen as attractive and the pressure to conform socially are power-ful reasons for weight control. The social importance placed on women's appearance can be so great that some women value weight loss above success in love or work (Charles & Kerr 1988; Wolf 1990). As Edwin Schur argues, 'physical appearance is much more central to evaluations of women than it is to evaluations of men; this emphasis implicitly devalues women's other qualities and accomplishments; women's "looks" thereby become a commodity and a key determinant of their "success" or "failure"' (1983, p. 68). Hesse-Biber (1991; 1996) argues that women are socialised to focus on physical appearance in order to receive social acceptance, while for men public achievement determines social worth and self-image. As Margaret Duncan states (1994, p. 50), women learn to 'compare their appearance with that of the patriarchal feminine ideal and thus become objects for their own gaze'.

Dieting and pursuit of the thin ideal can thus be viewed as a rational response by women striving for acceptance in the context of the dominant ideals of beauty, sexuality and femininity. The internalisation of patriarchal norms explains the active role women play in perpetuating the thin ideal (Bartky 1990). Women police their own bodies and the bodies of other women in a process of constant surveillance. In this way, the thin ideal is reinforced and perpetuated without coercion and often with women's consent. We have previously described this process of women's body monitoring as the 'body panopticon' effect (Germov & Williams 1999; see also Duncan 1994; Foucault 1979).

Our research has documented the myriad responses by women to the thin ideal (Germov & Williams 1996b). The benefit of a post-structuralist approach is that it sheds light on the active role that women play in the social construction of the thin ideal. While such an approach helps to explain the pervasiveness of the thin ideal, self-surveillance does not occur in a social vacuum and is reinforced by structural interests, such as the fashion, weight-loss, fitness, health and cosmetic industries.

Towards a synthesis of the structuralist and post-structuralist approaches

Both structuralist and post-structuralist perspectives are important in understanding the pressure on women to diet to attain the thin ideal—but can they be reconciled? On its own, neither perspective offers a complete explanation of why women diet. For example, structuralist explanations tend to imply that women are easily duped or even 'brainwashed' by the media, the fashion industry and men to succumb to the thin ideal. However, such an analysis ignores the fact that not all men act as oppressors of women (either consciously or implicitly) and that some women consciously and effectively resist the pressure to conform to the thin ideal. In an attempt to bridge these two approaches, we suggest that dieting and the thin ideal must be understood within a theoretical schema that acknowledges structural factors and female agency, but that avoids explanations of dieting behaviour as simply a matter of individual lifestyle choice. We have illustrated this model in Figure 15.6.

Lauren Williams and John Germov

Figure 15.6   The social and cultural reproduction of the thin ideal

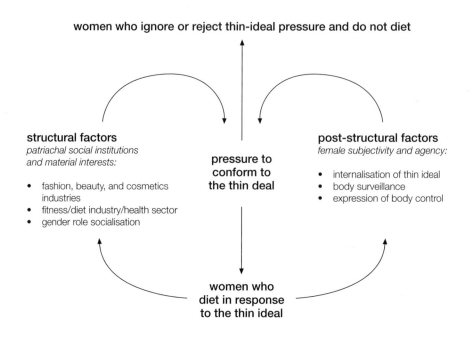

The starting point of Figure 15.6 is the pressure put on women in Western society to conform to the thin ideal. Women can respond to the pressure in one of two ways: by ignoring or actively rejecting the thin ideal, which takes them out of the cycle (as represented by the upward arrow); or, alternatively, by responding to the thin ideal by dieting, which results in gendered food and restrained eating practices. The lists of structural and post-structural factors summarise the key modes by which the pressure to conform to the thin ideal is produced and reproduced (the arrows indicate the direction of influence). Dieting behaviour reinforces both structural interests (for example, the dieting industry) and post-structural factors (for example, self-surveillance), which in turn reinforce pressure to conform to the thin ideal and dieting behaviour, and the cycle continues.

Challenges to the thin ideal

Incorporating the concept of female agency to understand the production of the thin ideal also allows for the possibility of women rejecting this ideal in favour of an alternative ideal—that of **body acceptance**. Not all women respond to the thin ideal by internalising it and making it an integral part of their identity. Nor do all women perpetuate the thin ideal by reinforcing it in their relationships with and evaluations of other women. Responses to the thin ideal can be divided into the categories listed in Table 15.2. This categorisation scheme has more to do with whether or not women choose to conform to the thin ideal, and with the subsequent effect on their eating behaviour, than it has to do with actual body weight. Category 1 refers to the thin ideal 'body conformers' who diet to lose weight, either permanently or on an 'on again, off again' basis, which often results in weight cycling. Women who diet or who consciously restrict their eating (by eating low-fat, low-calorie foods, for example) may be of any weight, but will probably tend to be thinner than other women. The women in category 4, whom we have called 'body acceptors', do not diet, possibly because they have failed to achieve their desired weight and have decided to be unrestrained eaters, or because they have consciously rejected the thin ideal and accepted body diversity. As a group, they will tend towards being heavier than the dieters. In category 3 are the 'weight maintainers', who have never had to diet to stay thin and are unrestrained eaters. These women are able to conform to the thin ideal easily. It is possible that if their weight were to increase, they would move to category 1. A further group are the 'health maintainers' (category 2), who do not pursue or conform to the thin ideal, but may seek to lose weight to improve their health or prevent the onset of disease (such as type 2 diabetes). Body accepting women move out of the cycle depicted in Figure 15.6, thereby challenging the dominance of the thin ideal. Enough individuals are choosing this option to constitute an emerging social movement, variously termed the 'anti-dieting', 'size acceptance' or 'fat rights' movement (Sobal 1999).

Table 15.2 Responses to the thin ideal

	Thin ideal acceptors	Thin ideal rejector
Diet to lose weight	*Category 1: Body conformers* Women who diet in pursuit of the thin ideal	*Category 2: Health maintainers* Women who diet for clear health benefits and not for aesthetic reasons
Do not diet	*Category 3: Weight maintainers* Women who are naturally slim and do not need to diet	*Category 4: Body acceptors* Women who accept body diversity and derive their self-identity from factors other than conforming to the thin ideal

Reflexive modernity, female identity and life politics

According to Anthony Giddens (1991), we live in an age of **reflexive modernity** in which social practices are increasingly questioned and changed as alternatives to past actions and beliefs come to light. The body, particularly the female body, has become a 'reflexive project', whereby the appearance of the body becomes a social marker of self-identity. The conscious monitoring and revision of appearance, behaviours and beliefs produces what Giddens refers to as **life politics**, defined as 'a politics of lifestyle' (1991, p. 214).

The life politics of body acceptance creates a bridge between the internal and external body—between self-identity and social identity. In an increasingly reflexive society, the conscious monitoring and revision of behaviours and beliefs creates the possibility of a socially reconstructed self-identity derived from life experiences and alternative body discourses. Furthermore, some women may translate their life politics of body acceptance into what Giddens (1991) refers to as **emancipatory politics**—that is, they may become body acceptance advocates and engage in public debate to undermine the dominance and salience of the thin ideal. For Giddens, emancipatory politics embodies a commitment to social justice and aims to reduce or eliminate discrimination and exploitation. Emancipatory body politics can be seen in the numerous groups and organisations that have formed to liberate women from the thin ideal. Representative organisations include the International Size Acceptance Association (ISAA) and the National Association to Advance Fat Acceptance (NAAFA), which disseminate information and publicity material to promote body diversity, and lobby governments and corporations about addressing size discrimination and **fatism** (Solovay 2000).

Critics of Giddens' notion of life politics and reflexivity argue that, when applied to women, such concepts tend to privilege self-determination and underestimate patriarchal constraints (McNay 2000; Frost 2001). Giddens does acknowledge the limits on lifestyle choice, saying that the existence of 'a multiplicity of choices is not to suppose that all choices are open to everyone … the selection or creation of lifestyles is influenced by group pressures and the visibility of role models, as well as by socioeconomic circumstances' (1991, p. 82).

Evidence of alternatives to the thin ideal

Few empirical studies have investigated women who have ceased dieting. Those studies that have been conducted suggest the ability of some women to resist the thin ideal involves personal reflection, and is mediated by the ageing process, life achievements and self-esteem (Blood 1996; 2005; Williams & Germov 2004; Tunaley et al. 1999; Paquette & Raine 2004). Jillian Tunaley and colleagues (1999) interviewed 12 women between 63 and 75 years of age and found that even though the women reported some body dissatisfaction, they tended to dismiss the social pressure to be thin by viewing weight gain as an 'inevitable' by-product of ageing and judging the pursuit of a body ideal to be of less importance than the pursuit of their own interests. Sylvia Blood interviewed six New Zealand women between the ages of 23 and 39 about why they stopped dieting and rejected 'the myth of the "ideal body"' (1996, p. 111). Blood found that the cessation of dieting tended to occur once women developed 'self-acceptance' and countered 'the self-condemnation of body size' through an awareness of the negative influence on body image of external factors such as the media (1996, p. 112). Marie-Claude Paquette and Kim Raine (2004) interviewed 44 Canadian women between 21 and 61 years of age to explore personal and socio-cultural influences on body image. They found that despite the powerful effect of the media and other influences, a proportion of the women had come to accept their bodies through a process of reflection and empowerment.

In qualitative research conducted with Australian women, we found that body acceptance can be the result of a history of failed dieting, or it can be based on the decision to end the pain of the dieting process and the obsession with one's body (Williams & Germov 2004). Participants were drawn from a large established national cohort of mid-aged women participating in the ALSWH (Brown et al. 1998). Twenty women (aged 47–51) who indicated in the 1996 ALSWH survey that they were satisfied with their weight and had not dieted to lose weight in the previous year were interviewed. The women were all in the medically defined 'healthy weight range' despite the fact that the study only deliberately excluded underweight women. The semi-structured interview protocol investigated the way the participants felt about their bodies and the factors influencing these body-image beliefs.

Although all participants had previously reported weight satisfaction and non-dieting behaviour in the earlier ALSWH survey, when interviewed it became apparent that they did not all reject the thin ideal (see Table 15.2). The 12 thin ideal conformers were divided into 'body conformers' (category 1 in Table 15.2) and 'weight maintainers' (category 3). The weight maintainers remained thin without dieting, had been 'naturally' thin all their lives; 'never having what you'd call a weight problem' as one participant put it. For the thin ideal conformers, maintaining a slim body was central to their self-identity. These women valued a general aesthetic preference for thinness and some even espoused victim-blaming attitudes towards those they deemed overweight.

The remaining eight women espoused attitudes that did not conform to the thin ideal and were identified as thin ideal rejectors; two of these eight indicated they would only diet to lose weight for health reasons and only if they gained a significant amount of weight, and were designated as 'health maintainers' (category 2); the remaining six were in category 4, 'body acceptors'. These women tended to value body diversity and derived their self-identity from factors other than conformity to the thin ideal including: self-acceptance based on life achievements, the influence of significant others, and non-discriminatory personal beliefs.

Among the body-accepting participants, self-identity was not based on 'body work' and thin-ideal conformity, but rather on life achievements and key life events. For these mid-age participants events such as motherhood, menopause, and workplace achievements were cited as fundamental influences on self-identity. As the women matured, self-identity was no longer derived from the 'external body', but rather focused on 'internal' factors such as self-esteem and self-worth derived from life achievements. These findings illustrate Giddens' (1991) reflexive self in action, as some women exercised their agency to construct an alternative life politics to counteract or override the influence of the thin ideal.

While life achievements were an alternative basis of self-identity for the body-accepting women in this study, life politics need not imply that voluntarism is

Lauren Williams and John Germov

the basis of body acceptance, because the experiences and choices of individuals are influenced by social practices. Participants commonly cited family members, and particularly partners, as either positive or negative influences on their body acceptance, highlighting that the formation of self-identity is a social process rather than solely a product of self-determination.

The final theme to emerge from the study was that of non-discriminatory beliefs about others. Participants' acceptance of their own bodies also tended to be extended to the bodies of others, and they supported body diversity as opposed to one ideal body type. A few participants also went further and drew a link between non-judgmental attitudes about physical features and non-discriminatory views regarding gender and ethnicity. Their acceptance of body diversity was characteristic of a broader tolerance of diversity and difference in society in line with Giddens' concept of emancipatory politics. This sheds light on how individuals' life politics can become the basis of social movements such as the fat-rights and anti-dieting movements.

Conclusion

This chapter has outlined the historical, structural and cultural factors that underlie the reasons why women diet and why the thin ideal is so pervasive. A critical conceptual framework was adopted to reconcile structuralist and post-structuralist approaches. Women are not merely victims of patriarchal and capitalist imperatives, nor are they simply free to adopt or reject the thin ideal as they please. Some women actively participate in the reproduction of the thin ideal, while others resist it by constructing alternative discourses, such as that of body acceptance. We argue for a nuanced approach that conceptualises a 'body project' that accounts for the influence of both social structure and agency on female identity. Raewyn Connell (2002, p. 47) refers to this process as **social embodiment**—that is, 'human social conduct in which bodies are both agents and objects'. While some women pursue the life politics of the thin ideal, albeit under significant social pressure, there is evidence that others construct their self-identity through alternative lifestyles. This framework attempts to move beyond both deterministic and voluntaristic assumptions of women's identity formation in order to understand how some women resist patriarchal social pressure and reject the thin ideal.

The empirical research conducted into body acceptance has shown that age and external influences affect body acceptance in women. We found that non-discriminatory attitudes contribute to the acceptance of the body in all its diversity. Such life politics or lifestyle factors, as Giddens states, create a set of routinised practices that 'give material form to a particular narrative of self-identity' (1991, p. 81). The anti-dieting and size-acceptance social movements, which have modelled themselves on the successful civil rights and women's liberation movements, provide an alternative form of social acceptance (of body diversity) by attempting to influence cultural and institutional practices. The rejection of the thin ideal and the promotion of body acceptance are key strategies through which body dissatisfaction and associated unnecessary and harmful dieting practices can be challenged. The extent to which health professionals will embrace this movement remains to be seen (see Box 15.3).

Responses of health professionals to body acceptance

In addition to activist organisations, some health professionals are also recommending body acceptance as part of a new health promotion paradigm (Parham 1996; 1999; Kassirer & Angell 1998; Herrin et al. 1999; Higgins & Gray 1999; Ikeda 2000; Ikeda et al. 1999; Jutel 2001; Miller & Jacob 2001; see Strain 1999 for a contrary view). These authors advocate an approach that does not equate thinness with health, nor fatness with increased risk of chronic disease. They argue that overweight people can be fit and healthy. While they do not dispute obesity-related health risks, they maintain that there is little evidence to support the position that weight loss per se improves health in overweight individuals. They note the continuing high failure rate of weight-loss diets; the rising prevalence of overweight, despite the widespread promotion of weight loss by health authorities; the detrimental effects of weight cycling; and the fact that chronic dieting is a risk factor for eating disorders.

Debate continues in the obesity literature over paradoxical empirical findings that suggest intentional weight loss is linked to increased mortality (Sørensen 2003; Yang et al. 2003). Given such a situation, some health professionals believe it is inappropriate to promote weight loss, particularly in the context of the social pressure of the thin ideal and the likelihood that many people use unhealthy practices to lose weight for aesthetic reasons. Dietitians such as Joanne Ikeda and Ellen Parham advocate alternative strategies to minimise health risks and promote positive self-esteem, body acceptance, healthy eating and moderate exercise, rather than dieting, weight loss and an idealised body size and shape—epitomised in the 10 basic tenets of size acceptance listed below. However, this is a contentious issue within the dietetic profession itself, with some dietitians opposing the promotion of body acceptance.

Ten basic tenets of size acceptance:

1. Human beings come in a variety of sizes and shapes. We celebrate this diversity as a positive characteristic of the human race.
2. There is no ideal body size, shape or weight that every individual should strive to achieve.

▶

BOX 15.3

Lauren Williams and John Germov

BOX 15.3 CONTINUED

3. Every body is a good body, whatever its size or shape.

4. Self-esteem and body image are strongly linked. Helping people feel good about their bodies, and about who they are, can help motivate and maintain healthy behaviours.

5. Appearance stereotyping is inherently unfair to the individual because it is based on superficial factors that the individual has little or no control over.

6. We respect the bodies of others even though they might be quite different from our own.

7. Each person is responsible for taking care of his/her body.

8. Good health is not defined by body size; it is a state of physical, mental and social well-being.

9. People of all sizes and shapes can reduce their risk of poor health by adopting a healthy lifestyle.

10. Health promotion programs should celebrate the benefits of a healthy lifestyle. Programs should be accepting of and sensitive to size diversity. They should promote body satisfaction and the achievement of realistic and attainable health goals without regard to weight change.

Source: Ikeda (2000)

Acknowledgments

The research reported in this chapter was supported by a grant awarded by the University of Newcastle, Australia. Thanks are due to Michelle Powers for her assistance in gathering and organising the qualitative body acceptance results into text, Jane Potter for research assistance and Jean Ball (data manager for the ALSWH project) for selecting the participants. We also thank the women themselves for giving so generously of their time and of themselves. The 10 basic tenets of size acceptance were developed by dietitians and nutritionists who are advocates of size acceptance; their efforts were coordinated by Joanne P. Ikeda, Department of Nutritional Sciences, University of California, Berkeley, USA.

SUMMARY OF MAIN POINTS

- A sexual division of dieting exists, in which dieting to lose weight is primarily a female act.
- The thin ideal has historical origins and is linked to events that have enhanced women's social status and power.

- Sociological explanations of why women diet can be divided into two broad categories: structuralist and post-structuralist.
- The representation of women as victims of patriarchal subordination has been successfully critiqued by post-structuralist feminist theorists through a renewed focus on women's agency and subjective experiences of femininity.
- An understanding of why women diet and of the persistence of the thin ideal requires a synthesis of structural and post-structural factors.
- Giddens' concepts of life politics and emancipatory politics provide a useful theoretical framework for understanding the interplay of structure and agency in the social construction of women's bodies and identities in Western society.
- Women react to the thin ideal in myriad ways—accepting, reinforcing and resisting the dominant discourse.
- Resistance of the thin ideal through body acceptance is an alternative gaining social momentum.

SOCIOLOGICAL REFLECTION

- Do you accept your own body? Do you judge other people's bodies?
- If you are a woman, reflect on where you fit into the schema presented in Table 15.2. Have you always been in this category, or have you changed the way you respond to your body? If so, what do you think caused that change?
- If you are male, what body-ideal pressures are you subject to? Are these pressures equivalent to the pressures on women to conform to the thin ideal?

DISCUSSION QUESTIONS

1. What are the differences between the structuralist and post-structuralist perspectives on the thin ideal?
2. How did the thin ideal originate, and why did it become so pervasive?
3. How do women perpetuate the thin ideal?
4. In what ways do you think women's and men's notions of body acceptance differ? What are some of the key factors that influence whether women and men accept their body?
5. Should health professionals in countries with a high prevalence of overweight and obesity promote body acceptance?
6. Discuss the potential of the size acceptance movement to dismantle the thin ideal. Do you think this could happen in your lifetime?

Lauren Williams and John Germov

Further investigation

1. Some authors argue that there is a parallel between Victorian attitudes to sex and modern attitudes to food, such that 'food rules have become as dour and inhibitory as the sex rules of the 19th century' (Seid 1994, p. 8). Discuss the implications of this quote with reference to gender and food.
2. The media is to blame for the thin ideal and the associated harmful dieting practices and eating disorders of many women. Discuss.
3. How have health professionals contributed to the reinforcement or dismantling of the thin ideal?
4. To what extent could the promotion of body acceptance challenge the thin ideal? What evidence have you seen that an alternative body ideal may be emerging?

FURTHER READING AND WEB RESOURCES

Books

Blood, S.K. 2005, *Body Work: The Social Construction of Women's Body Image*, Routledge, London.

Bordo, S. 1993, *Unbearable Weight: Feminism, Western Culture and the Body*, University of California Press, Berkeley.

Brownell, K.D., Puhl, R.M., Schwartz, M.B. & Rudd, L. (eds) 2005, *Weight Bias: Nature, Consequences, and Remedies*, Guilford Press, New York.

Davis, K. (ed.) 1997, *Embodied Practices: Feminist Perspectives on the Body*, Sage, London.

Fallon, P., Katzman, M.A. & Wooley, S.A. (eds) 1994, *Feminist Perspectives on Eating Disorders*, Guilford Press, New York.

Gimlin, D.L. 2002, *Body Work: Beauty and Self-Image in American Culture*, University of California Press, Berkeley.

Grogan, S. 1999, *Body Image: Understanding Body Dissatisfaction in Men, Women and Children*, Routledge, London.

Hesse-Biber, S. 1996, *Am I Thin Enough Yet? The Cult of Thinness and the Commercialization of Identity*, Oxford University Press, New York.

Schwartz, H. 1986, *Never Satisfied: A Cultural History of Diets, Fantasies and Fat*, The Free Press, New York.

Sobal, J. & Maurer, D. (eds) 1999, *Weighty Issues: Fatness and Thinness as Social Problems*, Aldine de Gruyter, New York.

Tebbel, C. 2000, *The Body Snatchers: How the Media Shapes Women*, Finch Publishing, Sydney.

Weitz, R. (ed.) 2003, *The Politics of Women's Bodies: Sexuality, Appearance, and Behavior*, 2nd edition, Oxford University Press, New York.

Articles and book chapters

Corrigan, A. & Meredyth, D. 1997, 'The Body Politic', in K. Pritchard Hughes (ed.), *Contemporary Australian Feminism 2*, 2nd edition, Longman, Melbourne.

Germov, J. & Williams, L. 1996, 'The Sexual Division of Dieting: Women's Voices', *Sociological Review*, vol. 44, no. 4, pp. 630–47.

Kassirer, J.P. & Angell, M. 1998, 'Losing Weight: An Ill-fated New Year's Resolution', *New England Journal of Medicine*, vol. 338, pp. 52–4.

Miller, W.C. & Jacob, A.V. 2001, 'The Health at Any Size Paradigm for Obesity Treatment: The Scientific Evidence', *Obesity Reviews*, vol. 2, pp. 37–45.

Parham, E.S. 1999, 'Promoting Body Size Acceptance in Weight Management Counseling', *Journal of the American Dietetic Association*, vol. 99, no. 8, pp. 920–6.

Williams, L., Germov, J. & Young, A. 2007, 'Preventing Weight Gain: A Population Cohort Study of the Nature and Effectiveness of Mid-age Women's Weight Control Practices', *International Journal of Obesity*, vol. 31, pp. 978–86.

Documentaries

Fat Files, 1999, BBC/Learning Channel Co-production, four episodes, 153 minutes.

Killing Us Softly 3: Advertising's Image of Women, 2000, Media Education Foundation, Northampton, Massachusetts, 35 minutes.

The Strength to Resist: The Media's Impact on Women and Girls, 2000, Cambridge Documentary Films, Cambridge, Massachusetts, 33 minutes.

Websites

About-Face: about-face.org/

Adios Barbie: www.adiosbarbie.com/

Health at Any Size Web Ring: http://d.webring.com/hub?ring=anysize

Healthy Weight Network: www.healthyweightnetwork.com/

International Size Acceptance Association: www.size-acceptance.org/

Mirror Mirror: www.mirrormirror.com.au

National Association to Advance Fat Acceptance: naafa.org/

Women's Health Australia—The Australian Longitudinal Study on Women's Health: www.alswh.org.au/

REFERENCES

AIHW—*see* Australian Institute of Health and Welfare.

Annandale, E. & Clarke, J. 1996, 'What is Gender? Feminist Theory and the Sociology of Human Reproduction', *Sociology of Health and Illness*, vol. 18, no. 1, pp. 17–44.

Australian Bureau of Statistics 1997, *National Nutrition Survey Selected Highlights, Australia 1995* (cat. no. 4802.0), Australian Bureau of Statistics, Canberra.

Australian Institute of Health and Welfare 2006, *Australia's Health 2006*, Australian Institute of Health and Welfare, Canberra.

Ball, K. & Kenardy, J. 2002, 'Body Weight, Body Image and Eating Behaviours: Relationships with Ethnicity and Acculturation in a Community Sample of Young Australian Women', *Eating Behaviors*, vol. 3, no. 3, pp. 205–16.

Banner, L.W. 1983, *American Beauty*, Knopf, New York.

Bartky, S.L. 1990, *Femininity and Domination: Studies in the Phenomenology of Oppression*, Routledge, New York.

Beller, A.S. 1977, *Fat and Thin: A Natural History of Obesity*, Farrar, Strauss & Giroux, New York.

Blood, S.K. 1996, 'The Dieting Dilemma: Factors Influencing Women's Decision to Give up Dieting', *Women & Therapy*, vol. 18, pp. 109–18.

—— 2005, *Body Work: The Social Construction of Women's Body Image*, Routledge, London.

Bordo, S. 1993, *Unbearable Weight: Feminism, Western Culture and the Body*, University of California Press, Berkeley.

Brown, W.J., Byles, J.E., Dobson, A.J., Lee, C., Mishra, G. & Scofield, M. 1998, 'Women's Health Australia: Recruitment for a National Longitudinal Cohort Study', *Women and Health*, vol. 28, pp. 23–40.

Brownell, K.D. & Rodin, J. 1994, 'The Dieting Maelstrom: Is It Possible and Advisable to Lose Weight?', *American Psychologist*, vol. 49, no. 9, pp. 781–91.

Burgoyne, J. & Clarke, D. 1983, 'You Are What You Eat: Food and Family Reconstruction', in A. Murcott (ed.), *The Sociology of Food and Eating*, Gower, Aldershot, UK.

Charles, N. & Kerr, M. 1988, *Women, Food and Families*, Manchester University Press, Manchester.

Connell, R.W. 2002, *Gender*, Polity Press, Cambridge.

Corrigan, A. & Meredyth, D. 1994, 'The Body Politic', in K. Pritchard Hughes (ed.), *Contemporary Australian Feminism*, Longman, Melbourne.

DeVault, M.L. 1991, *Feeding the Family: The Social Organization of Caring as Gendered Work*, University of Chicago Press, Chicago.

Duncan, M.C. 1994, 'The Politics of Women's Body Images and Practices: Foucault, the Panopticon and Shape Magazine', *Journal of Sport and Social Issues*, vol. 18, no. 1, pp. 48–65.

Dunstan, D., Zimmet, P., Welborn, T. et al. 2000, *Diabesity and Associated Disorders in Australia: The Final Report of the Australian Diabetes, Obesity and Lifestyle Study (AusDiab)*, International Diabetes Institute, Melbourne.

Ehrenreich, B. & English, D. 1979, *For Her Own Good: 150 Years of the Experts' Advice to Women*, Feminist Press, New York.

Faludi, S. 1991, *Backlash: The Undeclared War Against Women*, Chatto & Windus, London.

Ferguson, M. 1983, *Forever Feminine: Women's Magazines and the Cult of Femininity*, Heinemann, London.

Foucault, M. 1979, *Discipline and Punish*, Penguin Books, Harmondsworth.

French, S.A., Story, M., Neumark-Sztainer, D., Downes, B., Resnick, M. & Blum, R. 1997, 'Ethnic Differences in Psychosocial and Health Behavior Correlates of Dieting, Purging, and Binge Eating in a Population-based Sample of Adolescent Females', *International Journal of Eating Disorders*, vol. 22, no. 3, pp. 315–22.

Frost, L. 2001, *Young Women and the Body: A Feminist Sociology*, Palgrave, Hampshire.

Germov, J. & Williams, L. 1996a, 'The Sexual Division of Dieting: Women's Voices', *The Sociological Review*, vol. 44, no. 4, pp. 630–47.

—— 1996b, 'The Epidemic of Dieting Women: The Need for a Sociological Approach to Food and Nutrition', *Appetite*, vol. 27, pp. 97–108.

—— 1999, 'Dieting Women: Self-surveillance and the Body Panopticon', in J. Sobal & D. Maurer (eds), *Weighty Issues: Constructing Fatness and Thinness as Social Problems*, Aldine de Gruyter, New York, pp. 117–32.

Giddens, A. 1991, *Modernity and Self-identity*, Stanford University Press, California.

Groesz, L.M., Levine, M.P. & Murnen, S.K. 2002, 'The Effect of Experimental Presentation of Thin Media Images on Body Satisfaction: A Meta-analytic Review', *International Journal of Eating Disorders*, vol. 31, pp. 1–16.

Grogan, S. 1999, *Body Image: Understanding Body Dissatisfaction in Men, Women and Children*, Routledge, London.

Hepworth, J. 1999, *The Social Construction of Anorexia Nervosa*, Sage, London.

Herrin, M., Parham, E., Ikeda, J., White, A. & Branen, L. 1999, 'Alternative Viewpoint on National Institutes of Health Clinical Guidelines', *Journal of Nutrition Education*, vol. 31, no. 2, pp. 116–18.

Hesse-Biber, S. 1991, 'Women, Weight and Eating Disorders: A Socio-cultural and Political-economic Analysis', *Women's Studies International Forum*, vol. 14, no. 3, pp. 173–91.

—— 1996, *Am I Thin Enough Yet? The Cult of Thinness and the Commercialization of Identity*, Oxford University Press, New York.

Higgins, L. & Gray, W. 1999, 'What Do Anti-dieting Programs Achieve? A Review of Research', *Australian Journal of Nutrition and Dietetics*, vol. 56, no. 3, pp. 128–36.

Ikeda, J.P. 2000, 'Health Promotion: A Size Acceptance Approach', *Healthy Weight Journal*, January/February, pp. 10–12.

Ikeda, J.P., Hayes, D., Satter, E., Parham, E.S., Kratina, K., Woolsey, M., Lowey, M. & Tribole, E. 1999, 'A Commentary on the New Obesity Guidelines from NIH', *Journal of the American Dietetic Association*, vol. 99, no. 8, pp. 918–19.

Jutel, A. 2001, 'Does Size Really Matter? Weight and Values in Public Health', *Perspectives in Biology and Medicine*, vol. 44, no. 3, pp. 283–96.

Kassirer, J.P. & Angell, M. 1998, 'Losing Weight: An Ill-fated New Year's Resolution', *New England Journal of Medicine*, vol. 338, pp. 52–4.

McElhone, S., Kearney, J.M., Giachetti, I., Zunft, H.F. & Martínez, J.A. 1999, 'Body Image Perception in Relation to Recent Weight Changes and Strategies for Weight Loss in a Nationally Representative Sample in the European Union', *Public Health Nutrition*, vol. 2, pp. 143–51.

McKie, L.J., Wood, R.C. & Gregory, S. 1993, 'Women Defining Health: Food, Diet and Body Image', *Health Education Research*, vol. 8, no. 1, pp. 35–41.

Mennell, S. 1985, *All Manners of Food: Eating and Taste in England and France from the Middle Ages to the Present*, Basil Blackwell, Oxford.

Miller, W.C. & Jacob, A.V. 2001, 'The Health at Any Size Paradigm for Obesity Treatment: The Scientific Evidence', *Obesity Reviews*, vol. 2, pp. 37–45.

Morris, A., Cooper, T. & Cooper, P.J. 1989, 'The Changing Shape of Female Fashion Models', *International Journal of Eating Disorders*, vol. 8, pp. 593–6.

Murcott, A. 1983, 'Cooking and the Cooked: A Note on the Domestic Preparation of Meals', in A. Murcott (ed.), *The Sociology of Food and Eating*, Gower, Aldershot, UK.

National Heart Foundation 1990, *Risk Factor Prevalence Study: Survey No. 3 1989*, National Heart Foundation of Australia and Australian Institute of Health, Canberra.

New York Times Magazine, 27 May 1994, p. 22.

Norton, K.I., Olds, T.S., Olive, S. & Dank, S. 1996, 'Ken and Barbie at Life Size', *Sex Roles*, vol. 34, nos 3 & 4, pp. 287–94.

Nowak, M., Crawford, D. & Buttner, P. 2001, 'A Cross-sectional Study of Weight- and Shape-related Beliefs, Behaviours and Concerns of North Queensland Adolescents', *Australian Journal of Nutrition and Dietetics*, vol. 58, no. 3, pp. 174–81.

O'Brien, S. 1997, '"I Want to Be Just Like You"—Barbie Magazine and the Production of the Female Desiring Subject', *Journal of Interdisciplinary Gender Studies*, vol. 2, no. 2, pp. 51–66.

O'Dea, J. 1998, 'The Body Size Preferences of Underweight Young Women from Different Cultural Backgrounds', *Australian Journal of Nutrition and Dietetics*, vol. 55, no. 2, pp. 75–80.

Paquette, M. & Raine, K. 2004, 'Sociocultural Context of Women's Body Image', *Social Science and Medicine*, vol. 59, pp. 1047–58.

Parham, E.S. 1996, 'Is There a New Weight Paradigm?', *Nutrition Today*, vol. 31, pp. 155–61.

—— 1999, 'Promoting Body Size Acceptance in Weight Management Counselling', *Journal of the American Dietetic Association*, vol. 99, no. 8, pp. 920–5.

Parker, S., Nichter, M., Nichter, M., Vuckovic, N., Sims, C. & Rittenbaugh, C. 1995, 'Body Image and Weight Concerns among African American and White

Adolescent Females: Differences that Make a Difference', *Human Organization*, vol. 54, no. 2, pp. 103–14.

Rothblum, E.D. 1994, '"I'll Die for the Revolution but Don't Ask Me Not to Diet": Feminism and the Continuing Stigmatization of Obesity', in P. Fallon, M.A. Katzman & S.A. Wooley (eds), *Feminist Perspectives on Eating Disorders*, Guilford Press, New York.

Rubin, G. 1975, 'The Traffic in Women', in R.R. Rayna (ed.), *Toward an Anthropology of Women*, Monthly Review Press, New York, pp. 157–210.

Schur, E. 1983, *Labelling Women Deviant: Gender, Stigma, and Social Control*, Temple University Press, Philadelphia.

Schwartz, H. 1986, *Never Satisfied: A Cultural History of Diets, Fantasies and Fat*, The Free Press, New York.

Seid, R.P. 1994, 'Too "Close to the Bone": The Historical Context for Women's Obsession with Slenderness', in P. Fallon, M.A. Katzman & S.A. Wooley (eds), *Feminist Perspectives on Eating Disorders*, Guilford Press, New York.

Serdula, M.K., Mokdad, A.H., Williamson, D.F., Galuska, D.A., Mendlein, J. & Heath, G.W. 1999, 'Prevalence of Attempting Weight Loss and Strategies for Controlling Weight', *Journal of the American Medical Association*, vol. 282, pp. 1353–8.

Silverstein, B., Perdue, L., Peterson, B., Vogel, L. & Fantini, D.A. 1986, 'Possible Causes for the Thin Standard of Bodily Attractiveness for Women', *International Journal of Eating Disorders*, vol. 5, pp. 135–44.

Smith, B. 1998. Personal communication, 27 May.

Sobal, J. 1999, 'The Size Acceptance Movement and the Social Construction of Body Weight', in J. Sobal & D. Maurer (eds), *Weighty Issues: Fatness and Thinness as Social Problems*, Aldine de Gruyter, New York, pp. 183–205.

—— & Cassidy, C. 1987, 'Dieting Foods: Conceptualizations and Explanations', *Ecology of Food and Nutrition*, vol. 20, no. 2, pp. 89–96.

Solovay, S. 2000, *Tipping the Scales of Justice: Fighting Weight-based Discrimination*, Prometheus Books, New York.

Sørensen, T.I.A. 2003, 'Weight Loss Causes Increased Mortality: Pros', *Obesity Reviews*, vol. 4, pp. 3–7.

Strain, G.W. 1999, 'Response to Promoting Size Acceptance in Weight Management Counseling', *Journal of the American Dietetic Association*, vol. 99, no. 8 , pp. 926–8.

Tebbel, C. 2000, *The Body Snatchers: How the Media Shapes Women*, Finch Publishing, Sydney.

Tunaley, J.R., Walsh, S. & Nicholson, P. 1999, '"I'm Not Bad for my Age": The Meaning of Body Size and Eating in the Lives of Older Women', *Ageing and Society*, vol. 19, pp. 741–59.

Turner, B.S. 1992, *Regulating Bodies*, Routledge, London.

Wardle, J., Griffith, J., Johnson, F. & Rapoport, L. 2000, 'Intentional Weight Control and Food Choice Habits in a National Representative Sample of Adults in the UK', *International Journal of Obesity*, vol. 24, pp. 534–40.

Wearing, B. 1996, *Gender: The Pain and Pleasure of Difference*, Longman Australia, Melbourne.

Williams, L. & Germov, J. 2004, 'Body Acceptance: Exploring Women's Experiences', in J. Germov & L. Williams (eds), *A Sociology of Food and Nutrition: The Social Appetite*, 2nd edition, Oxford University Press, Melbourne, pp. 403–26.

Williams, L., Germov, J. & Young, A. 2007, 'Preventing Weight Gain: A Population Cohort Study of the Nature and Effectiveness of Mid-age Women's Weight Control Practices', *International Journal of Obesity*, vol. 31, pp. 978–86.

WHO—*see* World Health Organization.

Wolf, N. 1990, *The Beauty Myth*, Vintage, London.

World Health Organization 2000, *Obesity: Preventing and Managing the Global Epidemic*, World Health Organisation, Geneva.

Yang, D., Fontaine, K.R., Wang, C. & Allison, D.B. 2003, 'Weight Loss Causes Increased Mortality: Cons', *Obesity Reviews*, vol. 4, pp. 9–16.

CHAPTER 16

The Social Construction of Eating Disorders

Julie Hepworth

OVERVIEW

- What are eating disorders?
- What contribution does social science make to our understanding of eating disorders?
- What are some of the limitations of medical models of eating disorders?

The aim of this chapter is to provide an overview of the contribution of the social sciences to our understanding of the field commonly known as 'eating disorders'. Eating disorders, such as anorexia nervosa, bulimia nervosa, binge-eating disorders, and eating disorders not otherwise specified (EDNOS), are described in relation to the historical and social conditions that have shaped and defined them as biomedical and psychiatric phenomena. In addition, the psychological and cultural aspects of eating disorders are briefly discussed. While neurobiological and genetic research on the aetiological factors of eating disorders have attracted considerable interest over the last few years, these areas are not discussed in this chapter. Rather, the historical and social conditions that led to the discovery of anorexia nervosa are examined, as well as how bulimia nervosa was defined much later as a consequence of this earlier discovery. A social constructionist perspective is put forward as being valuable in developing alternative ways of thinking about eating disorders. The various social and cultural explanations proposed by feminist writers are described. Social constructionist and feminist approaches are then taken up later on in the chapter in a discussion of how social constructionism has informed some feminist criticism of biomedical models of eating disorders.

Key terms

anorexia nervosa

biomedical discourse

bulimia nervosa

culture-bound syndrome

eating disorders not
   otherwise specified
   (EDNOS)

feminism

patriarchy

post-structuralism

social constructionism

thin ideal

Introduction

Thus the discourse continues, debating whether and to what degree, and in what ways, the body is tomb or temple, loved or hated, personal or state property, machine or self.

Synnott 1993, p. 37

The field of eating disorders emerged in the late nineteenth century as a Western medical phenomenon that initially documented the clinical presentation of self-starvation, found almost exclusively in young, white, middle-class women. The current prevalence of eating disorders is difficult to estimate, because there are few full-syndrome eating disorders and a much greater number of women presenting with eating disorder symptoms. Susan Kashubeck-West and Laurie Mintz (2001) estimated, based on a close analysis of the current research and on information from the Diagnostic and Statistical Manual-1V (APA 1994), that full-syndrome eating disorders are rare—the prevalence of **anorexia nervosa** and **bulimia nervosa** are 0.5–1.0 per cent and 1–3 per cent respectively—although they are on the rise (see Boxes 16.1 and 16.2). The prevalence of **eating disorders not otherwise specified (EDNOS)** is estimated at 2–5 per cent. Many women (an estimated 19–32 per cent) suffer from only some eating disorder symptoms (Mulholland & Mintz 2001).

One of the major explanations of eating disorders is that changing cultural conditions give rise to concerns, particularly among women, about body size and shape. Cheryl Ritenbaugh (1982) proposed that obesity was a **culture-bound syndrome** and eating disorders are also culture-bound in the sense that they reflect the dominant ideals of women's slimness in Western societies. The responses made by the health-related professions to changing eating practices have also been linked to the cultural context of Western clinical treatment and management. As Western ideals of the slim female permeate other cultures, especially through mass media representations and changing social roles, these cultural ideals will influence non-Western women's behaviour by encouraging increased surveillance of the body. Indeed, eating disorders are increasingly becoming a global problem, with rising numbers of cases in non-Western countries worldwide—due not only to media representations of Western ideals but also to familial factors (such as intergenerational conflicts and confusion over racial identity), changes in dietary habits and increases in obesity (Nasser 1997). The rise in eating disorders among non-Western women is a result of the pressures of moving to the West and adapting to a new culture or, alternatively, of non-Western women's desire to conform to the norms and values of Western society, including those relating to body shape. However, more culturally sensitive measures of the prevalence of eating disorders are required, especially to

Diagnostic criteria for anorexia nervosa

BOX 16.1

A. Refusal to maintain body weight at or above a minimally normal weight for age and height (e.g. weight loss leading to maintenance of body weight less than 85% of that expected; or failure to make expected weight gain during period of growth, leading to body weight less than 85% of that expected).

B. Intense fear of gaining weight or becoming fat, even though underweight.

C. Disturbance in the way in which one's body weight or shape is experienced, undue influence of body weight or shape on self-evaluation, or denial of the seriousness of the current low body weight.

D. In postmenarcheal females, amenorrhoea, i.e., the absence of at least three consecutive menstrual cycles. (A woman is considered to have amenorrhoea if her periods occur only following hormone, e.g., estrogen, administration.)

Specific types:

- Restricting Type: during the current episode of anorexia nervosa, the person has not regularly engaged in binge-eating or purging behaviour (i.e., self-induced vomiting or the misuse of laxatives, diuretics, or enemas).

- Binge-Eating/Purging Type: during the current episode of anorexia nervosa, the person has regularly engaged in binge-eating or purging behaviour (i.e., self-induced vomiting or the misuse of laxatives, diuretics, or enemas).

Source: APA (2000)

facilitate more effective prevention and treatment of eating disorders in women of non-Western cultures who live in the West (Lake et al. 2000).

Also changing are the cultural representations and social conditions of men. Consequently, in the West, increasing numbers of men are being diagnosed with eating disorders. Males comprise approximately 10 per cent of individuals who present with anorexia nervosa and bulimia nervosa (APA 2000). The increasing problem of eating disorders in men is linked to the rise in media representations of the ideal male body, and the need to exercise to achieve the toned muscular appearance that typifies men's health magazines. While there is clear evidence of an increase in eating distress in males (Petrie & Rogers 2001), eating disorders are still overwhelmingly defined as female conditions and are associated with femininity (Gremillion 2001). For men, this definition of eating disorders as female conditions creates potential barriers to clinical diagnosis. Health professionals may not be as likely to associate symptoms in males with eating disorders, and there is a stigma

Julie Hepworth

BOX 16.2

Diagnostic criteria for bulimia nervosa

A. Recurrent episodes of binge eating. An episode of binge eating is characterised by both of the following:

1. Eating, in a discrete period of time (e.g., within any 2-hour period), an amount of food that is definitely larger than most people would eat during a similar period of time and under similar circumstances.

2. A sense of lack of control over eating during the episode (e.g., a feeling that one cannot stop eating or control what or how much one is eating).

B. Recurrent inappropriate compensatory behaviour in order to prevent weight gain, such as self-induced vomiting, misuse of laxatives, diuretics, enemas, or other medications, fasting, or excessive exercise.

C. The binge eating and inappropriate compensatory behaviour both occur, on average, at least twice a week for 3 months.

D. Self-evaluation is unduly influenced by body shape and weight.

E. The disturbance does not occur exclusively during episodes of anorexia nervosa.

Specific types:

*   Purging Type: during the current episode of bulimia nervosa, the person has regularly engaged in self-induced vomiting or the misuse of laxatives, diuretics, or enemas

*   Non-purging Type: during the current episode of bulimia nervosa, the person has used other inappropriate compensatory behaviours, such as fasting or excessive exercise, but has not regularly engaged in self-induced vomiting or the misuse of laxatives, diuretics, or enemas.

Source: APA (2000)

attached to eating disorders for males, who do not want to be perceived as suffering from a female condition (Hepworth 1999; Petrie & Rogers 2001).

The field of eating disorders is vast, in terms of both aetiological models and treatment approaches. While some explanations remain firmly situated within the disciplinary boundaries of medicine, dietetics and nutrition science, psychiatry or psychology, most researchers maintain there is multifactorial causation of eating disorders. Over the last 30 years, particularly within psychology, the contribution of social, cultural and familial factors to the onset and maintenance of eating disorders has gained recognition (Striegel-Moore & Cachelin 2001; Ogden 2003). Multifactorial models aim to explain the role played by these factors, and are commonly taught and used in such fields of medicine as primary care, in which eating disorders are understood as constituting more than just biological and pathological processes. These models take into account the multidimensional nature of eating disorders in a way that moves beyond the traditionally dominant **biomedical discourse**.

Interestingly, the last 150 years has not produced greater certainty about the nature of eating disorders. Rather, through the emergence of the social sciences in the twentieth century what has arisen instead is theoretical and explanatory diversity. The field has become vast, including both competing disciplinary and professional claims, as well as, more positively, interdisciplinary work on eating disorders and multiprofessional collaboration. Clearly, knowledge in this field has not progressed along a traditional linear route leading to increasing scientific certainty; rather, a number of approaches, including medical, **social constructionist** and **feminist** perspectives, have evolved, demonstrating the complexity of eating disorders. These three particular approaches to eating disorders are significant in that they constitute major strands of thought that have shaped current understanding. Through their examination, the field will be revealed as a contested domain in which different disciplines have made various claims to know the aetiological basis of eating disorders and the best treatments; the most long-standing claims being those made by clinical medicine.

Biomedical approaches to eating disorders

While research on eating disorders during the twentieth century has proliferated, a specific aetiology or clinical treatment for anorexia nervosa and bulimia nervosa has not been identified. Characterised still as psychiatric disorders in the DSM-IV-TR (APA 2000), eating disorders were historically defined by medical science and treated within the clinical domain. Current diagnostic and clinical management procedures share a number of key features with practices from over a hundred years ago: medical practitioners manage the conditions within primary care through regular consultations, weight monitoring and counselling, or in hospitals through refeeding programs together with psychotherapeutic interventions.

In order to understand the significance of biomedical approaches, it is important to know the basic historical background to the emergence of anorexia nervosa and bulimia nervosa as psychiatric disorders and their classification within the Diagnostic and Statistical Manual. The late-nineteenth-century definition of anorexia nervosa by Sir William Withey Gull was undoubtedly the defining moment when eating disorders became subsumed within biomedical science. Gull was an eminent British physician; he trained in medicine at Guy's hospital, London, and subsequently worked there as both practitioner and lecturer. Later, in 1872, his career reached its pinnacle when he was made Physician to Queen Victoria. Until the late 1800s, self-starvation had been largely understood through religious ideas about women's sainthood, such as in the case of the seventeenth-century figure of Jane Balan, who reportedly lived without nourishment for three years (cf. Morgan 1977); later accounts attributed fasting to an assumed 'negative spiritual state' and 'inherent wickedness' of women. The discovery of anorexia nervosa in 1874 firmly established self-starvation as a disease entity, as a biomedical condition, to be treated within the clinical domain. Julie Hepworth and Christine Griffin's (1990) critical examination of this discovery demonstrates how five key discourses—the femininity, medical-scientific, discovery, clinical and hysteria discourses—gave rise to the definition of anorexia nervosa, arguing instead how it was the social and cultural conditions of the period that had made this scientific discovery possible.

Here is a typical early case description of anorexia nervosa by Gull:

> Miss B., aged 18, was brought to me Oct. 8, 1868, as a case of latent tubercle. Her friends had been advised accordingly to take her for the coming winter to the South of Europe. The extremely emaciated look, much greater indeed than occurred for the most part in tubercular cases where patients are still going about, impressed me at once with the probability that I should find no visceral disease. Pulse 50, reps. 16. Physical examination of the chest and abdomen discovered nothing abnormal. All the viscera were apparently healthy. Notwithstanding the great emaciation and apparent weakness, there was a peculiar restlessness, difficult, I was informed, to control. The mother added, 'She is never tired.' Amenorrhoea since Christmas 1866. The clinical details of this case were in fact almost identical with the preceding one, even to the number of the pulse and respirations.

Gull 1874, pp. 23–4

With the publication of these kinds of clinical observations, physicians, particularly in Europe, the United States of America and Australia, began redefining self-starvation as diagnoses of anorexia nervosa in their patients. Following on from this, the search for the biological causation of anorexia nervosa dominated medical science and psychiatric thinking in this field for a number of decades. The discovery of anorexia nervosa was also influential in the subsequent definition of other eating disorders, especially bulimia nervosa.

The earliest English-language example of bulimia nervosa occurred in 1898 (Parry-Jones 1971) when bulimia nervosa was commonly associated with pituitary insufficiency (studied by Simmonds) from the 1900s onwards. 'Bulimia' comes from the Greek language and means ravenous hunger. One of the earliest clinical case descriptions is found in the work of Hilde Bruch (1974), who described a patient who binged and vomited. However, the term 'bulimia nervosa' was not defined until the late 1970s by Gerald Russell (1979), who acknowledged that bulimia nervosa was not a new disorder and that, indeed, there had been many case histories over the previous 60 years. Although not as much is known about bulimia nervosa as about anorexia nervosa, there are several key similarities and differences in relation to anorexia nervosa. Bulimia nervosa is regarded as often being a 'progression' from anorexia nervosa, and treatment outcomes are more optimistic than for anorexia nervosa. The close connection between the two conditions was recognised some time ago, when Marlene Boskind-White (Boskind-White & White 1987) coined the term 'bulimarexia' to refer to the condition of those people who presented with both anorexia nervosa and bulimia nervosa symptoms, also representing how people alternated between bingeing and fasting.

Bulimia nervosa was also primarily diagnosed in young women, and many of the assumptions and practices of biomedical discourse in relation to diagnosis and treatment were simply enlarged to accommodate what were considered to be new forms of disordered eating. Subsequent to the definition of bulimia nervosa, and notwithstanding the fact that anorexia and bulimia are considered the two major eating disorders, there were further conditions and syndromes, such as binge-eating disorder and EDNOS, that also became diagnostic categories within the field of eating disorders.

The nature of biomedical approaches, while having emerged from historical discourses of the nineteenth century, did begin to vary throughout the late twentieth century in the extent to which medicine included different psychological programs. Psychologists as well as other therapists working with medical practitioners have implemented an array of eating disorder programs that include both traditional one-to-one counselling as well as innovative approaches. The 'Food as Fuel' program in the USA is designed and run by Dr Louis Rappaport and includes carefully controlled medical evaluations combined with a cognitive–behavioural approach that aims to change the cognitive set of clients from a focus on food as the enemy to food as a resource that enables them to achieve physical goals through swimming, cycling, running or hiking (Rappaport 2007). One of the most famous programs, and to some extent controversial due to its alleged lack of medical involvement, is the Montreux Clinic, a residential therapeutic facility in Canada set up in 1993 by Peggy Claude-Pierre where patients are immersed in an environment of unconditional support. Interestingly, even though there is an ongoing shift in perspectives on eating disorders that includes a greater awareness of cultural and social factors, including the application of these perspectives to therapeutic programs, they nonetheless continue to be represented as disorders that are enigmatic and elusive. What precisely causes the onset and/or recovery from eating disorders has not been identified and, especially in relation to anorexia nervosa, eating disorders are regarded as intractable problems mostly associated with young women.

What biomedical approaches do not consider are the ways in which social and cultural conditions create subjectivity, sexuality and the body. Thus, the relationships between the social and cultural contexts of experience and individual behaviour remained poorly understood until the 1980s. These contexts are important to understanding eating disorders precisely because they reflect conflicts that individuals experience about changing societal norms and expectations. Biomedical approaches

Julie Hepworth

also do not take into account the dramatic economic, social and cultural changes in women's lives during the twentieth century that have given rise to contradictory demands, such as managing the dual roles of career and motherhood, and problematic values, such as the definition of women in terms of the **thin ideal** (Orbach 1986; see also Chapter 15). Through the definition of eating disorders as psychiatric categories, the complexity of social issues, particularly those faced by women and increasingly by men, are individualised as discrete conditions to be treated within the clinical domain and the social and cultural factors implicated in the onset and maintenance of eating disorders have remained largely unchallenged (Hepworth & Griffin 1995).

Social constructionist approaches to eating disorders

The dominance of the biomedical approach to eating disorders has been criticised by several authors, particularly those using social constructionist approaches since the 1980s. Social constructionism is not a unitary theory but rather is informed by numerous philosophical and theoretical approaches. Key social constructionist writings include the seminal work of Peter Berger and Thomas Luckmann (1967), as well as work by Kenneth Gergen (1985), Henriques and colleagues (1984) and Potter and Wetherell (1987). One of the most common approaches in social constructionism is informed by the work of French philosopher Michel Foucault (1974), who argues that discourses—regularly occurring systems of language—construct specific concepts. If we take this approach to the field of eating disorders, we can see how eating disorders are socially constructed concepts embedded within the historical, social and cultural conditions of the period in which they were defined. If we accept that knowledge is socially constructed, this also allows for the idea that during particular periods of history there are dominant discourses (such as biomedicine) and competing discourses (such as psychological and feminist explanations) that produce certain kinds of relationships and practices that are reproduced through the use of language. This is why language is central to any analysis in the social constructionist approach known as 'discourse analysis', though 'discourse analysis is best understood as a field of research rather than a single practice' (Taylor 2001, p. 5).

It is precisely by examining the language through which eating disorders emerged and through which treatment practices developed that it is possible to deconstruct or take apart the taken-for-granted meanings and assumptions of the field of eating disorders and identify possibilities for change. As Ludvilla Jordanova (1995) argues, social constructionism enables us to conceptualise, explain and interpret the processes through which scientific and medical ideas are shaped by given contexts. Psychological uses of social constructionism particularly emphasise the relationship between individual subjectivity and social processes. Discourse analysis provides us with the analytic tools to examine the structures within which certain concepts and conditions such as eating disorders emerged by analysing historical and institutional practices, and to examine the ways in which individual accounts of eating disorders are constructed and reproduced by the linguistic communities to which people belong, such as biomedicine.

Prior to **post-structural** interpretations, identity and self were regarded as being separable from social practices, an idea commonly referred to in psychology as 'individual–society dualism'. Identity responded to and was influenced by external events; although social and cultural pressures on women to be thin were external, they nevertheless underscored existing intrapsychic problems. In contrast, post-structural approaches maintain that the self is constituted by multiple identities, is constructed through specific social and cultural conditions and is not reified as an autonomous entity. Thus, the analysis and explanation of the relations between women, food and subjectivity focus on the intersections of these key areas that are represented through language.

What is particularly useful about feminist post-structural explanations of eating disorders is their capacity to represent the complex interrelations that constitute multifaceted phenomena. Indeed, a special issue of the *Journal of Community and Applied Social Psychology* is devoted to drawing on 'critical feminist, post-structuralist and discourse-orientated psychologies' to more fully explicate the relations between power, subjectivity and inequality that constitute existing cultural and social conditions of '(dis)orders of eating' (see Malson & Swann 1999). A further example of employing post-structural work is in the representation of the personal experience of eating disorders. In Squire's (2002, p. 61) compelling narrative of 'writing the bulimic body' she recounts a time when she searched for the words to represent her personal experience with bulimia because of it largely being:

> …untheorised, suffering at best a conflation with anorexia, a total silence or absence, or at worst existing as the repository of disgust and shame from all theoretical approaches, including feminism.

To some extent we can see a link between Squire's (2002) work and, as noted earlier in the section on biomedical approaches to eating disorders, the fact that not as much was known or written about bulimia historically as it evolved alongside a much more concentrated focus of clinical interest in anorexia nervosa.

Not least in the contribution of post-structural approaches to eating disorders is the work of American feminist Susan Bordo (1988; 1993). Women, food, sexuality and the body are fundamental to Bordo's writings. In 'Anorexia Nervosa and the Crystallization of Culture' (1988), Bordo argued that anorexia nervosa is a symptom of some of the 'multifaceted and heterogenous distress of our age'. She examined social and cultural images of the female body, 'the political anatomy', and identified slenderness as being significant to the relationship between women's subjectivity and media representations of women's bodies. Drawing on Foucault (1974), Bordo elaborated on a post-structural interpretation of anorexia nervosa by arguing that women achieve power through dieting and that this was a form of 'disciplinary practice' carried out by individual women on themselves in order to maintain and reproduce the thin ideal.

Using discourse analysis within a feminist framework enables a series of questions to be asked. In the earlier section on biomedical approaches to eating disorders, the historical and social conditions through which the discovery of anorexia nervosa was constructed were identified through post-structural analysis (Hepworth & Griffin 1990). Further to this, a post-structural approach demonstrated the ways in which health professionals take up and deploy discourses about eating disorders in various treatment arenas (see Hepworth 1999). In the next section the work of feminist authors from three different philosophical and theoretical backgrounds is discussed with specific reference to the ways in which they explained the onset of eating disorders that challenged the pathologising approach of some mainstream health care practitioners.

Feminist approaches to eating disorders

While it is important to recognise that feminist perspectives are informed by diverse theoretical frameworks, by different historical and cultural positions, and by the ethnicity of women, they share a common focus on women and power relations. These approaches privilege the experiences of women, and address various concerns about power in the onset, duration and treatment of eating disorders. Fundamental to feminist perspectives is the eschewing, to various degrees, of the medical model of eating disorders. The most common theoretical frameworks and backgrounds that inform feminist perspectives are psychoanalytic theory, existentialism, social and cultural theory, and post-structuralism. In the previous section on social constructionist approaches to eating disorders, examples of post-structural feminist approaches were discussed. This section focuses on early examples of feminist writing about eating disorders and selected examples of current feminist research in this area.

Feminist perspectives on eating disorders are mostly associated with work during the late 1970s and 1980s by psychoanalytic writers such as Orbach, work that included popular texts such as *Fat is a Feminist Issue* (Orbach 1978 & 1987). Orbach popularised social and cultural approaches to eating disorders, viewing body image as being defined and shaped by **patriarchy** in Western society and by patriarchal power relations. Women are thought to focus on food, eating, dieting and calorie counting in order to regain a sense of control over their lives and, to some extent, to reconcile contradictory beliefs about their social position. Two key themes were expounded through this feminist work: the processes of identity formation and the mother–daughter relationship. Early feminist work on eating disorders also included writing by women who had experienced eating disorders themselves and who wrote about their personal experiences by drawing on various theoretical perspectives, such as Kleinian psychoanalytic theory, in which the mother–daughter relationship is regarded as being fundamental to the conflict experienced in eating disorders (cf. Chernin 1986), and existentialism, which posits that it is a woman's 'being-in-the-world' that creates a sense of tension and conflicts with her developing sense of maturity and womanhood expressed through eating disorders (cf. Macleod 1981). The work of these particular writers was constituted as a series of first moves by feminists working around anorexia nervosa to locate eating disorders in a wider social, political and historical context (Hepworth & Griffin 1995).

Bruch (1974) is the key figure associated with an early broad interpretation of psychoanalytic theories and also became a significant figure in psychotherapy. Against earlier Freudian ideas about anorexia nervosa, she argued that even though the oral component was important, it was only one factor in the aetiology of anorexia nervosa among many others, such as family dynamics. Another main theme in psychoanalytic approaches was a focus on the mother–daughter relationship. Indeed, by the 1980s there was a shift away from 'oral impregnation theory' towards an exclusive focus on the mother–daughter relationship (Lawrence 1984). Issues relating to identification and separation in the psychosexual development of a young woman became paramount to clinical interventions using psychoanalytic ideas. Furthermore, the social and cultural identities of women, Chernin (1986) argued, constituted ambiguous roles for women, contributing to separation issues between daughter and mother.

Existential approaches to eating disorders focused mainly on female identity and its centrality to anorexia nervosa. Eating disorders were seen as a manifestation of a crisis about 'being-in-the-world'. Sheila MacLeod's (1981) own experience of anorexia nervosa is encapsulated in the statement 'I was free at last!' as she describes herself becoming a 'successful anorexic'. Earlier forms of an existential interpretation of anorexia nervosa are described in literature as asceticism, such as documented in Bell's (1985) book, *Holy Anorexia*.

Much of this early work has continued through the work of, for example, Katherine Zerbe (1993), who also maintains the significance of the mother–daughter relationship in the onset of a young woman's internal conflicts. On the one hand, a woman increasingly experiences the need to assert her individual identity and act upon the world, and on the other she desires the security offered by her mother. In early adulthood, it is argued by psychoanalytic-informed writers, a young woman can experience guilt at no longer requiring the security offered by her mother and fears about making her mother feel worthless. As Zerbe writes, 'Without individual

Julie Hepworth

susceptibility, liabilities imposed by society are less likely to take root' (1993, p. 10). These lines of feminist thought broaden our understanding of eating disorders by putting them in the contexts of familial relations, specifically the mother–daughter relationship, and women's social position, and influenced the later development of feminist treatment programs—see, for example, 'feminist group work with women with eating issues' (Black 2003). Yet, it is important to note that the contributions of Susie Orbach (1978), Kim Chernin (1986) and Sheila MacLeod (1981) were also caught in a discursive dilemma, in that the individual concepts and categorisation of eating disorders as psychiatric problems remained unchallenged (Hepworth & Griffin 1995).

It is precisely this long-standing problem of the individual level of explanation of eating disorders that social constructionism has challenged through, not least, combining feminist principles with post-structural approaches. In addition to the explanatory frameworks of eating disorders in relation to their historical emergence (see Hepworth & Griffin 1990; 1995), and clinical treatment (see Hepworth 1999), feminist post-structuralist writers have proposed new challenges to health care delivery. Drawing on Foucault, Ali (2002) maintains that empowering women has to involve a disengagement from the historical position of the passive eating disorder patient by women questioning contemporary health care practices and developing 'an emancipatory stance to knowledge-building'. While Ali (2002) acknowledges the tensions that exist in the treatment field towards encouraging patients to engage in health care activism when the patients may well be dealing with challenging mental health problems, her work does represent a new shift in focus in what she (2002, p. 240) refers to as 'the transformation of the survivor from patient to activist'.

Moreover, resistance to the role of passive patient is a theme increasingly evidenced by the upsurge in participation on pro-eating disorder internet sites. These sites have attracted significant media attention to the point of creating a 'media frenzy' focused on their dangers and the representation of young women as vulnerable and falling victim to the experience of online group participation. On the one hand, as Dias (2003) explains, pro-anorexia internet sites aspire to promote, support and discuss anorexia nervosa to the extent that it is considered a 'lifestyle' and not a disease. Clearly, there are inherent risks in using internet sites that include explicit details and encouragement of extreme weight loss. On the other, in a recent study of user participation of one pro-anorexia internet site it was precisely the perceived 'safety', 'coping function' and 'emotional support' while managing their weight that users experienced that maintained their participation (Mulveen & Hepworth 2006). While this research does not claim to be representative of all pro-anorexia internet sites, and participants reported the site to be unusual in that it demonstrated some responsibility towards the severity of its members' weight loss, the fact that participants were more comfortable describing their experience of disordered eating via this internet site than with some health professionals certainly indicates an area for mainstream health services to further address (Mulveen & Hepworth 2006).

Conclusion

Using a social constructionist approach, eating disorders and even the seemingly immutable empirical claims of medicine can be understood differently through their interpretation in relation to broader historical, cultural and social contexts. Also, through the delineation of competing explanations of eating disorders it is possible to examine the significance of cultural and social conditions in the construction of individual subjectivity. Examining these relationships from a constructionist perspective gives rise to alternative explanations both of why people develop eating disorders—see, for example, the work of American feminist writer Bordo (1993)—and how the field of eating disorders itself is embedded within historical and social structures of medicine and women's social position (Hepworth & Griffin 1990, 1995; Hepworth 1999).

This chapter has illustrated how the development of the social sciences has included a critical element that deconstructs taken-for-granted knowledge in the field of eating disorders. The range of biomedical theories that emerged from the late nineteenth century onwards assumed that young women had a propensity to develop nervous diseases and that hormonal and psychological changes predisposed them to develop eating disorders. This meant that it was assumed that eating disorders such as anorexia nervosa and bulimia nervosa had a pathological aetiology, thereby rendering them clinical entities to be medically managed within hospitals and/or by doctors in primary care. Alternatively, using a social constructionist perspective informed by post-structuralism, it is possible to see that these conditions only came about precisely because of the historical context and the social position of women over a hundred years ago.

The contribution of social constructionism to our understanding of the overarching importance of the structures of knowledge about eating disorders was further discussed in the chapter's later section on feminist approaches. These writers, using psychoanalytic, existential, social/cultural and post-structural explanations made considerable contributions throughout the 1980s and 1990s that challenged the dominance of biomedical explanations of eating disorders. Medical, social constructionist and feminist explanations, therefore, represent key movements in the knowledge about eating disorders. By considering these explanations, a broader contextualisation of eating disorders is possible, creating new opportunities to think about how knowledge in this field is reproduced, contested and evolves.

Julie Hepworth

SUMMARY OF MAIN POINTS

- The field of eating disorders originated in the medical discovery of anorexia nervosa in the late nineteenth century.
- A number of eating disorders and eating syndromes have been identified over the last hundred years, including bulimia nervosa, binge-eating syndrome and eating disorders not otherwise specified.
- Social constructionist approaches explain eating disorders in relation to the historical, cultural and social structures of knowledge.
- Social constructionist approaches maintain that individual subjectivity is created through the use and reproduction of language within specific contexts.
- Since the late 1970s, feminist writers have challenged the biomedical model, which explains eating disorders as resulting from hormonal, genetic or psychopathological dysfunction.
- Biomedical, social constructionist and feminist approaches produce different and conflicting explanations of eating disorders, and challenge us to think about new ways of practising in this field.
- Recent criticism of the passive role of the eating disorder patient has created alternative ways of thinking about young women and eating that focus on women's activism.

SOCIOLOGICAL REFLECTION

In 2006 Stanford University medical researchers published the results of a survey of 76 patients diagnosed with eating disorders and 106 parents in which 41 per cent of patients visited pro-recovery sites and 35.5 per cent visited pro-eating disorder sites, concluding that while visiting sites patients learned new techniques of disordered eating (Wilson et al. 2006). Given that eating disorders are intrinsically linked to changing economic, political, cultural and social conditions it seems unsurprising that the emergence of pro-eating disorder internet sites would interest some young women. Yet, these new forms of media create challenges for thinking about eating disorders and, in particular, how young women are positioned in the twenty-first century.

- To what extent do you consider young women at risk from pro-eating disorder internet sites?
- While women living in Western countries are particularly exposed to economic, political, cultural and social conditions that promote weight loss, why do only a small percentage of these women develop eating disorders?
- Drawing on social constructionist approaches, what alternative ways are there to represent young women's behaviour defined as eating disorders?

DISCUSSION QUESTIONS

1. In what ways do social constructionist approaches to eating disorders differ from biomedical approaches and some feminist approaches?
2. Discuss the contributions made by psychoanalytic, social and feminist theories to our understanding of eating disorders.
3. Identify three approaches to the explanation of eating disorders and the historical and social contexts in which they emerged.
4. To what extent are criticisms of the biomedical model of eating disorders justified? Reflect on the knowledge and information that you use in your answer.
5. What evidence is there that cultural pressures are a major contributory factor in the onset of anorexia nervosa and bulimia nervosa?

Further investigation

1. The prevalence of eating disorders is markedly different for females and males. What are the main reasons for this difference?
2. How can a social constructionist approach to eating disorders make an impact on practice?

FURTHER READING AND WEB RESOURCES

Books

Hepworth, J. 1999, *The Social Construction of Anorexia Nervosa*, Sage, London.

MacSween, M. 1993, *Anorexic Bodies: A Feminist and Sociological Perspective on Anorexia Nervosa*, Routledge, London.

Nasser, M., Katzman, M.A. & Gordon, R.A. (eds) 2001, *Eating Disorders and Cultures in Transition*, Brunner-Routledge, London.

Piran, N., Levine, M.P. & Steiner-Adair, C. (eds.) 1999, *Preventing Eating Disorders: A Handbook of Interventions and Special Challenges*, Brunner/Mazel, London.

Vandereycken, W. & Noordenbos, G. (eds.) 1998, *The Prevention of Eating Disorders*, Athlone Press, London.

Websites

Anorexia Nervosa and Related Eating Disorders (ANRED): www.anred.com

Eating Disorders Association: www.edauk.com

Eating Disorders Association: www.eda.org.au/home.htm

Health Education Board for Scotland—Talking About Eating Disorders: www.hebs. scot.nhs.uk

Julie Hepworth

REFERENCES

Ali, A. 2002, 'The Convergence of Foucault and Feminist Psychiatry: Exploring Emancipatory Knowledge-building', *Journal of Gender Studies*, vol. 11, no. 3, pp. 233–41.

American Psychiatric Association 1994, *Diagnostic and Statistical Manual of Mental Disorders (DSM-R)*, 4th edition, American Psychological Association, Washington, DC.

—— 2000, *Diagnostic and Statistical Manual of Mental Disorders (DSM-IV-TR)*, 4th edition, Text Revision, American Psychological Association, Washington, DC.

APA—*see* American Psychiatric Association.

Bell, R.M. 1985, *Holy Anorexia*, University of Chicago Press, Chicago.

Berger, P. & Luckmann, T. 1967, *The Social Construction of Reality*, Penguin, Harmondsworth.

Black, C. 2003, 'Creating Curative Communities: Feminist Group Work with Women with Eating Issues', *Australian Social Work*, vol. 56, no. 2, pp. 127–40.

Bordo, S. 1988, 'Anorexia Nervosa and the Crystallization of Culture', in I. Diamond & L. Quinby (eds), *Feminism and Foucault: Reflections on Resistance*, Northeastern University Press, Boston.

—— 1993, *Unbearable Weight: Feminism, Western Culture, and the Body*, University of California Press, Berkeley, CA.

Boskind-White, M. & White, W.C., Jr, 1987, *Bulimarexia: The Binge/Purge Cycle*, 2nd edition, Norton, New York.

Bruch, H. 1974, *Eating Disorders: Obesity, Anorexia Nervosa and the Person Within*, Routledge and Kegan Paul, London.

Chernin, K. 1986, *The Hungry Self: Daughters and Mothers, Eating and Identity*, Virago Press, London.

Dias, K. 2003, 'The ANA Sanctuary: Women's Pro-Anorexia Narratives in Cyberspace', *Journal of International Women's Studies*, vol. 4, no. 2, pp. 31–45.

Foucault, M. 1974, *The Archaeology of Knowledge*, Tavistock Press, London.

Gergen, K.J. 1985, 'The Social Constructionist Movement in Modern Psychology', *American Psychologist*, vol. 40, pp. 266–75.

Gremillion, H. 2001, 'In Fitness and in Health: Crafting Bodies in the Treatment of Anorexia Nervosa', *Signs: Journal of Women in Culture and Society*, vol. 27, no. 2, pp. 381–414.

Gull, W.W. 1874, 'Anorexia Nervosa (Apepsia Hysterica, Anorexia Hysterica)', *Transactions of the Clinical Society*, London, vol. 7, pp. 22–7.

Henriques, J.W., Hollway, C., Urwin, C., Venn, C. & Walkerdine, V. 1984, *Changing the Subject: Psychology, Social Regulation and Subjectivity*, Methuen, London.

Hepworth, J. 1999, *The Social Construction of Anorexia Nervosa*, Sage, London.

—— & Griffin, C. 1990, 'The Discovery of Anorexia Nervosa: Discourses of the Late 19th Century', *TEXT: The Journal of the Study of Discourse*, vol. 10, no. 4, pp. 321–38.

—— & Griffin, C. 1995, 'Conflicting Opinions? Anorexia Nervosa, Medicine and Feminism', in S. Wilkinson & C. Kitzinger (eds.), *Feminism and Discourse*, Sage, London.

Jordanova, L. 1995, 'The Social Construction of Medical Knowledge', *Social History of Medicine*, vol. 8, no. 4, pp. 361–81.

Kashubeck-West, S. & Mintz, L.B. 2001, 'Eating Disorders in Women: Etiology, Assessment and Treatment', *The Counselling Psychologist*, vol. 29, no. 5, pp. 627–34.

Lake, A.J., Staiger, P.K. & Glowinski, H. 2000, 'Effect of Western Culture on Women's Attitudes to Eating and Perceptions of Body Shape', *International Journal of Eating Disorders*, vol. 27, no. 1, pp. 83–9.

Lawrence, M. 1984, *The Anorexic Experience*, Women's Press, London.

MacLeod, S. 1981, *The Art of Starvation*, Virago, London.

Malson, H. & Swann, C. 1999, 'Prepared for Consumption: (Dis)orders of Eating and Embodiment', *Journal of Community & Applied Social Psychology*, vol. 9, pp. 397–405.

Morgan, H.G. 1977, 'Fasting Girls and Our Attitudes to Them', *British Medical Journal*, vol. 2, pp. 1652–5.

Mulholland, A.M. & Mintz, L.B. 2001, 'Prevalence of Eating Disorders among African American Women', *Journal of Counselling Psychology*, vol. 48, pp. 111–16.

Mulveen, R. & Hepworth, J. 2006, 'An Interpretative Phenomenological Analysis of Participation in a Pro-anorexia Internet Site and its Relationship to Disordered Eating', *Journal of Health Psychology*, vol. 11, no. 2, pp. 283–96.

Nasser, M. 1997, *Culture and Weight Consciousness*, Routledge, London.

Ogden, J. 2003, *The Psychology of Eating: From Healthy to Disordered Eating*, Blackwell, Oxford.

Orbach, S. 1986, *Hunger Strike: The Anorectic's Struggle as a Metaphor for Our Age*, Faber and Faber, London.

—— 1978, *Fat is a Feminist Issue*, Berkley, New York.

—— 1987, *Fat is a Feminist Issue II: A Program to Conquer Compulsive Eating*, Berkley, New York.

Parry-Jones, W.L. 1971, *The Trade in Lunacy: A Study of Private Madhouses in England in the Eighteenth and Nineteenth Centuries*, Routledge and Kegan Paul, London.

Petrie, T.A. & Rogers, R. 2001, 'Extending the Discussion of Eating Disorders to Include Men and Athletes', *The Counselling Psychologist*, vol. 29, no. 5, pp. 743–53.

Potter, J. & Wetherell, M. 1987, *Discourse and Social Psychology: Beyond Attitudes and Behaviour*, Sage, London.

Rappaport, L.J. 2007, Personal communication, 24 January.

Julie Hepworth

Ritenbaugh, C. 1982, 'Obesity as a Culture-bound Syndrome', *Culture, Medicine and Psychiatry*, vol. 6, pp. 347–61.

Russell, G.F.M. 1979, 'Bulimia Nervosa: An Ominous Variant of Anorexia Nervosa', *Psychological Medicine*, vol. 9, pp. 429–48.

Squire, S. 2002, 'The Personal and the Political: Writing the Theorist's Body', *Australian Feminist Studies*, vol. 17, no. 37, pp. 55–64.

Striegel-Moore, R.H. & Cachelin, F.M. 2001, 'Etiology of Eating Disorders in Women', *The Counselling Psychologist*, vol. 29, no. 5, pp. 635–61.

Synnott, A. 1993, *The Body Social: Symbolism, Self and Society*, Routledge, London.

Taylor, S. 2001, 'Locating and Conducting Discourse Analytic Research', in M. Wetherell, S. Taylor & S. Yates (eds), *Discourse as Data*, Open University Press, Milton Keynes.

Wilson, J.L., Peebles, R., Hardy, K.K. & Litt, I.F. 2006, 'Surfing for Thinness: A Pilot Study of Pro-Eating Disorder Web Site Usage in Adolescents with Eating Disorders', *Pediatrics*, vol. 118, no. 6, pp. 1635–43.

Zerbe, K.J. 1993, *The Body Betrayed: Women, Eating Disorders, and Treatment*, American Psychological Association, Washington, DC.

CHAPTER 17

Sociological Analysis of the Stigmatisation of Obesity

Jeffery Sobal

OVERVIEW

- Why is obesity stigmatised?
- What sociological approaches are useful in explaining the stigmatisation of obesity?
- How do individuals deal with the stigmatisation of obesity?

Stigmas are attributes of a person that are deeply discrediting, and obesity is highly stigmatised in contemporary post-industrial societies. Obesity is the condition of having high levels of stored body fat. Sociological work on the stigmatisation of obesity can be divided into two major streams: one focusing on documenting the presence, arenas, extent, and sources of stigmatisation, and the other examining strategies for managing and negotiating the stigma of obesity. Prejudice, labelling, stigmatisation and discrimination based on obesity are very widespread, and occur in many arenas of life (work, family, health and everyday interactions).

Obesity is stigmatised more than some conditions, but less than others. A variety of coping mechanisms are used by obese individuals, including denial, concealment, avoidance, mutual aid and redefinition of situations. Eating is an especially problematic act for obese individuals, because of the potential for stigmatisation. The coping strategies that obese people use to explain their food choices include providing several types of accounts, making disclaimers and discounting some eating behaviours. Obese individuals often adopt 'fat' identities as they deal with the stigmatisation of obesity. Sociologists have examined the stigmatisation of obesity from several mainstream disciplinary perspectives, and yet many aspects of the stigmatisation of obesity remain unresolved and need further attention.

Key terms

accounts	discounting	post-industrial society
attribution	functionalism	stigma
culture-bound syndrome	marginality	stigmatising act
deviant	master status	symbolic interactionism
disclaimer	obesity	

Introduction

A **stigma** is 'an attribute that is deeply discrediting' and that disqualifies a person from full social acceptance (Goffman 1963, p. 3). Stigmatised individuals are seen as blemished, disgraced, and tainted, and routine social interactions become problematic for them. Types of stigma include physical deformities, character blemishes and group stigmas (Goffman 1963). **Obesity** has become a stigma in contemporary post-industrial societies, and sociological perspectives on the stigmatisation of obesity will be the focus of this chapter.

It has been over 40 years since Erving Goffman (1963) brought the concept of stigma to the forefront of sociological attention with his classic book *Stigma: Notes on the Management of Spoiled Identity*. Since Goffman's insightful explication of the concept of stigma, the term and idea have diffused widely through sociology, other social sciences and wider public discourse (Page 1984; Ainlay et al. 1986; Falk 2001; Link & Phelan 2001), with psychologists showing particular interest (Jones et al. 1984; Herman et al. 1986; Heatherton et al. 2000).

In contemporary **post-industrial societies**, many conditions and characteristics are socially defined as **deviant** rather than being accepted as 'normal'. These conditions are viewed as marginal and labelled as 'deviant', and consequently are stigmatised. The **marginality** of an attribute is not necessarily based on its prevalence or functionality, but instead is based on the social norms and values attached to that particular trait or condition. Individuals who are marginal with respect to one attribute are not necessarily marginal in other respects (Sobal & Hinrichs 1986). Marginal conditions that are stigmatised in contemporary society include those that are medical (AIDS, cancer, leprosy, physical deformities, infertility, disability), economic (poverty, unemployment, use of welfare, homelessness), sociocultural (ethnicity, homosexuality, prostitution, criminality, illiteracy, substance abuse, divorce), and many other types of conditions. Obesity is a stigma that has received much attention from social scientists.

Obesity is the condition in which a person has a high level of stored body fat. The amount of body fat that people possess varies across a wide continuum. The leanest individuals carry only a few per cent of their total body weight as stored fat, while the majority of the fattest people's body weight is made up of stored fat. Cut-off points for defining obesity are not absolute and universally agreed upon, and many standards are used in practice (Dalton 1997). For sociological purposes, obesity can simply be considered as the condition in which an individual has relatively high amounts of body fat (Sobal & Devine 1997; Sobal 2001). Quantitative definitions that specify exactly the level of fat that constitutes obesity are often not necessary for examining sociological patterns and processes, despite their emphasis in biomedical work. A relative definition of obesity permits variation among different groups (such as dancers and construction workers) in their evaluations of how much body fat is excessive.

Public beliefs about the cause of obesity tend to focus on the assumption that obese people overeat and consume too much caloric energy, rather than on the role of low activity levels and low energy expenditure in producing obesity. In contemporary post-industrial societies, where the food system provides people with ample access to a wide variety of foods, many of which are high in fat and are calorically dense, there is a strong link between food, eating and weight. Post-industrial food systems add unnecessary calories at all stages (production, processing, distribution, acquisition, preparation and consumption) and are therefore labelled 'fattening food systems' (Sobal 2001). Sociologists have commented on how the social system provides easy access to high-calorie inexpensive food, with a consequently high prevalence of obesity and the parallel development of a fear of fatness (Mennell 1985; McIntosh 1996; Beardsworth & Keil 1997).

The stigmatisation of obesity reflects the extent to which high body weight is socially defined as either central or marginal to what is collectively agreed upon and accepted as 'normal' in society (or a portion of society). Thus a person with lower body weight than the average may be defined as socially normal, while someone with a body weight equally far above the average may be regarded as marginal and be stigmatised. Where negative and prejudicial attitudes about obesity exist, obesity is treated as a physical deformity, and obese people are discredited and discriminated against.

Cultural and historical factors

The cultural and historical location of the current stigmatisation of obesity is important to consider in order to gain a broader, relative perspective on how the stigma of obesity is socially constructed (Sobal 2001). Traditional societies, which have not been involved in the modernisation associated with the Industrial Revolution, tend to appreciate and value at least moderate, if not large, amounts of body fat (Brown & Konner 1987). Traditional cultures view stored body fat as a sign of health and wealth, particularly for women (Sobal & Stunkard 1989).

The harsher survival conditions of traditional societies mean that food supplies may be uncertain; moreover, concentrated fat sources are less available in their usual foods and their everyday life involves considerable energy expenditure. Consequently, people who can attain at least a moderate degree of fatness are viewed as attractive; they are clearly not afflicted by a wasting disease or intestinal parasites, and appear to have access to the social resources necessary to obtain food. Cross-cultural data about body preferences for women reveal that over 80 per cent of cultures for which body shape preference data are available prefer a plump shape (Anderson et al. 1992). The value of fatness in many African and Pacific cultures is evidenced by the existence of fattening huts (Brink 1989), in which women and

Jeffery Sobal

men engage in ritualistic ingestion of huge amounts of food and avoid activity to gain large amounts of weight to enhance their beauty and social status (Gaurine & Pollock 1995). The high prevalence of obesity and the strong rejection of body fat in Western, post-industrial nations are very different trends from most other cultures, and anthropologists have described obesity as a **culture-bound syndrome** unique to Western societies (Ritenbaugh 1982).

Historical changes in the evaluation and prevalence of obesity also provide important perspectives on the current patterns of stigmatisation of obesity. Like traditional cultures today and in the past, most Western societies until the late nineteenth century valued at least moderate levels of body fat (Brumberg 1988; Seid 1989; Stearns 1997). At the beginning of the twentieth century, a transformation in values relating to fatness was underway, as modern ideals of thinness were established, promulgated and widely applied (Stearns 1997). The emphasis on thinness intensified in the second half of the twentieth century, particularly for women. Evidence for this can be seen in the increasingly thinner body shapes of women in idealised social roles, such as beauty pageant winners (Garner et al. 1980; Wiseman et al. 1992) and fashion models (Morris et al. 1989). As pressures towards slimness escalated and intensified, fatness moved from being a social ideal to being rejected as a marginal, deviant and stigmatised attribute. Most concern about body weight is motivated by appearance, not health (Hayes & Ross 1987).

The stigma of obesity as a master status

Attribution of responsibility for a stigma is a crucial consideration: stigmas that are not considered the 'fault' of an individual are treated differently from those for which personal 'blame' can be attributed (DeJong 1980; 1993; DeJong & Kleck 1986; Weiner et al. 1988; Menec & Perry 1995). The causes of high body weight are currently not established with certainty, with claims and counterclaims about whether obesity is the result of overeating, lack of activity, or genetic or hormonal conditions (Saguy & Riley 2005; Sobal 1995). These disputes about the causes of obesity remain unresolved in the scientific and medical community, as well as among the general public. Stigmatising claims about gluttony and sloth are counterpoised with destigmatising claims about inheritance and metabolism. The general orientation in contemporary society is to hold obese individuals personally accountable for their size, and to discredit and reject them as personal failures.

An important aspect of stigma is that it is often incorporated into individuals' identities and involved in their self-evaluations. The impact of stigmas varies, with some stigmas being of only minor importance and others overwhelming a person and becoming a **master status** (Goffman 1963; Hiller 1981). Obese people are often characterised more by their size than by any of their other attributes, being described as simply 'fat' rather than being dealt with on the basis of other qualities. The effects of stigmatisation of obesity are often internalised, particularly by women (Crocker et al. 1993; Sobal & Devine 1997). Negative social stereotypes relating to obesity often become self-fulfilling prophecies for obese individuals.

Feminist analysis has shown that some stigmas, particularly obesity, are highly gendered (Yancey et al. 2006). Stigmatisation of obesity is much more problematic for women because they are evaluated more on the basis of their appearance and weight than are men (Millman 1980). The gendered nature of the stigmatisation of obesity makes weight much more important to women (Tiggemann & Rothblum 1988; Germov & Williams 1996; see also Chapter 15).

Ever since Steven Richardson and his colleagues' (1961) pioneering quantitative research and Werner Cahnman's (1968) interactionist analysis, sociologists have been examining the stigma of obesity. Sociological analysis of the stigma of obesity typically uses two mainstream theoretical perspectives—**functionalism** and **symbolic interactionism**—and has rarely applied other theoretical orientations, such as Marxism or rational choice theory (Cawley et al. 2006).

While a variety of research methods have been applied to the stigmatisation of obesity, the bulk of studies have used the two major sociological data-collection methods of surveys and participant observation. Functionalist analysis documents and describes as social facts the presence, arenas, extent and sources of the stigmatisation of obese individuals. This stream of analysis takes a positivist approach in examining stigma as a barrier to access to social roles and privileges. Analyses are often quantitative, using experiments or surveys to analyse the frequency and extent of stigmatisation.

Interactionist analysis examines the strategies that obese individuals use to manage their stigma and to negotiate their way in a world that values thinness. It does so while considering the construction of social definitions of obesity. These analyses follow the constructionist symbolic-interactionist tradition, often appealing to dramaturgical analyses grounded in the work of Goffman (1959; 1963). These investigations employ ethnographic techniques, such as participant observation and in-depth interviews, to investigate stigmatisation as a socially constructed, negotiated and managed process (Sobal & Maurer 1999a; 1999b). These two lines of analysis will be reviewed in the following two sections.

The presence, arenas, extent and sources of stigmatisation of obesity

Severe stigmatisation of obese people exists in contemporary post-industrial societies (Allon 1981; Sobal 1984a; 1991; Goode 1996), though some reviews suggest that the negative effects of the stigmatisation of obesity have not been clearly demonstrated

(Jarvie et al. 1983). In addition to establishing the presence of stigmatisation of obesity, studies have examined the arenas, extent and sources of stigmatisation.

Stigmatisation operates in many arenas, occurring broadly across most domains of an obese person's world—at work, at home, in public life and so on (Gortmaker et al. 1993; Carr & Friedman 2005). This observation supports the concept that obesity becomes a 'master status' (Goffman 1963) that pervades all aspects of life. Studies of stigmatisation have focused on some areas more than others, with much research having been carried out on stigmatisation in formal roles, such as that of employee. Less research has been done on stigmatisation in informal roles, such as that of friend. The major arenas in which stigmatisation of the obese has been documented are education and work, marriage and family, health and medical care, and interpersonal and social interactions.

Obese individuals in the United States of America are less favourably evaluated than thinner individuals for admission to the higher education that is essential for entry and advancement in many careers, and receive less financial support when they are admitted to college (Canning & Mayer 1966; Crandall 1991; 1995). People who are obese are also less successful in gaining employment and entering the labour force (Fikkan & Rothblum 2005). Obese individuals who do become employees receive lower wages than comparable co-workers, are less likely to receive promotions, and experience more discrimination on the job (Averett & Korenman 1996; Cawley 2003). Overall, stigmatisation of obese individuals consistently occurs across the span of educational and work roles.

Weight is an important criterion for dating and mate selection, and obese individuals (women in particular) have a more difficult time dating and finding marital partners than do thinner individuals (Cawley et al. 2005; Kallen & Doughty 1984; Sobal 1984b; Sobal et al. 1992; 1995; 2003; Gortmaker et al. 1993). Most obese people eventually marry, but their choice of partners is restricted because of their stigmatised condition (Garn et al. 1989a; 1989b). Obese women, once married, may feel they are unable to leave their marriage because they have less value on the marriage market (Cawley et al. 2005; Sobal et al. 1995). These research findings show that stigmatisation of obese individuals occurs in the entry into and maintenance of marital and family roles.

Health professionals frequently stigmatise obese individuals, holding prejudicial attitudes and exhibiting them in discriminatory actions. Health care professionals of many types (including physicians, nurses, counsellors, dietitians, psychologists, health administrators and others) at many stages of their careers (as students, interns, practitioners and educators) have negative attitudes and beliefs about obese individuals (Fabricatore et al. 2005). The antipathy exhibited by student health practitioners towards obese individuals suggests that their attitudes are based on wider societal values about obesity rather than on actual problems that they have experienced in dealing with obese clients. Prejudicial attitudes towards obese individuals among health care professionals translate into discrimination in the provision of health care services such as diagnosis and treatment (Allon 1979; Young & Powell 1985). Health care providers are not immune to the stigmatisation of obese individuals as they carry out their professional roles, providing unequal health care service on the basis of body weight.

The everyday interactions of obese individuals also may be hampered by stigmatisation (Pauley 1989; Sobal 2005). Compared with their thinner counterparts, obese individuals are discriminated against in basic transactions such as renting apartments (Karris 1977). Some investigations report that obese individuals have fewer friends (Strauss & Pollack 2003), although other studies find this not to be the case (Jarvie et al. 1983; Miller et al. 1995a). Overall, stigmatisation operates as a multidimensional burden on obese individuals, spanning work, family, health and interpersonal arenas.

A classic series of sociological investigations compared the stigmatisation of physical disabilities with the stigmatisation of obesity by showing participants a series of pictures of children with a variety of disabilities as well as pictures of an obese child and asking who they would prefer as a friend (Richardson et al. 1961; Goodman et al. 1963; Maddox & Liederman 1968; Richardson 1970; 1971). The striking findings revealed that both adults and children consistently preferred disabled people to obese people, providing clear evidence that obesity is more stigmatised than physical disabilities such as blindness, crippling diseases, amputations and facial disfigurements. A replication of these studies 40 years after the first ones showed that stigmatisation of obese children by other children had increased significantly over time in the USA (Latner & Stunkard 2003). However, in other cultures, such as Nepal, children reacted positively to the pictures of the obese child (Harper 1997).

Some broader comparative analyses of stigmatisation of different forms of deviant conditions have been done. Several studies reveal that obesity is seen as being as stigmatised as many other deviant conditions, such as AIDS, drug addiction, criminal behaviour and homosexuality (Spiegal & Keith-Spiegel 1973; Weiner et al. 1988; Schwarzer & Weiner 1990). Stigmatisation of obesity is more severe than that of eating disorders (Brotman et al. 1984; Sobal et al. 1995), although eating disorders are stigmatised and carry negative evaluations (Way 1995; Sobal & Bursztyn 1998). The stigma of obesity may combine with other stigmas, cumulating to produce 'double jeopardy' in discrimination (NaPier et al. 2005). While legal measures and social norms have greatly reduced the stigmatisation of many racial, religious, gender and sexual groups, prejudice against and derogation of obese individuals are tolerated and even treated as socially acceptable (Stunkard & Sobal 1995; Solovay 2000).

Myriad sources of stigmatisation permeate the lives of obese individuals. In interpersonal interactions, obese individuals are stigmatised by others in a variety of social roles and relationships. The public at large stigmatises obese individuals in informal interactions of many types (Sobal 2005). The mass media stigmatise obese individuals actively by negatively representing those large people who do appear on television, and passively by not including large people in television, film and other media in numbers proportional to their presence in the general population (Fouts & Burggraf 1999; Fouts & Vaughan 2002; Wykes & Gunter 2005). The mass media also present extremely thin people as the ideal, which leads to negative comparisons of obese individuals with media images (Silverstein et al. 1986; Myers & Biocca 1992; Waller et al. 1994). In summary, stigmatisation of obese individuals exists, is prevalent and often intense, occurs in multifaceted ways, and emanates from a variety of sources.

Coping with the stigma of obesity

Goffman (1963) used the concept of stigma within a broad theoretical examination of interpersonal interaction processes, revealing the development and management of deviant identities. The development of the concept of stigma complemented his other sociological work on the presentation of self, dramaturgical role analysis and impression management (Goffman 1959; 1961; Ditton 1980; Drew & Wootton 1988). Based on the perspectives used by Goffman, many sociologists and psychologists have examined how obese individuals who are stigmatised construct their identities and manage their interactions with others so as to cope with the stigma of obesity (Puhl & Brownell 2003) situated within social categories (Kusow 2004).

Stigmatising acts can be verbal (such as teasing, joking and negative comments) or non-verbal (such as staring, making gestures and avoiding a person). Stigmatisation can be active (operating through overt negative behaviours) or passive (occurring through avoidance of interactions with stigmatised individuals).

Everyday life involves the performance of a variety of activities, with individuals operating as actors presenting themselves to actual or imagined others who constitute audiences for their behaviour (Goffman 1959). Stigmatised individuals recognise that their performance of various tasks may be disrupted by negative treatment as a result of their stigma, and attempt to prevent or deal with problems resulting from their stigma. Obese people are treated negatively in social interactions because of their body size and develop many strategies for dealing with the stigmatising acts of others (Sobal 1991; Brownell et al. 2005).

Gaining and maintaining acceptance is a central feature of a stigmatised person's life. Although legitimacy in interpersonal interactions may be claimed by individuals, it is conferred by others (Elliott et al. 1990). A variety of coping mechanisms exist for individuals with various types of stigma. These include denial, concealment, avoidance, mutual aid, redefinition of situations, and others (Elliott et al. 1990; Puhl & Brownell 2003; 2006).

Some obese people, particularly men, use denial to deal with interactional challenges associated with their body weight (Millman 1980). By denying that they are 'really' fat, or denying that the fat they have is their fault, they effectively ignore the stigma of obesity; this strategy offers one way of coping for particular individuals in specific situations. This type of management of stigmatising acts typically involves claims that large size or weight is caused by muscle, large bones or genetics.

Concealment is a form of strategic impression management whereby a stigma is hidden, disguised or modified to make it less obtrusive and therefore less likely to be attended to or focused on in a social encounter. Many obese individuals make considerable efforts in concealment, including hiding parts of their bodies by wearing loose or heavy clothing to mask their size. One form of concealment is deflection or distraction, whereby other aspects of appearance, such as hair or jewellery, are used to draw attention away from an obese person's body. 'Passing' occurs when stigmatised individuals successfully conceal their stigma and are accepted as 'normal' (Goffman 1963); passing as 'normal' may or may not be possible for an obese individual in face-to-face interaction, depending on the extent of their weight and their ability to conceal it.

Avoidance and withdrawal are common methods of coping with stigmatisation. Many stigmatised individuals arrange their lives so as to avoid or minimise stigmatising contacts, because of uncertainty about how 'normals' will receive and deal with them (Goffman 1963). Many obese individuals practise selective or widespread avoidance of social settings and individuals where they perceive a likelihood of being stigmatised. This involves outright refusal to enter some situations, particularly those in which their entire body will be on display, such as on a beach, at a swimming pool or in a locker room. Management of the frequency, content and extent of interactions with particular individuals is another form of avoidance, with obese individuals eschewing contact with people who have stigmatised them in the past or who are thought to be likely to engage in future stigmatising acts. Self-segregation (Schur 1979) occurs where stigmatised individuals interact with, and accept as 'insiders', only those who are obese or are 'wise' (Goffman 1963) to the plight of overweight people.

By redefining situations, a stigmatised person can steer the topic or subject of interactions away from a stigmatised condition to other more neutral or safe areas. Obese individuals often develop strategies for deflecting or shifting the focus of interactions away from their size to other topics (Sobal 1991). The threat of stigmatisation leads some obese individuals to present themselves in a comedic role, using humour to facilitate and negotiate interactions with people who could potentially discredit them because of their size.

Mutual aid is a strategy whereby communities of stigmatised individuals form to share feelings and resources and provide social support for one another (Goffman 1963). Mutual aid ranges from the exchange of stories and ideas between obese friends to the establishment of national or international organisations to promote size acceptance (Sobal 1999). While the manifest goal of weight-loss programs is to become thinner through diet and exercise, the latent services often sought and provided through such groups are the sharing of emotional support and the exchange of coping strategies for dealing with being overweight (Allon 1975; Laslett & Warren 1975).

Collective behaviour often results from the establishment of advocacy groups and organisations, and the size acceptance movement has established itself as an important force in contemporary public discourse on obesity (Sobal 1995; 1999). Many large people rebel against sizeism, fatism or weightism and celebrate their bodies (Joanisse & Synnott 1999; Braziel & LeBesco 2001).

Eating is an especially problematic act for obese people (English 1991), because it carries so much potential for critique and criticism by others (Zdrodowski 1996). Several sociological concepts help us to identify some of the special coping methods used by stigmatised individuals when their eating behaviours are scrutinised by others. Even when an obese person eats the same things as a 'normal'-weight companion, the obese person faces the threat of being criticised for overeating. Stigmatising acts include challenges to, and criticisms of, the eating behaviours of obese individuals. Obese people may avoid food events entirely as a way of coping with the threat of being discredited. Alternatively, they may attend but eat nothing, or they may eat selectively and be prepared to explain their food choices.

Obese individuals may defend the legitimacy of their eating behaviour by providing what Scott and Lyman (1963) term '**accounts**' (English 1991; Orbuch 1997). Accounts can be divided into justifications and excuses (Scott & Lyman 1963). Justifications accept responsibility but deny the negative qualities of the behaviour, as when an obese person eating confectionery claims that it is the only thing that they have eaten all day. Excuses admit the negative qualities of an action, but deny responsibility, and there are several types. Accident excuses deny fault because a behaviour was beyond personal control, as when an obese individual eating ice-cream claims that it was the only food available. Defensibility excuses state that insufficient information was available, as when an obese person claims to have believed that the food being eaten was a reduced-calorie version. Biological-drive excuses explain actions in terms of a lack of control over a behaviour, as when an obese person claims that hormones led him or her to eat a particular item.

There are other ways of managing eating related to accounts. **Disclaimers** (Hewett & Stokes 1975) anticipate challenges to legitimacy, as in claims by obese people that they have adhered to a restricted diet earlier in anticipation of a particular food event. **Discounting** (Pestello 1991) includes several strategies. Coercion discounting occurs when a violation of personal principles is outside a person's control, as when an obese person claims that someone else prepared high-calorie foods for them. Exception discounting involves compromises that are seen as serving a greater purpose, as when an obese person claims not to have wanted to offend someone by refusing to eat high-calorie ceremonial foods that were specially prepared. Denial discounting makes no admission of a behaviour or its meaning, as when an obese person eats what is served at a dinner and makes no comments or explanations about the food.

Concealment discounting entails accepting responsibility for a behaviour but denying that the behaviour is negative, as when an obese person reports having eaten a chocolate dessert but claims that the chocolate prevents other food cravings. All of these techniques are used to socially manage eating. They help obese individuals to negotiate a path through potentially precarious social interactions and to ward off threats to their selves.

Often obese individuals develop a 'fat identity' as they accept their weight and as they establish and elaborate a social self that incorporates weight as a personal attribute (McLorg & Taub 1987; O'Brien & Bankston 1990; Degher & Hughes 1991; Hughes & Degher 1993). Attempts to lose weight also involve aspiration to a new, thinner identity. Many obese people perceive this as the attainment of a 'normal' weight status, which will free them from stigmatisation. Often people who do change their weight have to reconcile their social identity with their body size (English 1993; Rubin et al. 1993). Thinner identities may be seen as desirable in that they avoid stigmatisation, but they may also carry undesirable consequences, such as the need to deal with unwanted sexual advances, which did not occur before (Sobal 1984a).

While obese individuals suffer from stigmatisation in contemporary post-industrial society (Millman 1980), they employ many strategies to cope with their stigma and to establish functional life patterns in spite of negative societal attitudes towards them. Psychological strategies are used to compensate for stigma (Miller et al. 1995b; Puhl & Brownell 2006), and social relationships are established to buffer against negative experiences (Millman 1980).

Organisations and groups help to empower individuals by validating and valorising their struggles against the weight prejudices of many people in the wider society (Sobal 1999). Struggles with negative attitudes and with social avoidance and ostracism are often required throughout an obese individual's life, requiring coping efforts that deeply shape their identities. Sociological analyses that examine how obese individuals construct, negotiate and manage their lives provide a portrait of the stigmatisation of obesity that differs from, but complements, work describing the prevalence and types of stigmatisation.

Conclusion

Over the past 40 years, stigma has emerged as an important sociological concept, grounded in the pioneering work of Erving Goffman (1963). The concept of stigma has been widely applied to a variety of conditions, stretching and testing the boundaries of its conceptual coverage. Obesity was mentioned as a stigmatised condition in Goffman's seminal book, and it remains a clear case of a stigma in contemporary society.

The examination and elaboration of the concept of stigmatisation in relation to obesity has involved some work in a positivist tradition in psychological social psychology and functionalist sociology. Simultaneously, constructionist work based in the symbolic interactionist tradition of sociological social psychology continued the lines of analysis begun by Goffman. The existing literature on the stigma of obesity reflects a consensus in some areas, but leaves other aspects of the topic to be addressed in future investigations.

Obesity has become a highly stigmatised condition in contemporary post-industrial societies, with obese individuals being labelled negatively and risking a variety of defiling and degrading prejudicial attitudes and discriminatory actions. The social position of obesity relative to other deviant conditions is not currently very clear.

Obese individuals employ several types of coping mechanisms to manage their social interactions with others. However, the frequency and success of different strategies for coping with the stigmatisation of obesity have not been thoroughly researched. Clearly, obesity is a stigma in contemporary society, but it is not clear how obese people can most effectively deal with this stigma.

SUMMARY OF MAIN POINTS

- Stigmas are discrediting attributes, and obesity is often stigmatised in post-industrial societies.
- Stigmatisation of obesity is widespread, frequent and often severe.
- Stigmatisation of obesity occurs in work, family, health and everyday arenas.
- The mechanisms used to cope with the stigmatisation of obesity include denial, concealment, avoidance, mutual aid and redefinition of situations.
- Eating is problematic for obese individuals, who use accounts, disclaimers and discounting to explain their food choices.

SOCIOLOGICAL REFLECTION

- To what extent is obesity biological, psychological, social, economic, political and cultural?
- Which parts of society are more or less responsible for preventing and managing obesity: individuals using personal will power, governments using political will, companies/corporations using industrial will, or others?
- Under what conditions, and how much, does stigmatisation deter obesity and prevent health problems? In contrast, how, for whom, where, when and how much does stigmatisation harm obese individuals, their families, their friends and the larger society?

DISCUSSION QUESTIONS

1. How is the stigmatisation of obesity similar to and different from the stigmatisation of other 'deviant' attributes?
2. How would obese individuals be treated in a culture that did not stigmatise either fatness or thinness, or in a culture that highly valued fatness?
3. What types or categories of people in society are least likely to stigmatise obese individuals, and what types are most likely to do so?
4. How do different approaches to sociological analysis (such as functionalist theory using quantitative methods, or symbolic interactionist theory using qualitative methods) provide both incompatible and compatible perspectives on the stigmatisation of obesity?
5. How could society change in order to reduce stigmatisation of obese individuals, and how can obese individuals better deal with stigmatisation?

Further investigation

1. Describe and discuss the medicalisation of obesity.
2. Discuss how the stigmatisation of obesity differs between women and men.

FURTHER READING AND WEB RESOURCES

Books

Brownell, K.D., Puhl, R.M, Schwartz, M.B. & Rudd, L. (eds) 2005, *Weight Bias: Nature, Consequences, and Remedies*, Guilford Press, New York.

Bryant, C.D. (ed.) 1990, *Deviant Behavior: Readings in the Sociology of Norm Violations*, Hemisphere, New York.

Gaurine, I. & Pollock, N.J. (eds) 1995, *Social Aspects of Obesity*, Gordon & Breach, New York.

Goffman, E. 1963, *Stigma: Notes on the Management of Spoiled Identity*, Simon & Schuster, New York.

Maurer, D. & Sobal, J. (eds) 1995, *Eating Agendas: Food and Nutrition as Social Problems*, Aldine de Gruyter, New York.

Millman, M. 1980, *Such a Pretty Face: Being Fat in America*, Norton, New York.

Sobal, J. & Maurer, D. (eds) 1999, *Interpreting Weight: The Social Management of Fatness and Thinness*, Aldine de Gruyter, Hawthorne, New York State.

—— (eds) 1999, *Weighty Issues: The Construction of Fatness and Thinness as Social Problems*, Aldine de Gruyter, Hawthorne, New York State.

Jeffery Sobal

Websites

International Size Acceptance Association: www.size-acceptance.org/
National Association to Advance Fat Acceptance: naafa.org/

REFERENCES

Ainlay, S.C., Becker, G. & Coleman, L.M. (eds) 1986, *The Dilemma of Difference: A Multidisciplinary View of Stigma*, Plenum, New York.

Allon, N. 1975, 'Latent Social Services of Group Dieting', *Social Problems*, vol. 23, pp. 59–69.

—— 1979, 'Self-Perceptions of the Stigma of Overweight in Relationship to Weight-losing Patterns', *American Journal of Clinical Nutrition*, vol. 32, pp. 4770–80.

—— 1981, 'The Stigma of Overweight in Everyday Life', in B.J. Wolman (ed.), *Psychological Aspects of Obesity: A Handbook*, Van Nostrand Reinhold, New York, pp. 130–74.

Anderson, J.L., Crawford, C.B., Nadeau, J. & Lindberg, T. 1992, 'Was the Duchess of Windsor Right? A Cross-cultural Review of the Socioecology of Ideals of Female Body Shape', *Ethnology and Sociobiology*, vol. 13, pp. 197–227.

Averett, S. & Korenman, S. 1996, 'The Economic Reality of the Beauty Myth', *Journal of Human Resources*, vol. 31, pp. 304–30.

Beardsworth, A. & Keil, T. 1997, *Sociology on the Menu: An Invitation to the Study of Food and Society*, Routledge, London.

Braziel, J.E. & LeBesco, K. 2001, *Bodies Out of Bounds: Fatness and Transgressions*, University of California Press, Berkeley, California.

Brink, P.J. 1989, 'The Fattening Room among the Annang of Nigeria. Anthropological Approaches to Nursing Research', *Medical Anthropology*, vol. 12, pp. 131–43.

Brotman, A.W., Stern, T.A. & Herzog, D.B. 1984, 'Emotional Reactions of House Officers to Patients with Anorexia Nervosa, Diabetes, and Obesity', *International Journal of Eating Disorders*, vol. 3, pp. 71–7.

Brown, P.J. & Konner, M. 1987, 'An Anthropological Perspective on Obesity', *Annals of the New York Academy of Sciences*, vol. 499, pp. 29–46.

Brownell, K.D., Puhl, R.M., Schwartz, M.B. & Rudd, L. (eds) 2005, *Weight Bias: Nature, Consequences, and Remedies*, Guilford Press, New York.

Brumberg, J. 1988, *Fasting Girls: The History of Anorexia Nervosa*, Harvard University Press, Cambridge, Massachusetts.

Cahnman, W.J. 1968, 'The Stigma of Obesity', *Sociological Quarterly*, vol. 9, pp. 282–99.

Canning, H. & Mayer, J. 1966, 'Obesity: Its Possible Effect on College Acceptance', *New England Journal of Medicine*, vol. 275, pp. 1172–4.

Carr, D. & Friedman, M.A. 2005, 'Is Obesity Stigmatizing? Body Weight, Perceived Discrimination, and Psychological Well-Being in the United States', *Journal of Health and Social Behavior*, vol. 46, pp. 244–59.

Cawley, J. 2003, 'What Explains Race and Gender Differences in the Relationship between Obesity and Wages?', *Gender Issues*, vol. 21, pp. 30–47.

Cawley, J., Joyner, K. & Sobal, J. 2006, 'Size Matters: The Influence of Adolescents' Weight and Height on Dating and Sex', *Rationality and Society*, vol. 18, pp. 67–94.

Crandall, C.S. 1991, 'Do Heavyweight Students Have More Difficulty Paying for College?', *Personality and Social Psychology Bulletin*, vol. 17, pp. 606–11.

—— 1995, 'Do Parents Discriminate Against Their Heavyweight Daughters?', *Personality and Social Psychology Bulletin*, vol. 21, pp. 724–35.

Crocker, J., Cornwall, B. & Major, B. 1993, 'The Stigma of Overweight: Affective Consequences of Attributional Ambiguity', *Journal of Personality and Social Psychology*, vol. 64, pp. 67–70.

Dalton, S. 1997, 'Body Weight Terminology, Definitions, and Measurement', in S. Dalton (ed.), *Overweight and Weight Management*, Aspen Publishers, Gaithersburg, Maryland, pp. 1–38.

Degher, D. & Hughes, G. 1991, 'The Identity Change Process: A Field Study of Obesity', *Deviant Behavior*, vol. 12, pp. 385–401.

DeJong, W. 1980, 'The Stigma of Obesity: Consequences of Naive Assumptions Concerning the Causes of Physical Deviance', *Journal of Health and Social Behavior*, vol. 21, pp. 75–85.

—— 1993, 'Obesity as a Characterological Stigma: The Issue of Responsibility and Judgments in Task Performance', *Psychological Reports*, vol. 73, pp. 963–70.

DeJong, W. & Kleck, R.E. 1986, 'The Social Psychological Effects of Overweight', in C.P. Herman, M.P. Zanna and E.T. Higgins (eds), *Physical Appearance, Stigma, and Social Behavior: The Ontario Symposium*, vol. 3, Lawrence Erlbaum Associates, Hillsdale, New Jersey, pp. 65–87.

Ditton, J. (ed.) 1980, *The View from Goffman*, St Martin's, New York.

Drew, P. & Wootton, A. (eds) 1988, *Erving Goffman: Exploring the Interaction Order*, Northeastern University Press, Boston.

Elliott, G.C., Ziegler, H.L., Altman, B.M. & Scott, D.R. 1990, 'Understanding Stigma: Dimensions of Deviance and Coping', in C.D. Bryant (ed.), *Deviant Behavior: Readings in the Sociology of Norm Violations*, Hemisphere, New York, pp. 423–43.

English, C. 1991, 'Food is My Best Friend: Self-justifications and Weight-loss Efforts', *Research in the Sociology of Health Care*, vol. 9, pp. 335–45.

—— 1993, 'Gaining and Losing Weight: Identity Transformations', *Deviant Behavior*, vol. 14, pp. 227–41.

Fabricatore, A.N., Wadden, T.A. & Foster, G.D. 2005, 'Bias in Health Care Settings', in K.D. Brownell, R.M. Puhl, M.B. Schwartz & L. Rudd (eds), *Weight Bias: Nature, Consequences, and Remedies*, Guilford Press, New York, pp. 29–41.

Falk, G. 2001, *Stigma: How We Treat Outsiders*, Prometheus Books, Amherst, New York State.

Fikkan, J. & Rothblum, E. 2005, 'Weight Bias in Employment,' in K.D. Brownell, R.M. Puhl, M.B. Schwartz & L. Rudd (eds), *Weight Bias: Nature, Consequences, and Remedies*, Guilford Press, New York, pp. 15–28.

Fouts, G. & Burggraf, K. 1999, 'Television Situation Comedies: Female Body Images and Verbal Reinforcements', *Sex Roles*, vol. 40, pp. 473–81.

Fouts, G. & Vaughan, K. 2002, 'Television Situation Comedies: Male Weight, Negative References, and Audience Reactions', *Sex Roles*, vol. 46, pp. 439–42.

Garn, S., Sullivan, T.V. & Hawthorne, V.M. 1989a, 'The Education of One Spouse and the Fatness of the Other Spouse', *American Journal of Human Biology*, vol. 1, pp. 233–8.

—— 1989b, 'Educational Level, Fatness, and Fatness Differences between Husbands and Wives', *American Journal of Clinical Nutrition*, vol. 50, pp. 740–5.

Garner, D.M., Garfinkel, P.E., Schwartz, D. & Thompson, M. 1980, 'Cultural Expectations of Thinness in Women', *Psychological Reports*, vol. 47, pp. 483–91.

Gaurine, I. & Pollock, N.J. (eds) 1995, *Social Aspects of Obesity*, Gordon & Breach, New York.

Germov, J. & Williams, L. 1996, 'The Sexual Division of Dieting: Women's Voices', *Sociological Review*, vol. 44, pp. 630–47.

Goffman, E. 1959, *The Presentation of Self in Everyday Life*, Anchor, New York.

—— 1961, *Asylums*, Doubleday, New York.

—— 1963, *Stigma: Notes on the Management of Spoiled Identity*, Simon & Schuster, New York.

Goode, E. 1996, 'The Stigma of Obesity', in E. Goode (ed.), *Social Deviance*, Allyn & Bacon, Boston, pp. 332–40.

Goodman, N., Richardson, S.A., Dombusch, S. & Hastort, A.H. 1963, 'Variant Reactions to Physical Disabilities', *American Sociological Review*, vol. 28, pp. 429–35.

Gortmaker, S.L., Must, A., Perrin, J.M., Sobol, A.M. & Dietz, W.H. 1993, 'Social and Economic Consequences of Overweight in Adolescence and Young Adulthood', *New England Journal of Medicine*, vol. 329, pp. 1008–12.

Harper, D.C. 1997, 'Children's Attitudes toward Physical Disability in Nepal: A Field Study', *Journal of Cross-cultural Psychology*, vol. 28, pp. 710–29.

Hayes, D. & Ross, C.E. 1987, 'Concern with Appearance, Health Beliefs, and Eating Habits', *Journal of Health and Social Behavior*, vol. 28, pp. 120–30.

Heatherton, T.F., Kleck, R.E., Hebl, M.R. & Hull, J.G. 2000, *The Social Psychology of Stigma*, Guilford Press, New York.

Herman, C.P., Zanna, M.P. & Higgins, E.T. (eds) 1986, *Physical Appearance, Stigma, and Social Behavior: The Ontario Symposium*, vol. 3, Lawrence Erlbaum Associates, Hillsdale, New Jersey.

Hewett, J.P. & Stokes, R. 1975, 'Disclaimers', *American Sociological Review*, vol. 40, pp. 1–11.

Hiller, D.V. 1981, 'The Salience of Overweight in Personality Characterization', *Journal of Personality*, vol. 108, pp. 233–40.

Hughes, G. & Degher, D. 1993, 'Coping with Deviant Identity', *Deviant Behavior*, vol. 14, pp. 297–315.

Jarvie, G.J., Lahey, B., Graziano, W. & Framer, E. 1983, 'Childhood Obesity: What We Know and What We Don't Know', *Developmental Review*, vol. 2, pp. 237–73.

Joanisse, L. & Synnott, A. 1999, 'Fighting Back: Reactions and Resistance to the Stigma of Obesity', in J. Sobal & D. Maurer (eds), *Interpreting Weight: The Social Management of Fatness and Thinness*, Aldine de Gruyter, Hawthorne, New York State, pp. 49–70.

Jones, E.E., Fanna, A., Hastort, A.H., Markus, H., Miller, D.T. & Scott, R.A. 1984, *Social Stigma: The Psychology of Marked Relationships*, W.H. Freeman & Company, New York.

Kallen, D. & Doughty, A. 1984, 'The Relationship of Weight, the Self Perception of Weight, and Self Esteem in Courtship Behavior', *Marriage and Family Review*, vol. 7, pp. 93–114.

Karris, L. 1977, 'Prejudice Against Obese Renters', *Journal of Social Psychology*, vol. 101, pp. 159–60.

Kusow, A.M. 2004, 'Contesting Stigma: On Goffman's Assumptions of Normative Order,' *Symbolic Interaction*, vol. 27, pp. 179–97.

Laslett, B. & Warren, C.A.B. 1975, 'Losing Weight: The Organizational Promotion of Behavior Change', *Social Problems*, vol. 23, pp. 69–80.

Latner, J.D. & Stunkard, A.J. 2003, 'Getting Worse: The Stigmatization of Obese Children', *Obesity Research*, vol. 11, pp. 452–6.

Link, B.G. & Phelan, J.C. 2001, 'Conceptualizing Stigma', *Annual Review of Sociology*, vol. 27, pp. 363–85.

Maddox, G.L. & Liederman, V.R. 1968, 'Overweight as Social Deviance and Disability', *Journal of Health and Social Behavior*, vol. 9, pp. 287–98.

McIntosh, W.A. 1996, *Sociologies of Food and Nutrition*, Plenum, New York.

McLorg, P.A. & Taub, D.E. 1987, 'Anorexia and Bulimia: The Development of Deviant Identities', *Deviant Behavior*, vol. 8, pp. 177–89.

Menec, V.H. & Perry, R.P. 1995, 'Reactions to Stigmas: The Effects of Targets' Age and Controllability of Stigmas', *Journal of Aging and Health*, vol. 7, pp. 365–83.

Mennell, S. 1985, *All Manners of Food: Eating and Taste in England and France from the Middle Ages to the Present*, Blackwell, Oxford.

Miller, C.T., Rothblum, E.D., Brand, P.A. & Felicio, D.M. 1995a, 'Do Obese Women Have Poorer Social Relationships than Nonobese Women? Reports by Self, Friends, and Coworkers', *Journal of Personality*, vol. 63, pp. 65–85.

Miller, C.T., Rothblum, E.D., Felicio, D.M. & Brand, P.A. 1995b, 'Compensating for Stigma: Obese and Nonobese Women's Reactions to Being Visible', *Personality and Social Psychology Bulletin*, pp. 1093–106.

Millman, M. 1980, *Such a Pretty Face: Being Fat in America*, Norton, New York.

Morris, A., Cooper, T. & Cooper, P.J. 1989, 'The Changing Shape of Female Fashion Models', *International Journal of Eating Disorders*, pp. 593–6.

Myers, P.N. & Biocca, F.A. 1992, 'The Elastic Body Image: The Effect of Television Advertising and Programming on Body Image Distortions of Young Women', *Journal of Communication*, vol. 42, pp. 108–33.

NaPier, E.A., Meyer, M.H. & Hymes, C.L. 2005, 'Old and Overweight: Another Kind of Double Jeopardy?', *Generations*, vol. 29, pp. 31–6.

O'Brien, M.S. & Bankston, W.B. 1990, 'The Moral Career of the Reformed Compulsive Eater: A Study of Conversion to Charismatic Conformity', in C.D. Bryant (ed.), *Deviant Behavior: Readings in the Sociology of Norm Violations*, Hemisphere, New York, pp. 774–83.

Orbuch, T.L. 1997, 'People's Accounts Count: The Sociology of Accounts', *Annual Review of Sociology*, vol. 23, pp. 455–78.

Page, R.M. 1984, *Stigma*, Routledge and Kegan Paul, Boston.

Pauley, L.L. 1989, 'Customer Weight as a Variable in Salespersons' Response Time', *Journal of Social Psychology*, vol. 129, pp. 713–14.

Pestello, F. 1991, 'Discounting', *Journal of Contemporary Ethnography*, vol. 20, pp. 27–46.

Puhl, R. & Brownell, K.D. 2003, 'Ways of Coping with Obesity Stigma: Review and Conceptual Analysis', *Eating Behaviors*, vol. 4, pp. 53–78.

—— 2006, 'Confronting and Coping with Weight Stigma: An Investigation of Overweight and Obese Adults,' *Obesity*, vol. 14, pp. 1802–15.

Richardson, S.A. 1970, 'Age and Sex Differences in Values toward Physical Handicaps', *Journal of Health and Social Behavior*, vol. 11, pp. 207–14.

—— 1971, 'Research Report: Handicap, Appearance, and Stigma', *Social Science and Medicine*, vol. 5, pp. 621–8.

——, Hastorf, A.H., Goodman, N. & Dornbusch, S.M. 1961, 'Cultural Uniformity in Reaction to Physical Disabilities', *American Sociological Review*, vol. 26, pp. 241–7.

Ritenbaugh, C. 1982, 'Obesity as a Culture-bound Syndrome', *Culture, Medicine and Psychiatry*, vol. 6, pp. 347–61.

Rubin, N., Shmilovitz, C. & Weiss, M. 1993, 'From Fat to Thin: Informal Rites Affirming Identity Change', *Symbolic Interaction*, vol. 16, pp. 1–17.

Saguy, A.C. & Riley, K.W. 2005, 'Weighing Both Sides: Morality, Mortality, and Framing Contests over Obesity,' *Journal of Health Politics, Policy and Law*, vol. 30, pp. 869–921.

Schur, E. 1979, *Interpreting Deviance*, Harper & Row, New York.

Schwarzer, R. & Weiner, B. 1990, 'Die Wirkung von Kontrollierbarkeit und Bewaltigungs-verhalten auf Emotionen und Sociale Unterstutzung', *Zeitschrift fur Socialpsychologie*, vol. 21, pp. 118–25.

Scott M.B. & Lyman, S. 1963, 'Accounts', *American Sociological Review*, vol. 33, pp. 44–62.

Seid, R.P. 1989, *Never Too Thin*, Prentice-Hall, New York.

Silverstein, B., Perdue, L., Peterson, B. & Kelly, E. 1986, 'The Role of the Mass Media in Promoting a Thin Standard of Bodily Attractiveness for Women', *Sex Roles*, vol. 14, pp. 519–33.

Sobal, J. 1984a, 'Group Dieting, the Stigma of Obesity, and Overweight Adolescents: Contributions of Natalie Allon to the Sociology of Obesity', *Marriage and Family Review*, vol. 7, pp. 9–20.

—— 1984b, 'Marriage, Obesity and Dieting', *Marriage and Family Review*, vol. 7, pp. 115–40.

—— 1991, 'Obesity and Nutritional Sociology: A Model for Coping with the Stigma of Obesity', *Clinical Sociology Review*, vol. 9, pp. 125–41.

—— 1995, 'The Medicalization and Demedicalization of Obesity', in D. Maurer & J. Sobal (eds), *Eating Agendas: Food and Nutrition as Social Problems*, Aldine de Gruyter, Hawthorne, New York State, pp. 79–90.

—— 1999, 'The Size Acceptance Movement and the Social Construction of Body Weight', in J. Sobal & D. Maurer (eds), *Weighty Issues: Fatness and Thinness as Social Problems*, Aldine de Gruyter, Hawthorne, New York State, pp. 231–49.

—— 2001, 'Social and Cultural Influences on Obesity', in P. Bjorntorp (ed.), *International Textbook of Obesity*, John Wiley and Sons, London, pp. 305–22.

—— 2005, 'Social Consequences of Weight Bias by Partners, Friends, and Strangers', in K.D. Brownell, R.M. Puhl, M.B. Schwartz & L. Rudd (eds), *Weight Bias: Nature, Consequences, and Remedies*, Guilford Press, New York, pp. 150–64.

—— & Bursztyn, M. 1998, 'Dating People with Anorexia Nervosa and Bulimia: Attitudes and Beliefs of University Students', *Women and Health*, vol. 27, no. 3, pp. 73–88.

—— & Devine, C. 1997, 'Social Aspects of Obesity: Influences, Consequences, Assessments, and Interventions', in S. Dalton (ed.), *Overweight and Weight Management*, Aspen Publishers, Gaithersburg, Maryland, pp. 289–308.

—— & Hinrichs, D. 1986, 'Bias against "Marginal" Individuals in Jury Wheel Selection', *Journal of Criminal Justice*, vol. 14, pp. 71–89.

—— & Maurer, D. 1999 (eds), *Interpreting Weight: The Social Management of Fatness and Thinness*, Aldine de Gruyter, Hawthorne, New York State.

—— & Maurer, D. (eds) 1999, *Weighty Issues: The Construction of Fatness and Thinness as Social Problems*, Aldine de Gruyter, Hawthorne, New York State.

—— & Stunkard, A.J. 1989, 'Socioeconomic Status and Obesity: A Review of the Literature', *Psychological Bulletin*, vol. 105, pp. 260–75.

——, Nicolopoulos, V. & Lee, J. 1995, 'Attitudes about Weight and Dating among Secondary School Students', *International Journal of Obesity*, vol. 19, pp. 376–81.

——, Rauschenbach, B. & Frongillo, E. 1992, 'Marital Status, Fatness, and Obesity', *Social Science and Medicine*, vol. 35, pp. 915–23.

——, Rauschenbach, B.S. & Frongillo, E.A. 2003, 'Marital Changes and Body Weight Changes: A US Longitudinal Analysis', *Social Science and Medicine*, vol. 56, pp. 1543–55.

Solovay, J.D. 2000, *Tipping the Scales of Justice: Fighting Weight-based Discrimination*, Prometheus Books, Amherst, New York State.

Spiegal, D. & Keith-Spiegel, P. 1973, *Outsiders USA*, Rinehart Press, San Francisco, pp. 570–3.

Stearns, P.N. 1997, *Fat History: Bodies and Beauty in the Modern West*, New York University Press, New York.

Strauss, R.S. & Pollack, H.A. 2003, 'Social Marginalization of Overweight Children,' *Archives of Pediatrics and Adolescent Medicine*, vol. 157, pp. 746–52.

Stunkard, A.J. & Sobal, J. 1995, 'Psychosocial Consequences of Obesity', in K.D. Brownell & C.G. Fairburn (eds), *Eating Disorders and Obesity*, Guilford Press, New York, pp. 417–21.

Tiggemann, M. & Rothblum, E.D. 1988, 'Gender Differences in Social Consequences of Perceived Overweight in the United States and Australia', *Sex Roles*, vol. 18, pp. 75–86.

Waller, G., Shaw, J., Hamilton, K., Baldwin, G., Harding, T. & Sumner, T. 1994, 'Beauty is in the Eye of the Beholder: Media Influences on the Psychopathology of Eating Problems', *Appetite*, vol. 23, p. 287.

Way, K. 1995, 'Never Too Rich … or Too Thin: The Role of Stigma in the Social Construction of Anorexia Nervosa', in D. Maurer & J. Sobal (eds), *Eating Agendas: Food and Nutrition as Social Problems*, Aldine de Gruyter, Hawthorne, New York State, pp. 91–113.

Weiner, B., Perry, R.P. & Magnusson, J. 1988, 'An Attributional Analysis of Reactions to Stigmas', *Journal of Personality and Social Psychology*, vol. 55, pp. 738–48.

Wiseman, C.V., Gray, J.J., Mosimann, J.E. & Ahrens, A.H. 1992, 'Cultural Expectations of Thinness in Women: An Update', *International Journal of Eating Disorders*, vol. 11, pp. 85–9.

Wykes, M. & Gunter, B. 2005, *The Media and Body Image*, Sage: Thousand Oaks, CA.

Yancey, A.K, Leslie, J. & Abel, E.K. 2006, 'Obesity at the Crossroads: Feminist and Public Health Perspectives,' *Signs*, vol. 31, pp. 425–43.

Young, L.M. & Powell, B. 1985, 'The Effects of Obesity on the Clinical Judgements of Mental Health Professionals', *Journal of Health and Social Behavior*, vol. 26, pp. 233–46.

Zdrodowski, D. 1996, 'Eating Out: The Experience of Eating in Public for the "Overweight" Woman', *Women's Studies International Forum*, vol. 19, pp. 665–74.

Glossary

accounts

Specific claims about the reasons for particular behaviours, used to manage interactions and to gain or maintain acceptance.

activities of daily living

Activities considered fundamental to an individual's independent existence, including getting out of bed, cooking and eating food, and shopping for groceries.

ageism

Discrimination based on age.

agency

The ability of people, individually and collectively, to influence their own lives and the society in which they live.

agribusiness

The complete operations performed in producing agricultural commodities, including farming, manufacturing, handling, storing, processing and distributing.

agri-food

The industries involved in the production of food.

agroforestry

To establish tree plantations on a farm so as to mix forestry with cropping and grazing.

alienated labour/alienation

'Alienation' is a Marxist term that refers to the experience of people who have to work for a monetary wage to live. They are alienated from—have no control over—their conditions of work, the process of production, what they produce, and the ownership and distribution of their products.

anorexia nervosa

A complex eating disorder in which a person severely restricts food consumption to lose or maintain body weight, to such an extent that it is detrimental to normal physiological functioning and life-threatening.

anti-vivisection

A movement that is against the use of animals for laboratory experiments.

appropriationism

The use of manufactured inputs in agriculture (seeds, fertilisers, machinery, etc.) produced by off-farm transnational industries. Compare with *substitutionism*.

attribution

Ascribing a characteristic, quality or causation to some factor.

biological determinism

An unproven belief that individual, group and organisational behaviours are ultimately determined by biology.

biomedicine/biomedical model

The conventional approach to medicine in Western societies, based on the diagnosis and explanation of illness as a malfunction of one of the body's biological mechanisms. This approach underpins most health professions and health services, which focus on treating individuals and generally marginalise social, economic and environmental factors. In terms of diet, eating is conceptualised as a process of sustaining the body as a biological organism by using the nutrients that medical science considers most effective.

biotechnology

The use of molecular biology and genetic engineering to modify plants and animals, including humans, at the molecular level.

body acceptance

A set of beliefs held by those who have a positive body image. These beliefs support body diversity in the community by rejecting conformity to the thin ideal. Also referred to as 'size acceptance', which is promoted by social movements that aim to counteract prejudice and discrimination based on body size and shape. See also *body image, fatism* and *thin ideal*.

body image

The image an individual has of their own body. Body image depends on both the actual shape and size of the body as well as the affective component of how that body is perceived in relation to body expectations. Thus, if the body expectations held by an individual are unrealistic, it is possible for that individual to have a negative body image despite having a body that others would envy.

body mass index (BMI)

A measure of body weight used in the health sciences to determine the prevalence in the population of underweight, overweight and obesity. BMI is derived by dividing a person's weight in kilograms by their height in metres squared. The World Health Organization has defined the following weight ranges for women and men:

<18.50	Underweight
18.50–24.99	Normal range
25.00–29.99	Grade I overweight
30.00–34.99	Grade IIa overweight
35.00–39.99	Grade IIb overweight
40+	Grade III overweight

A measure equal to or above 30 is also referred to as 'obese'.

bulimia nervosa

An eating disorder indicated by repeated episodes of binge eating and purging. A person with bulimia nervosa will consume large amounts of food in a short period of time, usually experienced as a lack of control over eating, and will then try to prevent weight gain through self-induced vomiting, misuse of laxatives and medications, fasting or excessive exercise.

capitalism

An economic and social system based on the private accumulation of wealth; a system in which a relatively small capitalist class owns almost all the productive property of a society.

cash crops

Crops produced to be exchanged for cash.

civilising process/civilising of appetite

The 'civilising process' is a concept coined by Norbert Elias to refer to the never-ending social process by which external forms of social control of people's behaviour are replaced by internalised forms of moral self-control. Stephen Mennell has applied this idea to food habits, using the term 'civilising of appetite'.

class (or social class)

A concept used by sociologists to refer to a position in a system of structured inequality based on the unequal distribution of power, wealth, income and status. People who share a social class typically share similar life chances.

Commodity Systems Analysis (CSA)

Developed by William Friedland, this analytical framework identifies a wide range of factors that contribute to the production of commodities, including production practices, technology, farm and factory labour processes, marketing, distribution networks and the retail sector.

competencies

'Competence' is the ability to perform activities to the expected professional standard in the workplace. 'Competency standards' are the level of expertise required for professional practice in terms of the unique role and employment context of a particular profession.

conspicuous consumption

Coined by Thorstein Veblen, this term refers to overt displays of wealth by which the upper class demonstrates its social status.

continuing competency development

The process of further skill and knowledge development, after an initial professional qualification has been obtained. This usually occurs in the workplace.

cooperative

An enterprise in which ownership is shared by all members for mutual benefit.

cosmopolitanism

The global hybridisation of cultures, tastes and cuisines caused by the globalisation of the media, trade and travel.

culinary tourism

The promotion of gastronomic experiences, events and products (such as food festivals and regional foodstuffs) as a key feature of the travel experience.

cultural capital

A concept that implies that culture can be treated like an economic asset upon which social hierarchies are founded.

cultural economy

An analytical framework that avoids privileging cultural or economic factors by drawing on both, and examining how these factors interact, to understand the way markets and organisations operate.

culture

The values, assumptions, and beliefs shared by a group of people, which structure the behaviour of group members from birth until death.

culture-bound syndrome

A health or medical condition that only occurs in particular cultures and is not universal, or culture-free.

deviance

Behaviour that violates social expectations about what is normal.

dietary guidelines

Principles of nutrition advice for policy makers and health professionals.

Dietary Guidelines for Australians

Dietary advice for the Australian population. The guidelines aim to reverse those trends in the Australian diet that contribute to chronic disease and disorders.

dietitian

A university-trained health professional with expertise on the relationship between food and health, particularly in terms of illness prevention and treatment for individuals and communities.

disabilities

Limitations on the ability to fulfil role obligations as a result of physical impairments; impairments include limited motion of limbs and generalised muscular weakness, which are usually the result of injury or illness.

disclaimer

An explanation provided in anticipation of challenges to a person's or a behaviour's legitimacy.

discounting

A set of techniques for dealing with violations of personal principles without threatening internal self-definitions or identity.

DNA

Deoxyribonucleic acid: the molecule within cells that transmits hereditary information.

eating disorders

Generic term for the cluster of disorders including anorexia nervosa, bulimia nervosa, and eating disorders not otherwise specified.

eating disorders not otherwise specified (EDNOS)

Eating disorders that do not fall within the definition of anorexia nervosa or of bulimia nervosa, in terms of severity or range of symptoms, but that nonetheless may include elements of each.

emancipatory politics

A term used by Anthony Giddens to refer to a value-based commitment to reducing or eliminating inequality, discrimination and exploitation. See also *life politics*.

epidemiology

The statistical study of patterns of disease in the population. Originally focused on epidemics, or infectious diseases, it now covers non-infectious conditions. Social epidemiology is a subfield, aligned with sociology, which focuses on the social determinants of illness.

ethical responsibilities

Obligations that individuals are required to fulfil on the basis of their cultural or societal position. For example, individuals who are parents have ethical responsibilities concerning the duty of care for their children; these responsibilities form the standards by which individuals judge themselves to be 'good' parents.

ethics

Socially or culturally patterned codes of conduct that oblige individuals to act in particular ways.

fatism

Discrimination against people with high levels of body fat.

feminism/feminist

A broad social and political movement based on a belief in equality of the sexes and advocating the removal of all forms of discrimination against women. A feminist is one who subscribes to, and may act upon, a body of theory that seeks to explain the subordinate position of women in society.

flexible accumulation

A general term, often used interchangeably or in conjunction with 'flexible specialisation' and 'flexible production', denoting changes in work organisation. Specifically, it refers to a mode of capital accumulation by corporations that is characterised by an ability to respond quickly to competition and consumer demand by flexibly managing employment (using contract, part-time or casual labour), by developing staff multiskilling and task flexibility, and by using new technologies that allow production processes to be changed quickly.

food forest

Tree crops and other perennials provide most carbohydrates.

food guides

Advice about healthful diets for the general public.

food safety

The 'safety' of food for human consumption—safe food is free from biological and chemical contaminants (due to food handling, production or storage) that have the potential to cause illness.

food security/insecurity

'Food security' is the availability of affordable, nutritious and culturally acceptable food. 'Food insecurity' is a state of regular hunger and fear of starvation.

food sovereignty

Goal of global small farmer movement; government policy giving priority to local food production and ensuring the right to wholesome food, fair wages for workers and fair prices for producers; domestic control of natural and genetic resources such as seeds.

food system

All the factors that comprise processes of food production, distribution and consumption—from the paddock and fisheries to the plate—such as agriculture and agri-business, government regulation, marketing, retail preparation and sales.

food use

A term proposed by Anne Murcott in preference to 'food consumption' to distinguish sociological concerns about the social organisation of food from the nutritional meaning of consumption as eating and the economic meaning of consumption as (food) purchasing.

foodways

Habits and practices relating to food acquisition, food preparation, food storage, distribution of food among family members, meal and snack patterns, food combinations, uses of food, beliefs about food, and identification of core, secondary and peripheral foods in the diet.

Foucaultian perspective

A theoretical approach drawn from the work of French social theorist Michel Foucault (1926–84). A Foucaultian (pronounced 'Foo-co-shian') perspective entails a focus on how power is exercised in a multitude of indirect and self-induced forms, particularly in terms of the social control of people's behaviour.

frame

Refers to unconscious assumptions about causation and meaning that shape our perceptions, choices and what we believe to be possible; similar to worldview, belief system or ideology.

functional foods/nutraceuticals

Food products that allegedly deliver a health benefit beyond just providing nutrients.

functionalism

Also known as 'structural functionalism', 'consensus theory' or 'systems theory', this theoretical perspective focuses on how social structures function to maintain social order, based on the assumption that a society is a system of integrated parts, each of which has certain requirements that must be fulfilled for social order to be maintained. Key functionalist theorists include Emile Durkheim (1858–1917), Talcott Parsons (1902–79), Robert Merton (1910–2003) and Jeffrey Alexander (1947–).

fusion food

A general term to refer to the combination of different cultural food traditions resulting in innovative cuisines.

gender socialisation

The process by which males and females learn the socially constructed behaviour patterns of masculinity and femininity (the cultural values that dictate how men and women should behave).

genetic engineering (or genetic modification)

The alteration of the DNA in plants, animals and humans to perform new functions, by rearranging or deleting existing genes or inserting genetic material from another species.

genetically modified organisms (GMOs)

Plants, animals and micro-organisms that have had their DNA altered by human intervention.

genetic modification

See *genetic engineering*.

gift economy

A proposed utopia in which goods and services are produced by collectives of people and either consumed by the collective or given to other community groups or to the community at large. There is no money and no wage labour in a gift economy: community groups have effective ownership of productive property; individuals, families or households have effective ownership of personal property.

globalisation

Political, social, economic and cultural developments—such as the growth of multinational companies, information technology and international agencies— that result in people's lives being increasingly influenced by global, rather than national or local, factors.

Global South, Global North

Terms gaining use because they are seen as more neutral than previous terms: underdeveloped and developed; non-industrial, industrial; poor, wealthy; third world, first world.

global warming

Climate change caused by human activities—mainly carbon dioxide from burnt fossil fuels and destroyed forests.

government/governmentality

In general sociological terms, 'government' is understood as a wide range of practices, strategies, techniques and programs that influence the beliefs and conduct of the population, rather than simply as a set of centralised state bureaucracies.

Green Revolution

A term used to refer to certain technological developments in agricultural production that increased productivity and were heralded as possible solutions to world hunger (such as hybrid seeds, irrigation, mechanisation, synthetic fertilisers and pest control agents made largely from fossil fuels). Many of the intensive farming methods that were developed and continue to be used have been criticised for damaging the environment.

habitus

An expanded notion of habit, 'habitus' refers to the internalised and taken-for-granted personal dispositions we all possess, such as our accent, gestures, and preferences in food, fashion and entertainment (among other things).

haute cuisine

Translates from French as 'high cooking', and refers to the cooking of the grand and expensive restaurants, which became characterised by elaborately presented and rich meals in small portions and numerous courses.

health claim

In the context of food products, this term refers to a statement of the impact of a food, or food ingredient, on a person's health.

healthism

An extreme concern with personal health, which is becoming increasingly common.

health promotion

Any combination of education interventions and related organisational, economic and political interventions designed to promote behavioural and environmental changes conducive to good health. This may cover a variety of strategies, including legislation, health education, community development and advocacy. See also *public health nutrition* and *population health*.

horizontal integration

The purchasing by a company of similar companies to form a larger organisation and reduce competition (for example, a flour mill purchasing another flour mill). Compare with *vertical integration*.

ideological contest

Conflict between different views of social processes, which reflect the goals and interests of different groups and organisations (for example, public health professionals or food producers).

identity

A person's self-conception or self-definition. See also *social identity*.

individualism

In sociology, the belief that we can explain social phenomena in terms of individual ideas, attributes and behaviour.

just-in-time (JIT)

A system of managing production so that goods are produced as needed to meet market demand by keeping only a minimal amount of stock warehoused.

life chances

The probability of people realising their lifestyle choices.

life choices

People's choices in their selection of lifestyle.

life politics

A term used by Anthony Giddens to refer to life decisions or lifestyle choices that affect the formation of self-identity, which occurs as a reflexive process in the context of the dynamic nature of social life. See also *emancipatory politics*.

marginality

The socially constructed definition of a characteristic as 'out of the mainstream' or 'abnormal'.

master status

The dominant social label applied to an individual, according to which the individual is automatically attributed with a host of stereotyped personality traits commonly associated with the particular status (for example, criminal or homosexual) irrespective of the person's individual personality.

maternal ideal

The social construction of the female body that reinforces the desirability of the physiological changes of pregnancy. To conform to the maternal ideal, women should have a large body size when pregnant (as opposed to the thin ideal of female beauty that dominates most Western societies).

McDonaldisation

A term coined by George Ritzer to expand Max Weber's notion of rationalisation; defined as the standardisation of work processes through rules and regulations based on increased monitoring and evaluation of individual performance, akin to the uniformity and control measures used by fast-food chains.

medical–food–industrial complex

A term adapted from Vincente Navarro and colleagues' (1998) 'medical-industrial complex', coined in 1967 and popularised by Arnold S. Relman (1980); refers to the combination of manufacturing interests, medical scientists and government agencies that have a vested interest in the development and introduction of functional foods for the purpose of profit maximisation.

medical model

See *biomedicine/biomedical model*.

medicalisation

The process by which the influence of medicine is expanded by defining non-medical problems as medical problems, usually in terms of illnesses, disorders or syndromes.

microcredit

System for lending very small amounts to low-income people for income-generating purposes, and where financial collateral is not required.

'modern' foods

Those foods for which overall consumption is increasing and that are consumed more by high-status groups than by low-status groups.

modernity

A particular view of society that is founded upon rational thought and the belief that objective realities can be discovered and understood through rational and scientific means—a view rejected by postmodernists. Anthony Giddens has referred to contemporary society in developed countries as high or late modernity, reflecting the advanced and dominant nature of rational and scientific views.

molecular nutrition

The study of the chemical constituents of food and their impact on the physiological functioning of the body.

monoculture

The use of a piece of land to produce a single crop.

monopsonic power

The ability to influence a market based on there being only one provider of goods and services.

multinational oligopolies

The control of markets by a small number of international companies, which often have a budget larger than that of many small countries. Such companies are able to act together in pursuit of their mutual vested interests, via price-fixing arrangements, limiting competitors' access to markets, and gaining government concessions (tax breaks, subsidies and favourable legislation), thereby limiting competition (particularly from local producers).

muscular ideal

The social construction of the male body that reinforces the desirability of a large, muscular body as epitomising masculinity.

neo-liberalism

A philosophy based on the primacy of individual rights and minimal state intervention. Sometimes used interchangeably with economic rationalism/liberalism.

neo-Marxism

See *Marxism*.

neural tube defects

Defects in the development of the spinal cord and brain in an embryo, resulting in conditions such as spinal bifida, cleft lip, cleft palate and the failure of brain development (anencephaly).

new nutrition science

A multifactorial approach to the study of nutrition that blends the traditional biological focus with sociological and ecological perspectives.

normality

Behaviours, procedures and practices that conform to certain socially or culturally patterned standards or goals.

novel food

Defined by Standard 1.5.1 of the Australia New Zealand Food Standards Code as 'a non-traditional food for which there is insufficient knowledge in the broad community to enable safe use in the form or context in which it is presented'.

nutraceuticals

See *functional foods/nutraceuticals*.

nutrient standards

Levels of intake of single nutrients that meet the needs of most healthy individuals in a population.

nutrigenomics

The study of the relationship between human nutrition, genetics and health.

nutritional risk

Factors thought to increase the probability that an individual will develop undernutrition or malnutrition; risk factors include social isolation and disabilities such as difficulty chewing or swallowing food.

obesity

The condition of having a high level of stored body fat.

oil crunch

Also known as the oil peak or big rollover, it refers to oil prices rising drastically as oilfields run out and demand increases.

one-rule economy

An economy driven by the principle that a successful society depends on business decisions based solely on what brings the highest return to shareholders.

organics

Agriculture that makes no use of artificial (synthetic) chemicals for fertilisers, pesticides or herbicides.

pacifism

Opposition to war and violence in general.

participatory budgeting

Government processes involving citizen volunteers in a series of face-to-face deliberations to select priorities for using a portion of tax revenues.

patriarchy
> A system of power through which males dominate households. The term is used more broadly by feminists to refer to the pre-eminence of patriarchal power throughout society, which functions to subordinate women and children.

permaculture
> A specific system of permanent, sustainable agriculture and settlement design.

phytosterols
> Chemicals derived from plants that have biological activity in humans.

polyculture
> The use of a piece of land to produce a diversity of crops.

population health
> The collective health status of a specified population; also referred to as public health. A public health approach aims to assess and improve the health status of large groups of people, rather than focusing on the health of individuals at high risk. The strategies used to promote the health of populations are those that tend to have broad effects, such as policy development (for example, legislation for a safe food supply).

post-industrial society
> A society in which information replaces property as the prime source of power and social control; in such societies, professionals become powerful social groups and employment is increasingly in service industries rather than manufacturing industries.

postmodern society
> A debated concept in sociology that characterises contemporary society as one in which many social institutions, including the state, have lost their power to determine social outcomes. There are no longer clear paths for the individual to influence events by participating in such institutions as political parties, unions, or professional bodies. The result is a society that becomes fragmented as a result of a high level of social differentiation and cultural diversity.

post-structuralism
> A term, often used interchangeably with *postmodernism*, which refers to a perspective that is opposed to the view that social structure determines human action, and that emphasises the local, the specific and the contingent in social life.

primary prevention
> Efforts to improve health or prevent disease in those who are essentially well—for example, providing health-promoting foods in school canteens to keep children healthy and prevent the development of coronary heart disease and diabetes in later life.

probiotic
> Beneficial bacteria that can aid the digestive system.

public health nutrition

A population approach to preventing diet-related health problems that addresses the influence of food production, distribution and consumption on the nutritional status of the population at large and specific subgroups in particular (such as children, the disadvantaged and indigenous groups).

public health nutritionist

A professional employed as part of the public health workforce whose efforts are aimed at preventing nutrition-related problems in populations. The majority of public health nutritionists in Australia are dietitians. See also *dietitian* and *public health nutrition*.

rationalisation

See *McDonaldisation*.

reductionist

In the context of health, refers to an assumption that health and illness can be reduced to biological factors.

reflexive modernity

A term coined by Ulrich Beck and Anthony Giddens to refer to the present social era in developed societies, in which social practices are open to reflection, questioning and change, and therefore in which social traditions no longer dictate people's lifestyles.

risk discourse

'Risk' refers to danger and risk discourse is often used in health promotion messages warning people that certain actions (such as eating foods high in saturated fat and sugar) involve significant risks to their health.

risk factors

Conditions that are thought to increase an individual's susceptibility to illness or disease—for example, abuse of alcohol, poor diet or smoking.

risk society

A term coined by Ulrich Beck (1992) to describe the centrality of risk calculations in people's lives in Western society, whereby the key social problems today are unanticipated hazards, such as the risks of food poisoning, pollution and environmental degradation.

role

Behavioural expectations (including duties and rights) associated with a position in society.

ruralisation

A process of relocating urban populations to agricultural regions so that all food is produced and consumed locally.

salinity/salinisation

Agricultural processes that bring salts in the soil to the surface, making the land unfit for agricultural use.

size acceptance

See *body acceptance*.

social appetite

The social patterns of food production, distribution and consumption.

social class

See *class*.

social control

Mechanisms that aim to induce conformity, or at least to manage or minimise deviant behaviour.

social constructionism

The theory that people actively construct reality and its associated meanings, so that nothing is 'natural' or inevitable and notions of normality/abnormality, right/wrong and health/illness are subjective human creations that should not be taken for granted.

social differentiation

A trend towards social diversity based on the creation of social distinction and self-identity through particular consumption choices and through group membership.

social embodiment

Refers to the experience of one's body as both a social artefact/object and as a corporeal entity.

social identity

A person's understanding of themself and how others perceive them reflects social processes and experiences, such as nationality, religion and social status. See also *identity*.

social isolation

The condition in which an individual both lives alone and has little social contact with other people.

social network

The persons with whom an individual normally has the most contact. These can include friends, immediate family members, more distant relatives, neighbours, co-workers, fellow members of voluntary organisations and fellow church members.

social structure

The recurring patterns of social interaction by which people are related to each other through social institutions and social groups.

social support

Instrumental aid (goods and services) and expressive aid (companionship, comfort and advice about personal matters) provided by members of a social network.

socialism

A political ideology and system of government with numerous variations, based on the elimination of social inequality, the promotion of altruistic values, and the replacement of private wealth accumulation with state ownership and/or distribution of economic resources.

socio-ecological model

Derived from the broad field of human ecology, which studies the links between human interaction, social organisation and ecology. When applied to public health, this model explores the determinants of health within a social, economic and geographic context, rather than simply examining the contribution of medical factors (as in the biomedical model).

socioeconomic status (SES)

A measure of social status based on the statistical grouping of people into high-, medium- and low-SES groups according to certain criteria (usually a composite index of income, occupation and education); used to gauge social and economic inequalities.

sociological imagination

A term coined by Charles Wright Mills (1959) to describe the sociological approach to the analysis of issues. We see the world through a sociological imagination, or think sociologically, when we make a link between personal troubles and public issues.

speciesism

A term coined by Peter Singer to describe the form of discrimination where one species allows their own interests to justify causing pain and suffering to another species.

status

The respect or prestige associated with a particular position in society.

stigma

An attribute of a person that is deeply discrediting and that disqualifies that person from full social acceptance.

stigmatising act

An act of a 'normal' individual that devalues another person, in the process of stigmatisation.

structuralism

A view maintaining that individuals' actions and beliefs are primarily determined by the society in which they live, emphasising that language, culture and economic organisation pre-exist the individual and limit the possibilities for thought and action.

structure/agency debate

A key debate in sociology regarding the extent to which human behaviour is determined by the social structure.

substitutionism

The replacement of costly and/or unreliably supplied inputs with 'generic ingredients' in the food processing industry (for example, sugar from cornstarch rather than cane). Compare with *appropriationism*.

sustainable farming agriculture

Any system of plant and animal production that can satisfy human food needs and maintain or enhance natural resources by maximising the use of renewable resources, conserving and efficiently using non-renewable resources, and ensuring that the environmental impact of agricultural processes is minimised, so that affected ecological systems survive and prosper. Also known as agroecology.

symbolic interactionism

A theoretical perspective that focuses on agency and how people construct, interpret and give meaning to their behaviour through interaction with others. Rather than large social structures, small-scale, face-to-face symbolic interactions are studied, as social life is viewed as the cumulative product of human action, interaction and interpretation. Key symbolic interactionist theorists include George Herbert Mead (1863–1931), Charles Cooley (1864–1929), Howard Becker (1928–), Erving Goffman (1922–82) and Herbert Blumer (1900–87), who coined the term in 1937.

technologies of government

A range of institutions operating outside state bureaucracy that are able to exert control over the population.

thin ideal

The dominant aesthetic ideal of female beauty in Western societies, which refers to the social desirability of a thin body shape.

time famine

A general term used to refer to the pressure on people's time use in contemporary social life. Being 'time poor' is a common complaint, as people deal with increasingly complex and fast-paced lifestyles, particularly when combining long (and possibly odd) working hours, study, and family and social life.

transgenic organisms

Organisms created through the transferral of genetic information from one species to another by combining DNA molecules from, for example, a plant and/or an animal into a single 'recombinant' strand to produce a change in the genetic make-up (for example, transgenic pigs with human growth hormone).

transnational corporations (TNCs)

Refers to companies that have operations in more than one country and no clearly identifiable country as a home base. Often used in preference to the superseded term 'multinational corporations', which tended to refer to companies primarily based in one country, but with subsidiary operations in other countries. See also *multinational oligopolies*.

unproblematised

Treated as natural and therefore not requiring research or examination.

vegetarianism

The practice of voluntarily refraining from eating meat, chicken or fish and the beliefs underpinning this practice. There are many variations, but the major subcategories include lacto-vegetarian (dairy food is still consumed), ovo-vegetarian (eggs are consumed) and vegan (abstinence from eating and sometimes from wearing all animal products).

vertical integration

The purchase by a company of dissimilar companies that can form strategic production linkages (for example, a flour mill purchasing a biscuit or bread manufacturer or a supermarket chain) with the aim of expanding sales and profits. Compare with *horizontal integration*.

Index